Biomedical Visualization

Volume 10

Series Editor

Paul M. Rea, Anatomy Facility, School of Medicine, Dentistry and Nursing, College of Medical, Veterinary and Life Sciences, University of Glasgow, Glasgow, UK

Aims and Scope

The Biomedical Visualization book series invites contributions related to visualization and imaging in the biomedical sciences and related fields such as medicine, dentistry, veterinary surgery, informatics, and the allied health professions.

This can encompass work in image analysis, workflow methodologies, photogrammetry in science, animations, digital reconstructions and applications, big data and visualizations, educational methodologies, usability and evaluations, augmented and virtual reality, and 3D and 4D technologies, including 3D printing, as well as informatics, e-tutorials, MOOCs, HCI and public engagement. It can be from macroscopic to microscopic but show how we can view data and information related to the biomedical field in a much more accessible, innovative and engaging way using technology.

This series is intended for researchers, clinicians, students, and teaching staff in biomedical and medical schools who use and develop visualization and imaging techniques in medical education, patient care, and biomedical and medical research.

Peer review description:

Proposal review

The book proposal developed by the invited volume editors is reviewed by the series editors and in-house editors at Springer to meet the scope of the series. Editors can make suggestions for content changes and contributing authors at this stage, which are then included in the proposal.

Manuscript review

1st round of revision: Submitted manuscripts are first reviewed by the volume editor(s), who are expert(s) in the field of the volume. In cases of particular concern, a system of single-blind review is applied, in which independent external experts who know the identity of the authors can be asked for advice.

2nd round of revision: The manuscripts approved by the volume editor(s) then undergo a technical review by Springer and are then forwarded to the series editor for additional content review.

Type of review: The review of manuscripts by the volume editor(s) and series editor includes a check for the scientific soundness and coherence of the manuscript, and adherence to the guidelines for the Biomedical Visualization series regarding style, content, and level of writing. The authors are asked to address any recommended revisions and resubmit to the editors. The resubmitted manuscripts are again reviewed by the volume editor and series editor and, once approved, sent to Springer. The technical review by Springer comprises a plagiarism check, a check for completeness of the chapter, and an assessment of its compliance with Springer's and the series' guidelines for chapter authors.

Volume and series editors jointly decide on the suitability of the manuscript for the *Biomedical Visualization* series based on their reviews.

The book series *Biomedical Visualization* publishes only solicited contributions, which are invited by the volume or series editors.

Johann Malawana
Arian Arjomandi Rad
Robert Vardanyan • George Miller
Editors

Artificial Intelligence in Healthcare and Biomedical Visualization

Springer

Editors
Johann Malawana
School of Medicine and Dentistry
University of Lancashire
Preston, UK

Robert Vardanyan
Department of Neurosurgery
John Radcliffe Hospital, Oxford
University Hospitals NHS Foundation Trust
Oxford, UK

Arian Arjomandi Rad
Department of Cardiothoracic Surgery
John Radcliffe Hospital, Oxford
University Hospitals NHS Foundation Trust
Oxford, UK

George Miller
Exmouth Business Centre
The Healthcare Leadership Academy, Suite 30
Exmouth, UK

ISSN 2731-6130 ISSN 2731-6149 (electronic)
Biomedical Visualization
ISBN 978-3-032-06519-3 ISBN 978-3-032-06520-9 (eBook)
https://doi.org/10.1007/978-3-032-06520-9

Cover Illustration: Catherine MacRobbie

This Springer imprint is published by the registered company Springer Nature Switzerland AG
The registered company address is: Gewerbestrasse 11, 6330 Cham, Switzerland

Preface

Healthcare is at a transformative juncture, where the convergence of advanced technology and medical practice offers unprecedented opportunities to revolutionize patient outcomes and streamline healthcare systems. Artificial Intelligence (AI) has emerged as a pivotal force, capable of addressing some of the most intricate and persistent challenges in contemporary healthcare. From alleviating global workforce shortages to enabling hyper-personalized treatment plans, AI is fundamentally reshaping how diseases are diagnosed, treated, and managed. Complementing these advancements is the field of biomedical visualization, which has unlocked powerful new tools for interpreting complex medical data, offering clinicians and researchers actionable insights that were previously unattainable.

Why AI in Healthcare Matters

Globally, healthcare systems face a convergence of crises—aging populations, increasing chronic disease burdens, soaring costs, and critical workforce shortages. By 2030, the World Health Organization predicts a shortfall of 18 million healthcare workers, which will further strain already overburdened systems. Simultaneously, the exponential growth in medical data—doubling every 73 days—renders it virtually impossible for practitioners to remain fully informed without advanced technological support. AI offers innovative solutions to these challenges, providing tools that optimize workflows, enhance diagnostic accuracy, and deliver tailored treatments to patients even in resource-constrained settings. However, the widespread integration of AI also introduces significant ethical, regulatory, and practical complexities, requiring a concerted effort from policymakers, clinicians, and technologists to navigate these challenges responsibly.

Purpose of the Book

This book serves as a comprehensive guide to understanding the transformative integration of AI into healthcare. It convenes experts across diverse fields to explore how AI and biomedical visualization are revolutionizing medical practice and research. Through detailed case studies, robust evidence-based analyses, and forward-looking perspectives, the book aims to equip readers with the knowledge and tools necessary to harness AI responsibly and effectively. By contextualizing AI's applications within current healthcare challenges, this book aspires to bridge the gap between technological potential and practical implementation.

Cohesive Themes in AI and Healthcare

The transformative potential of AI in healthcare cannot be overstated, and this book organizes its insights into interrelated themes to provide a comprehensive understanding of its applications. At its core, the text explores how AI integrates with key areas such as diagnostic precision, medical training, telemedicine, global healthcare disparities, and future innovations. Central to these discussions is the recognition of AI's reliance on robust data, advanced algorithms, and interdisciplinary collaboration to achieve meaningful outcomes. By exploring these themes in depth, the book illustrates AI's far-reaching implications across clinical, educational, and operational settings in medicine.

AI and Data-Driven Medicine

AI thrives on data, transforming vast amounts of unstructured medical information into actionable insights. The book explores how diverse datasets, including genomic sequences, diagnostic imaging, and electronic health records, are harnessed to train machine learning models capable of enhancing diagnostic accuracy, streamlining workflows, and predicting patient outcomes.

Education and Training: A Paradigm Shift

Medical education is undergoing a seismic shift as AI enables personalized learning and competency-based training. The book examines how technologies like virtual reality and AI-driven simulations are redefining how clinicians are trained, offering immersive environments that replicate real-world challenges while providing tailored feedback to improve skill acquisition and decision-making.

Equitable Healthcare Access Through AI

In regions where resources are scarce, AI holds the promise of bridging gaps in healthcare delivery. The book highlights how telemedicine, remote monitoring, and AI-driven diagnostic tools are making high-quality healthcare accessible to underserved populations, particularly in low- and middle-income countries. By addressing these disparities, AI has the potential to democratize healthcare and improve global health outcomes.

Pioneering Frontiers: Space Medicine and Beyond

The unique challenges posed by space exploration demand innovative solutions, and AI is at the forefront of addressing these needs. From autonomous health systems to predictive analytics for astronaut well-being, the book delves into how AI is shaping the future of space medicine, offering insights that may one day benefit terrestrial healthcare as well.

Ethical Imperatives and Responsible AI

Ethical considerations are woven throughout the text, emphasizing the importance of transparency, accountability, and inclusivity in AI development. Discussions on algorithmic bias, data privacy, and the moral implications of automation provide a balanced perspective on the opportunities and challenges AI presents. By prioritizing these principles, the book advocates for a responsible approach to innovation.

Overarching Vision

The integration of AI and biomedical visualization into healthcare holds the promise of a more efficient, equitable, and innovative future. By streamlining complex workflows, improving diagnostic accuracy, and personalizing care, AI is poised to address some of the most enduring challenges in medicine. However, realizing this vision demands interdisciplinary collaboration, rigorous ethical oversight, and a commitment to ensuring equitable access to technological advancements. This book underscores the necessity of balancing technological progress with the humanistic values that underpin healthcare.

Ethical and Practical Considerations

While the potential of AI in healthcare is immense, its adoption must be approached with caution and responsibility. Addressing critical concerns such as algorithmic bias, data privacy, and the reliability of AI systems is essential to maintaining trust and ensuring patient safety. This book emphasizes the importance of navigating these challenges thoughtfully, advocating for ethical frameworks that prioritize transparency, accountability, and inclusivity.

Reading Guidance

Designed for a diverse audience that includes clinicians, researchers, students, and policymakers, this book offers a comprehensive exploration of AI's role in healthcare. Readers are encouraged to engage with the themes sequentially to appreciate the narrative progression or focus on specific sections that align with their professional interests and expertise. Each chapter contributes to a cohesive and interdisciplinary discourse on the transformative potential of AI in medicine.

Conclusion

AI and biomedical visualization are redefining the boundaries of modern healthcare, offering tools to address longstanding challenges and ushering in an era of unprecedented innovation. By embracing these technologies responsibly, we can bridge gaps in care, enhance patient outcomes, and shape a future where innovation and compassion coexist. This book invites readers to delve into the transformative potential of AI in medicine, fostering a deeper understanding of its applications, challenges, and opportunities.

Oxford, UK

Arian Arjomandi Rad
Robert Vardanyan

Contents

Editors and Contributors

About the Series Editor

Paul M. Rea is an internationally recognized leading expert, in the applications of digital technologies to biomedical/medical visualization in education, clinical settings, and industry linked research. Initially he trained in Medicine, undertaking roles in general medicine, paediatric surgery, and emergency medicine, followed by a period as a pathologist. He then changed direction, pursuing a clinical anatomy educator role as Full Professor of Digital and Anatomical Education. It was in academia he realized the potential digital technologies had for education, simulation, training, and public/civic engagement. He led the strategic partnership with the School of Simulation and Technology (SIT), the Glasgow School of Art (GSA), and founded the MSc Medical Visualisation and Human Anatomy, following significant grant funded research. This degree improved graduate employability and had significant high-profile media coverage. He was the founding and now Series Editor (Editor-in-Chief equivalent) for the internationally acclaimed Biomedical Visualization book series with Springer Nature. He holds strategic leadership roles for innovation, engagement, and enterprise; body donation; education; and previously project management for large-scale infrastructural developments. He is a Licensed Teacher of Anatomy, licensed by the Scottish government, and has held this role for 19 years.

He is also the Director of Innovation, Engagement and Enterprise within the School of Medicine, Dentistry and Nursing, a role he has held since August 2022. He is responsible for leading, delivering, and managing the three pillars of the strategy: driving innovation and enterprise; employability for careers and growing entrepreneurs; and regional economic and societal impact.

About the Volume Editors

Johann Malawana is the CEO of Medics Academy, Managing Director of The Healthcare Leadership Academy (HLA), and the Associate Dean—Innovation at the School of Medicine and Dentistry, the University of

Lancashire. He has a focus on Innovation, Entrepreneurship, Leadership of Health Systems, and Technology Enhanced Learning.

Arian Arjomandi Rad is the Research Director at The Healthcare Leadership Academy and currently a cardiothoracic surgery nationally appointed trainee in Oxford. He graduated from Imperial College London, with a degree in Medicine and Surgery. He also obtained a degree in Management from Imperial College London Business School. He is a PhD candidate in Cardiothoracic Surgery at the University of Maastricht, School for Cardiovascular Diseases. He has a strong interest in Cardiothoracic Surgery, with a particular focus on academic cardiac surgery, mitral valve surgery, left ventricular assist devices, and mechanical circulatory support. He holds a particular passion for innovation, leadership, and research with interests spanning the intersection of surgery, medical technology, and digital health. Over his short career, he has published over 90 papers, served as editor for 2 books, held over 40 national and international presentations, and received 13 academic awards/prizes, including The Diana Legacy Award for his research and volunteering activities.

Robert Vardanyan is a neurosurgical nationally appointed trainee in the Severn deanery. Graduated from Imperial College School of Medicine and Imperial College Business School, his professional life has been dedicated to excelling in academic neurosciences, operative neurosurgery, and surgical research.

He has achieved 50 publications and presented at more than 70 national and international academic forums, all while developing his clinical and operative abilities into a devoted neurosurgical resident. His academic contributions are further demonstrated by his co-authorship of various educational resources, including two textbooks on the Objective Structured Practical Examinations for undergraduate medical education. He is also a co-director of the HLA Research Masterclass Course with Dr Arjomandi Rad, aimed at fostering research skills among students and professionals worldwide.

Additionally, his involvement in Bioethics and Diploma in the Philosophy of Medicine have allowed him to explore and contribute to the application of bioethics in everyday clinical practice, particularly, with regard to artificial intelligence-enabled healthcare and surgery.

George Miller is an Emergency Medicine Doctor. The Executive Committee takes responsibility for the day-to-day running of the HLA, and George also separately chairs the HLA Research Collaborative. He is also an Honorary University Lecturer, a Fellow of the Institute of Leadership and Management, and a lead for the Intermediate Leadership Programme.

In addition to his work at the HLA, he is a President at Amnesty International and sits on the International Advisory Council at Action Against Hunger.

He was one of the top scoring applicants for the AFP, CST, and Public Health Training across the country, and he has presented national courses on 'Success in Medical School', 'Preparing for the AFP', and 'Preparing for the PSA'. He has conducted his policy research at the Department of Social Policy and Intervention, University of Oxford.

Contributors

Ezgi Aldemir Department of Trauma and Orthopaedics, Jersey General Hospital, St Helier, Jersey

Aws Al-Omari Department of Neurosurgery, Oxford University Hospital NHS Trust, Oxford, UK

Arian Arjomandi Rad Department of Cardiothoracic Surgery, Maastricht University Medical Center, Maastricht, The Netherlands

Department of Cardiothoracic Surgery, John Radcliffe Hospital, Oxford University Hospitals NHS Foundation Trust, Oxford, UK

Thanos Athanasiou Department of Surgery and Cancer, Imperial College London, London, UK

Carla Bloom Department of Trauma and Orthopaedics, Jersey General Hospital, St Helier, Jersey

Emma Cox Medics.Academy, London, UK

Leila Ellis University of Bristol, Bristol, UK

Susan Honeyman Department of Neurosurgery, John Radcliffe Hospital, Oxford University Hospitals NHS Foundation Trust, Oxford, UK

Anam Jawaid Department of Trauma and Orthopaedic Surgery, The Dudley Group NHS Foundation Trust, Dudley, UK

Aida Kafai Golahmadi The Whittington Hospital, London, UK

Yusuf Karmali Medics.Academy, Kings College Hospital NHS Trust, London, UK

Hiba Khan Medics.Academy and The School of Medicine, University of Central Lancashire, Preston, UK

Souradip Mookerjee University of Cambridge, Cambridge, United Kingdom

Peyman Sardari Nia Department of Cardiothoracic Surgery, Maastricht University Medical Center, Maastricht, The Netherlands

Pedra Rabiee The Healthcare Leadership Academy, London, UK

Viraj Shah Department of Medicine, Faculty of Medicine, Imperial College London, London, UK

Hariharan Subbiah Ponniah Department of Medicine, Faculty of Medicine, Imperial College London, London, UK

Abdullah Tahir Department of Trauma and Orthopaedic Surgery, University Hospitals of North Midlands, Stoke-On-Trent, UK

Robert Vardanyan Department of Neurosurgery, John Radcliffe Hospital, Oxford University Hospitals NHS Foundation Trust, Oxford, UK

The Anatomy of Medical Data

1

Souradip Mookerjee

Abstract

This chapter offers a comprehensive exploration of the diverse spectrum of medical data types, including medical imaging, genomics, and electronic health records (EHRs). In doing so, it delves into the anatomy of these data sources and examines their relevance in machine learning applied to clinical decision-making and medical research. Emphasizing the importance of effective data visualization techniques, the chapter highlights how advanced analytics—such as machine learning and artificial intelligence—can be leveraged to uncover new insights, enhance predictive capabilities, and optimize treatment strategies, topics which will be expanded upon in subsequent chapters.

By taking a first-principles approach, the chapter investigates how data is derived from the human body, starting at the molecular level and gradually zooming out to the cellular, organ, multi-organ, whole organism, and inter-organism levels. This reductionist framework assumes that a healthy state results from the optimal configuration and location of every molecule. The chapter explores the tools available for interrogating these data at each level, with an emphasis on the time-series nature of the data across these scales, thus constructing a mental framework that can be extended to consider future yet-unknown data sources about the human body. In addition, it explores how effective visualization tools are integral to transforming raw data into actionable knowledge, enabling clinicians to make informed decisions and researchers to draw meaningful conclusions.

Finally, the chapter concludes with a discussion on the practicalities and challenges associated with analysing complex medical data, particularly regarding the integration of these diverse data sources and the future of medical data science.

Keywords

Medical data · Imaging · Genomics · Electronic health records · Data visualization

1.1 Introduction

In the modern era of healthcare, data is not just abundant—it can also be transformative. If data represents the ways in which we can describe the world around us, the modern age allows us to describe the human body in ever more sophisti-

S. Mookerjee (✉)
University of Cambridge, Cambridge, United Kingdom
e-mail: sm2030@cantab.ac.uk

J. Malawana et al. (eds.), *Artificial Intelligence in Healthcare and Biomedical Visualization*, Biomedical Visualization 10, https://doi.org/10.1007/978-3-032-06520-9_1

cated detail. Medical data has always been the cornerstone of evidence-based clinical practice and research, and from the sequences of our genomes to the detailed images of our organs and tissues, this has never been more important.

As the digital age progresses, health data systems have evolved, integrating a vast array of information from electronic health records (EHRs), diagnostic imaging, clinical outcomes, laboratory results, and genomic sequences. The goal of modern healthcare is not only to capture and store these data but to analyse and interpret them in ways that can significantly improve patient care. Understanding how to work with and interpret these diverse data types is essential for anyone involved in clinical decision-making or health-related research.

Unlike other areas of machine learning, it can often be difficult to obtain structured, labelled data at scale in medicine due to the human capital required for such labelling, the inherently unstructured formats in which this data is often captured and the ethical and legal implications of collecting this form of data at scale (Ghassemi et al. 2020). Thus, this area of artificial intelligence research and development raises interesting and novel challenges for both the clinician and researcher.

In this chapter, we will explore the anatomy of different medical data types and emphasize the importance of effective data visualization techniques. With the help of advanced analytics, including machine learning and artificial intelligence, medical data can be leveraged to uncover new insights, enhance predictive capabilities, and optimize treatment strategies, which will be expanded upon in the following chapters. We will also explore how effective visualization tools are integral to transforming raw data into actionable knowledge, enabling clinicians to make informed decisions and researchers to derive meaningful conclusions.

By taking a first principles approach to understanding the sources of data that can arise from the human body and the different types of data that may be derived from each level, we can understand how each type of medical data relates to one another, and how future data sources may fit within this framework. We will take a reductionist approach to the human body by assuming that if every molecule is in the optimal configuration and location, then this will result in a healthy person. We will examine the tools that are available to us to interrogate this information, starting from the molecular level, and slowly zooming out to the cellular level, organ level, multi-organ level, whole organism level, and inter-organism level. We will also see that all the data obtainable at each of these levels form a time series. Finally, we will finish on the practicalities of these data formats and challenges in analysing them.

1.2 Molecular Data: Genes, Proteins, and Regulatory Networks

The closest we can get to reading the molecular states and positions of every cell in the body is at the genomic level. Every cell contains the same genomic material as every other cell from birth (Wabl et al. 1975). Mutations in these genes give rise to normal variation, as well as pathological variants. However, this is not the end of the story—these genes may interact with one another (the phenomenon of epistasis and recessive/dominant alleles), have gene dosage effects, and be silenced depending on which cell type the genome is found within (epigenetics) (Trerotola et al. 2015). In a clinical setting, the depth and complexity of all this biological information is not routinely captured, although it can be in a research setting (e.g., through techniques such as single-cell RNA sequencing [scRNAseq], chromatin immunoprecipitation [ChIP], bisulphite sequencing, and more). The source of the genetic material being sequenced may arise from the DNA, RNA, or focussed sequencing based on only the expressed parts of the genome (exome).

The most widely used techniques to collect genomic data at present are Sanger sequencing, single nucleotide polymorphism (SNP) phenotyping, and whole genome sequencing. Sanger sequencing is the oldest and lowest throughput methodology of the above techniques, which makes it less suited for machine learning applications due to the sparsity and low volume of data generated.

Single nucleotide polymorphisms (SNPs) are the most common type of genetic variation found in the human genome, occurring when a single nucleotide (A, T, C, or G) in the DNA sequence is altered. The study of how specific SNPs are associated with observable traits is a process known as SNP phenotyping. Although capturing only a subset of possible mutations (i.e. only single point mutations, and not copy number variations, indels, or other more exotic genetic alterations), they have been useful because it is not necessary for any particular SNP to have a direct relation to a gene of interest. It is only necessary for a SNP to be associated with a particular allele (e.g. through a close proximity on the genome) such that the SNP and the actual mutation of interest are transmitted together down the germline without being separated away through recombination—the probability of recombination separating a SNP from a mutant allele increases as the SNP is further away from the allele in the chromosome (Balagué-Dobón et al. 2022).

This allows a panel of selected SNPs to be a useful marker for measuring (at low resolution) which alleles a certain individual is carrying, without needing to sequence the entire genome. Crucially, this allows a crude amount of information to be collected about an individual's genome cheaply and thus at scale across a large population. Services such as 23andme and other consumer genetic testing organizations often use this technique to inform their clients about their ancestry, disease risk profiles, and more by associating which combination of SNPs correlates with which disease profiles and ancestries (Lu et al. 2021). Blood and tissue banks often use this technique to identify the tissue types and other factors to be able to identify compatible donors and recipients.

More recently, as the cost of sequencing whole genomes has dropped exponentially from the circa \$300 M required to sequence the first human genome in 2001 to the ~£600 it takes in 2023, whole genome sequence (and consequently, exome sequencing) data has become much more widely available (National Human Genome Research Institute 2023). This has been made possible using next-generation sequencing technology, which splits apart a genome into many small fragments, which are all sequenced in parallel, and the original sequence is then reconstructed computationally by aligning these fragments to a "reference" genome. Variants are then called by identifying differences between the reconstructed genome and the reference genome. It is important to note that variants here are neither normal nor abnormal, as the reference genome was itself constructed from an "imperfect" human; it may therefore be possible that certain variants may be protective, and others may be detrimental. It may be that combinations of such variants have an additive predictive ability over any individual variant (Slatko et al. 2018).

The data from these next-generation sequencing techniques often arrives as a FASTA or FASTQ format file. This is a text file containing the reads from each of these short sequences. The FASTA file, while fundamental for storing raw sequencing reads, is only the beginning of the data analysis pipeline. These raw reads must first undergo quality control (QC), a critical step that ensures the accuracy and reliability of the sequencing data. Common QC processes include removing low-quality reads, trimming adapter sequences, and filtering out contaminants. Tools such as FastQC and Trimmomatic are widely used for this purpose (Leipzig 2017).

Once the raw reads have been pre-processed, the next step is alignment. Here, each sequence read is mapped to a reference genome using alignment tools like BWA (Burrows-Wheeler Aligner) or Bowtie. These tools determine the most likely position of each read within the genome, creating a SAM/BAM file—a binary format that records how each read aligns to the reference genome.

After alignment, variant calling is performed to identify differences between the sequenced genome and the reference genome. This step relies on algorithms that distinguish true variants (e.g. single nucleotide polymorphisms, insertions, and deletions) from sequencing errors. Variant calling tools like GATK (Genome Analysis Toolkit) and FreeBayes are commonly employed to generate VCF (Variant Call Format) files, which catalogue the identified variants along with their positions and quality scores.

At this stage, the VCF file serves as the foundation for downstream analyses. Researchers can annotate variants to determine their functional impact using tools like ANNOVAR or VEP (Variant Effect Predictor). Annotation provides insights into whether variants occur in coding or non-coding regions, whether they cause missense or nonsense mutations, and their potential association with disease risk or protective effects, or provide further input for machine learning models.

All these forms of data are useful in machine learning analysis, with both supervised and unsupervised techniques. Sequence data may be used, for example, in tissue classification, protein structure prediction, single-cell RNA sequence classification, and more (Auslander et al. 2021). This data can be visualised and expressed in the form of text (e.g. the raw sequences), images (e.g. expression maps, ChIP maps), as well as higher dimensional, more abstract embedding formats (e.g. a vector containing the expression values for all the genes in a cell). This allows for the use of many different machine learning approaches, based on the representation chosen.

1.3 Cellular Data Can Be Collected Through Blood Testing

As we zoom out from the genome level, there is a wealth of information that can be collected about an individual cell, reflecting the many diverse cellular functions. At a fundamental level, each cell metabolizes oxygen and glucose into energy, producing carbon dioxide and water as byproducts. This process, known as cellular respiration, is tightly regulated and can become dysregulated in metabolic conditions such as diabetes. High-throughput monitoring of this process has been made possible through tools like continuous glucose monitors (CGMs). These devices provide real-time blood glucose data and are often paired with detailed food logs to correlate dietary intake with glucose responses. The resulting time-series data can be analysed using machine learning algorithms to detect patterns, predict glucose spikes, and optimize dietary and treatment recommendations for individuals with diabetes or pre-diabetes.

In addition to glucose monitoring, blood tests such as the full blood count (FBC) provide a snapshot of cellular health and function. An FBC measures the concentration and proportions of red blood cells, white blood cells, and platelets. Machine learning models can leverage FBC data to identify trends over time that might predict conditions such as iron deficiency anaemia, infections, or even early-stage cancers based on abnormalities in white blood cell subtypes (Santos-Silva et al. 2024).

Beyond the FBC, blood tests like C-reactive protein (CRP) and erythrocyte sedimentation rate (ESR) are widely used as markers of inflammation. Elevated CRP levels, for example, are associated with infections, autoimmune diseases, and cardiovascular events. In machine learning applications, longitudinal CRP data can be combined with other clinical and genomic datasets to develop models for predicting disease flare-ups in rheumatoid arthritis or identifying individuals at higher risk for myocardial infarction (Momtazmanesh et al. 2022).

Lipid panels, which measure total cholesterol, HDL, LDL, and triglyceride levels, are another routine blood test with significant relevance in predictive modelling. These tests are key biomarkers for cardiovascular risk stratification. By training machine learning algorithms on lipid data combined with other features like age, lifestyle factors, and genetics, predictive models can estimate a patient's risk of heart disease or stroke and guide early interventions (Liu et al. 2025).

Similarly, kidney function tests, such as serum creatinine and blood urea nitrogen (BUN), are essential for assessing renal health. Abnormal trends in these biomarkers can be detected early using machine learning, enabling prediction and monitoring of chronic kidney disease (CKD) progression. For instance, models trained on historical patient data can identify subtle changes in creatinine levels, providing clinicians with early warning systems for CKD risk.

Blood-based biomarkers are also revolutionizing the field of oncology. Tests measuring circulating tumour markers like CA-125 (for ovarian cancer) or PSA (prostate-specific antigen for prostate cancer) are routinely used for screening and disease monitoring. Advanced multi-omics approaches allow the measurement of thousands of metabolites, proteins, and cytokines from a single blood or fluid sample, allowing for the discovery of new biomarkers through large-scale data analysis. Proteomic and metabolomic data, when analysed using machine learning techniques, enable the discovery of novel biomarkers for diseases such as Alzheimer's, sepsis, or autoimmune disorders. For example, machine learning algorithms trained on complex proteomic data can identify signatures indicative of early neurodegeneration years before clinical symptoms manifest (Gogishvili et al. 2023).

The crucial element to the utility of these tests is their ability to be collected cheaply at scale, which allows for large datasets to be amassed with relative speed. Additionally, non-invasive technologies like photoplethysmography (PPG)—which measure blood volume changes using optical sensors, often via wearable devices—are emerging as important tools for capturing cellular-level data. PPG signals, which are routinely collected by smartwatches and fitness trackers, can be analysed with machine learning to predict a variety of health metrics. For example, PPG-derived features like pulse rate variability and waveform morphology have been shown to predict diabetes risk, with studies demonstrating strong correlations between abnormal PPG signals and impaired glucose metabolism (Avram et al. 2020). Similarly, PPG data has been used to identify vascular ageing and cardiovascular disease risk, which are reflected in PPG waveforms (Dall'Olio et al. 2020; Weng et al. 2024). These non-invasive insights open new avenues for continuous health monitoring, enabling the identification of at-risk individuals without the need for traditional blood tests.

Taken together, blood tests and non-invasive technologies like PPG generate a broad array of cellular and biochemical data that provide actionable insights into cellular physiology. Machine learning algorithms are increasingly able to harness this rich dataset to identify patterns, biomarkers, and predictive models that improve disease diagnosis, treatment personalization, and prognosis. By analysing vast quantities of blood test and PPG data over time, these technologies have the potential to revolutionize precision medicine and enable earlier, data-driven interventions.

1.4 Organ-Level Data Can Be Collected Through Imaging

Imaging is a critical source of macroscopic data in medicine, providing detailed anatomical and functional insights that are invaluable for clinical decision-making about organs and organ systems. These imaging studies are also a rich resource for machine learning (ML) projects, with their ability to identify patterns, anomalies, and predictive biomarkers at scale. Again, the key to a good imaging modality is the ability to collect this form of data in a high-throughput manner quickly across many patients at scale. Many modalities fit this description and, as such, are uniquely suited for analysis through machine learning techniques.

1.4.1 X-Ray Imaging

X-rays are the simplest and most ubiquitous form of medical imaging. They produce two-dimensional representations of dense structures, such as bones, and are widely used in emergency departments, outpatient clinics, and routine screenings. Hospital systems often store millions of X-ray images—virtually every patient passing through an emergency department may have an X-ray taken, making these datasets a readily available resource for machine learning. ML algorithms, such as convolutional neural networks (CNNs), have already demonstrated high accuracy in identifying pneumonia, fractures, and other abnormalities from X-ray images (Najjar and Najjar 2023).

1.4.2 Computed Tomography (CT) and Magnetic Resonance Imaging (MRI)

CT scans go beyond two-dimensional images by producing detailed cross-sectional views of the body through the use of X-ray technology. These slices can be reconstructed into three-dimensional models, providing deeper insights into soft tissue, bones, and organs. CT scans are particularly useful in diagnosing conditions such as traumatic injuries, tumours, and vascular diseases. These 3D reconstructions can then be fed into machine learning models for training, for classification, segmentation and risk prediction (Bellens et al. 2024).

MRI, on the other hand, uses magnetic fields and radio waves to generate high-resolution images of soft tissues, making it the gold standard for imaging the brain, muscles, ligaments, and organs. For example, MRI is extensively used to detect and monitor neurological disorders like multiple sclerosis or brain tumours. Machine learning algorithms can analyse MRI data to segment tissues, identify lesions, and even predict disease progression, as seen in applications for Alzheimer's disease and spinal injuries (Shah and Shah 2024).

1.4.3 Ultrasound

Ultrasound imaging is a non-invasive technique that uses high-frequency sound waves to create real-time images of organs, blood flow, and developing foetuses during pregnancy. While ultrasound offers significant advantages in portability and real-time imaging, it also presents challenges due to operator-dependent variability and inconsistent imaging angles. These issues can, however, be mitigated through standardized imaging protocols. For example, the four-chamber heart view is a common, reproducible ultrasound standard used in cardiac imaging (Gudigar et al. 2022). Machine learning can be applied to ultrasound data to detect cardiac abnormalities, fatal growth patterns, and even early signs of liver disease. For example, the EchoNet dataset provides over 10,000 apical 4-chamber views of the heart for use in training various models (Ouyang et al. 2020).

1.4.4 Emerging Imaging Modalities

Newer imaging technologies, such as functional MRI (fMRI), positron emission tomography (PET), and hybrid imaging systems (e.g. PET-CT), offer insights into not only the anatomical but also the functional and metabolic states of tissues. These imaging modalities produce highly complex data that are particularly suited for advanced machine learning techniques, enabling applications such as early cancer detection, brain activity mapping, and precision therapy planning (Fallahpoor et al. 2024; Wei and Naqa 2020). These emerging imaging modalities in machine learning are especially exciting due to the possibility of combining structural information with functional and biochemical data of tissues in situ.

1.4.5 Photography in Dermatology and Ophthalmology

Not all imaging modalities need to require expensive equipment—as photography becomes more accessible and cheaper to perform, this can be an especially cheap high-throughput imaging modality. In dermatology, for example, photographic data plays a crucial role in identifying and tracking skin conditions. High-quality images of the skin can be used to detect melanomas, eczema, and psoriasis through computer-aided diagnostic systems. Machine learning models trained on large datasets of dermatological images have achieved dermatologist-level accuracy in detecting skin cancers, making them a powerful tool for screening and triage (Chan et al. 2020; Jeong et al. 2023).

As well as photography of the skin, it is also possible to obtain retinal photographs, upon which many diseases paint their various clinical signs, such as hypertension, atherosclerosis, and diabetes. This data is also cheap to collect at scale and use in medical machine learning pipelines. As well as regular photography, optical coherence tomography can also be a powerful functional imaging technique that can be obtained at scale to identify both ophthalmological and systemic signs of disease (Kulyabin et al. 2024; Leandro et al. 2023).

1.4.6 Beyond Visual Data: Heart Sounds and Audio Systems

Radiological imaging is not the only source of macroscopic data about organ systems. Audio systems, such as digital stethoscopes, can capture heart sounds and lung sounds, which provide functional data about the cardiovascular and respiratory systems, and electrocardiograms (ECG) can aid in providing important diagnostic data about the electrical activity of the heart. Machine learning models can analyse this audio data to detect anomalies like murmurs, arrhythmias, and signs of chronic obstructive pulmonary disease (COPD). Combining these audio inputs with imaging data can offer a holistic, multimodal approach to diagnosis (Bachtiger et al. 2022; Huang et al. 2023).

1.4.7 Standardization and Formatting of Imaging Data for Machine Learning

Medical imaging data is typically stored in standardized formats to ensure compatibility across devices, systems, and software. For example, Digital imaging and communications in medicine (DICOM) is the most common format for radiological imaging data. DICOM files contain both the image data and metadata, such as patient information, imaging parameters, and timestamps, which can be invaluable for machine learning pipelines. Neuroimaging informatics technology initiative (NIfTI) is another imaging format primarily used for MRI and CT scans; this format is popular in neuroimaging research because it allows for multi-dimensional data storage. Regular images can be held in commonly available formats such as JPEG for photographs or PNG for diagrams, but one should always note the level of compression applied and image resolution in case of image artefacts from this processing step which may interfere with the accuracy of the machine learning models downstream. Storing and managing these large volumes of imaging data often requires robust infrastructure, such as picture archiving and communication systems (PACS), and cloud-based solutions for secure, scalable access.

1.4.8 Challenges in Medical Imaging Data

Medical imaging data presents a variety of challenges that can significantly impact the effectiveness of machine learning (ML) models. One major issue lies in noise and artifacts. Images often contain inconsistencies and disturbances, such as those caused by patient movement, improper calibration of medical equipment, or operator-related variability—particularly prevalent in modalities like ultrasound. For ML models to produce reliable results, they must be robust enough to identify and filter out such noise without compromising critical information.

Another challenge stems from resolution and data quality. The variability in image resolution across different scanning equipment or imaging environments can influence the accuracy of ML model outputs. For instance, while high-resolution MRIs provide rich, detailed insights into anatomical structures, lower-quality scans might obscure crucial details. To address this, pre-processing techniques such as image enhancement or advanced super-resolution algorithms often need to be employed to standardize and improve data quality.

Equally complex is the issue of registration and alignment. In longitudinal studies or multimodality imaging—such as PET-CT fusions—it is essential to align images acquired at different time points or from different modalities. This alignment ensures that meaningful comparisons can be made. However, achieving precise image registration across such datasets can be particularly challenging due to anatomical variability or imaging distortions.

Finally, the interpretation and labelling of medical imaging data pose a significant hurdle. Annotating these datasets typically requires the expertise of trained radiologists, a process that is both time-intensive and resource-heavy. Machine learning models, especially those reliant on supervised learning techniques, require large volumes of accurately labelled data to perform optimally. Producing these high-quality datasets can be prohibitively expensive and laborious, creating a bottleneck in the development and deployment of robust ML solutions in medical imaging.

By addressing these key challenges—noise, resolution, alignment, and labelling—researchers can enhance the reliability and scalability of ML models, ultimately improving diagnostic capabilities and patient care outcomes.

1.5 Interorganism-Level Data Is Often Much More Unstructured

Interorganism level data encompasses information that arises from interactions between individuals or individuals and their broader environments. Unlike cellular or macroscopic data, this data is inherently more unstructured, nuanced, and challenging to quantify. It often captures behavioural, psychological, and social determinants of health that are increasingly recognized as critical factors in understanding overall well-being and disease outcomes. Advances in machine learning have enabled researchers to parse patterns from this unstructured data, turning it into actionable insights.

One prominent example of interorganism data is psychiatric data, which often relies on behavioural observations, patient self-reports, and clinician evaluations. Psychiatric conditions like depression, anxiety, and schizophrenia frequently lack clear biological markers, making diagnosis dependent on subjective or semi-structured assessments. However, with the integration of technology, new avenues for objective data collection have emerged. Speech and voice patterns, for instance, can provide subtle indicators of psychiatric states. Prosody—the rhythm, tone, and stress in speech—has been shown to change with mental health conditions. Machine learning algorithms can analyse these prosodic features to detect emotional distress, suicidal ideation, or cognitive decline (Ben Moshe et al. 2024; Wasserzug et al. 2023). For example, slower speech rates, reduced pitch variation, and monotone delivery are commonly observed in patients with severe depression, whereas manic states may be associated with increased speech rate and irregular pauses. These subtle changes, imperceptible to the human ear, can be quantified and used as biomarkers for early detection and monitoring of psychiatric disorders.

In addition to direct clinical data, social media data has emerged as a unique, large-scale source of interorganism-level information. Platforms like Twitter, Facebook, and Reddit provide an unprecedented lens into human behaviour, emotions, and societal trends (Ahmed et al. 2022). Posts, comments, and even emojis can be analysed to detect mental health concerns, monitor population-level disease outbreaks, and study the influence of social determinants of health. For example, machine learning models trained on language patterns have successfully identified signs of depression, anxiety, and loneliness based on the frequency of negative sentiment, self-referential language, and expressions of isolation. Social media data can also help track real-time trends in public health crises, such as vaccination hesitancy, misinformation spread, and emotional responses to major events like pandemics or natural disasters (Bar-Lev et al. 2021).

Social determinants of health—factors such as socioeconomic status, education, living conditions, and social support—represent another crucial category of interorganism level data. These determinants influence health outcomes as much as genetic predispositions or lifestyle behaviours, yet they are often poorly captured in traditional medical datasets. Machine learning models can leverage diverse sources of information, including census data, geolocation information, and environmental exposure data, to uncover how social factors drive health disparities. For example, models that integrate neighbourhood-level data can predict rates of chronic illnesses such as diabetes or cardiovascular disease, identify food deserts where access to healthy food is limited, or pinpoint regions with poor air quality that exacerbate respiratory conditions (Segar et al. 2022).

Further extending the scope of interorganism data, wearable devices and mobile applications now capture real-time behavioural signals that reflect interactions with the external world. Smartphone sensors, such as GPS, accelerometers, and microphones, can monitor mobility patterns, activity levels, and social engagement. These data streams are particularly relevant for studying psychiatric conditions and neurodegenerative diseases. For example, reduced mobility and social isolation detected via phone data can act as early warning signs for depression or cognitive decline. Similarly, continuous monitoring of speech and social interactions can provide critical insights into conditions like autism spectrum disorder (ASD) and Parkinson's disease (Hsu et al. 2024; Iaboni et al. 2022; Varghese et al. 2024).

Finally, interorganism data extends to environmental and external stimuli that affect human biology and behaviour. Prospective studies have shown that factors such as air pollution, noise exposure, and even urban design can influence mental and physical health. Machine learning models that combine environmental data with individual-level health outcomes can highlight hidden associations, such as increased psychiatric hospital admissions in high-noise areas or heightened asthma rates in industrial regions (Chen et al. 2024; Lee et al. 2022).

While rich in potential, analysing interorganism-level data presents unique challenges. The data is often unstructured, noisy, and context-dependent, making it difficult to draw standardized conclusions. Language and prosody analyses, for instance, must account for linguistic, cultural, and individual variations. Social media data also raises ethical considerations surrounding privacy, consent, and the risk of algorithmic bias. Nonetheless, the integration of interorganism data with other health information—such as genomic, macroscopic, and cellular data—can enable a more comprehensive understanding of health, disease, and human behaviour. Machine learning provides the tools to uncover hidden patterns, transforming this unstructured and complex data into meaningful predictions and interventions that address the broader determinants of health.

1.6 Time Series of the Above Is Often Present Within Medical Records

Medical records are a rich and evolving source of time series data, capturing a patient's health journey over days, months, or even years. This temporal nature allows clinicians and machine learning models to detect patterns, predict outcomes, and enable proactive interventions. At the heart of these records lies the Electronic Health Record (EHR) system, which organizes vast amounts of structured and unstructured clinical data across multiple encounters with the healthcare system.

1.6.1 Structure of EHRs: Standardized Data and Unstructured Notes

Electronic Health Records contain two primary types of data: structured data and unstructured data. Structured data includes standardized fields such as diagnoses, medications, laboratory results, and vital signs. These entries often follow controlled vocabularies or clinical coding systems, such as SNOMED CT (Systematized Nomenclature of Medicine), ICD (International Classification of Diseases), or RxNorm for medications. This structured approach ensures consistency across healthcare systems and simplifies downstream analysis.

In contrast, unstructured data consists of free-text clinical notes—narratives written by healthcare providers during patient encounters. These notes include patient histories, physician observations, discharge summaries, and surgical reports. Unstructured data often represents the richest sources of information in healthcare, but it is also the most difficult to process. To unlock the potential of unstructured data, advanced techniques in machine learning, natural language processing, and image analysis are required. For example, NLP can be used to extract key medical concepts, diagnoses, or medications from physician notes, while deep learning algorithms can help classify and analyse medical images.

While they are rich in information, their unstructured nature poses challenges for computational analysis. Here, natural language processing (NLP) techniques are instrumental, extracting valuable insights by converting free text into machine-readable formats. For example, models can identify diagnoses, treatment plans, and adverse events hidden within clinical notes, enabling better decision support (Gao et al. 2022; Noaeen et al. 2023).

1.6.2 Clinical Data Types in EHRs

EHRs encompass a variety of clinical data types that evolve over time, making them ideal for time series analysis. Diagnoses represent chronological records of conditions diagnosed over multiple visits. Machine learning models can use this data to predict disease trajectories and comorbidities. Medications, including prescriptions, dosages, and adherence timelines, provide valuable insights into treatment responses and risks of adverse drug interactions. Time series models, for instance, can predict medication non-adherence based on patterns of missed refills. Laboratory results, such as regular lab tests like blood glucose, liver function, and kidney markers, can reveal trends indicative of underlying conditions or treatment effectiveness. Vital signs, including measurements like blood pressure, heart rate, and respiratory rate, offer real-time indicators of a patient's stability or deterioration. These values are especially valuable in intensive care settings for predicting critical events such as sepsis or cardiac arrest.

Time series data within EHRs allows clinicians and machine learning algorithms to model changes over time. For instance, hospital systems can analyse length of stay (LOS) data to predict discharge timelines, optimize bed management, and reduce resource strain. Similarly, ICU datasets like MIMIC (Medical Information Mart for Intensive Care) provide granular, time-stamped clinical data that have been widely used to develop predictive models for mortality, organ failure, and early warning systems (Johnson et al. 2023).

1.6.3 Interoperability of EHRs: Standards and APIs

To fully harness time series data across healthcare systems, interoperability—the seamless exchange of health information between systems—is essential. Standardized frameworks such as FHIR (Fast Healthcare Interoperability Resources) have emerged as critical tools for structuring and exchanging healthcare data. FHIR, in particular, provides a modern API-based approach that allows secure, real-time data access, enabling healthcare applications to retrieve and process patient records efficiently (Rigas et al. 2024).

In the UK, electronic healthcare systems such as S1 (SystmOne), and EMIS have established APIs that allow for data sharing between general practitioners, hospitals, and third-party systems (e.g. GP Connect, Interface Mechanism 1). These interfaces provide access to time series data, such as patient medications, immunizations, and visit histories, ensuring continuity of care and enabling data-driven analysis across providers (Sullivan et al. 2023).

1.6.4 Analysing Time Series Data for Decision Support and Predictive Modelling

The temporal structure of EHR data makes it particularly well-suited for decision support systems and predictive modelling. Machine learning techniques like recurrent neural networks (RNNs) and transformers are adept at analysing time series patterns to predict outcomes such as disease progression, hospital readmission, or risk of adverse events. For example, medication data can be used for predicting drug adherence, side effects, or therapy effectiveness based on historical prescriptions, length of stay can be used to model patient discharge timelines based on vitals, diagnosis, and treatment history, and using time-stamped vital signs and lab results to detect early signs of sepsis in ICU settings (Bohlmann et al. 2021).

Additionally, wearable devices and home monitoring systems now feed real-time data streams, such as heart rate, blood glucose, and blood pressure, directly into EHRs. These continuous measurements enrich time series data, providing opportunities for earlier detection of deteriorating health and remote management of chronic diseases (Sabry et al. 2022).

1.6.5 Challenges of EHR Time Series Data

Despite its vast potential, time series data in EHRs poses unique challenges. Data fragmentation across different healthcare providers and systems can result in incomplete records, limiting the accuracy of models. Data may also suffer from noise, such as irregular time gaps between measurements, inconsistencies in clinical coding, or human errors during data entry. Moreover, the integration of structured and unstructured data requires sophisticated pipelines capable of harmonizing disparate sources.

However, advancements in machine learning, combined with standardized frameworks like FHIR and NLP techniques for free-text analysis, are steadily overcoming these hurdles. The ability to analyse EHR time series data is transforming patient care by enabling early intervention, resource optimization, and more precise predictions of patient outcomes. As healthcare systems continue to digitize and integrate, time series data will play a central role in driving data-driven medicine forward.

1.7 Data Visualization Techniques

Data visualization enables healthcare professionals to make sense of large, complex datasets. By presenting data in an easily digestible format, such as graphs or maps, healthcare providers can quickly identify patterns, trends, and anomalies that may be overlooked in a sea of numbers. In an industry where decisions need to be made rapidly—whether diagnosing patients, monitoring disease outbreaks, or managing hospital resources—visualization aids in streamlining these processes.

In healthcare, visualizations are crucial for improving patient outcomes. Data visualization helps in tracking patient vitals, diagnostic results, and treatment progress. By displaying this information visually, healthcare providers can identify subtle changes in a patient's condition that might require immediate attention. In the same way, visualizing medical data can help a machine learning practitioner identify useful data sources, identify clusters within high-dimensional datasets of relevance and provide a structured transformation to allow machine learning models to more easily identify trends in data. For example, raw pixel data in a one-dimensional matrix without positional information is infinitely less useful than structured two-dimensional pixel data representing an image, and audio data in the form of raw sound values is far less useful than an audio spectrogram constructed from this data, to which a convolutional neural network can be applied to.

1.8 Challenges in Medical Data

The proliferation of digital health technologies has resulted in the generation of vast amounts of medical data, from electronic health records (EHRs) and diagnostic images to wearable devices and genomics. While these data have the potential to improve patient outcomes, healthcare efficiency, and medical research, they also introduce several challenges. These challenges range from privacy concerns and data security issues to biases in data analysis and the complexities of managing both structured and unstructured data.

One of the most significant challenges in managing medical data is ensuring its privacy and security. Medical data is inherently sensitive, and any compromise can have serious consequences for both patients and healthcare providers. Legal frameworks, such as the Health Insurance Portability and Accountability Act (HIPAA) in the United States and the General Data Protection Regulation (GDPR) in the UK and European Union, have been developed to regulate the collection, storage, and sharing of medical data to protect patients' privacy.

HIPAA, enacted in 1996, governs the confidentiality, security, and transmission of health data. The law applies to healthcare providers, insurers, and their business associates. One of its key provisions is the Privacy Rule, which regulates the use and disclosure of Protected Health Information (PHI), ensuring that patients' personal health data remains confidential. Another important aspect is the Security Rule, which establishes standards for securing electronic health data. It requires healthcare providers to implement safeguards to protect data integrity and confidentiality. Additionally, the Breach Notification Rule mandates that healthcare organizations notify individuals if their data is compromised. HIPAA violations can lead to significant fines and loss of reputation, highlighting the critical need for robust data security measures in healthcare.

The GDPR, enforced in 2018, provides guidelines for data privacy and protection within the European Union. It has significant implications for how medical data is managed, both within the EU and by organizations outside the EU that process data of EU citizens. One of its key provisions is the requirement for consent, meaning patients must provide explicit consent for their data to be used, with the ability to withdraw consent at any time. Another critical aspect is the Right to be Forgotten, which allows patients to request that their personal data be deleted, giving them greater control over their health information. The GDPR also emphasizes data minimization, ensuring that only data necessary for a specific purpose is collected and stored, thereby reducing the risk of over-collection and misuse.

Both HIPAA and GDPR aim to balance the need for medical data to improve healthcare outcomes with the protection of patient privacy. However, healthcare providers must navigate these complex regulations, often finding it challenging to stay compliant in an increasingly digital healthcare environment.

Beyond legal regulations, there are ethical concerns surrounding medical data, such as the risk of dehumanization, where patients' health is reduced to a set of numbers and algorithms. Ethical challenges also arise in data sharing, especially when using data for research without patient consent. The use of patient data for secondary purposes, like research or marketing, raises questions about ownership and control. Ensuring that ethical principles guide the use of medical data is essential for maintaining patient trust.

Bias in medical data can significantly affect healthcare outcomes, leading to disparities in diagnosis, treatment, and care. One common source of bias is sampling bias, which occurs when data is not representative of the general population. This can result in underrepresentation of certain groups, leading to skewed results. For example, many clinical trials have historically included predominantly white male participants, limiting the applicability of findings to other demographic groups.

Algorithmic bias is another concern, as machine learning models used in healthcare are only as reliable as the data they are trained on (Gianfrancesco et al. 2018). If the training data contains biases—such as the underrepresentation of specific ethnic groups or genders—these biases can be perpetuated in the model's predictions. Additionally, data collection bias can arise when healthcare providers make subjective decisions influenced by their own biases or stereotypes, resulting in skewed records.

Bias in medical data undermines the validity of research and clinical decisions while exacerbating health inequalities. Addressing this issue requires a comprehensive approach, including diversifying data sources, improving data collection methods, and developing more inclusive algorithms.

Data quality is a significant concern in healthcare, as missing, incomplete, or noisy data can distort analysis, leading to incorrect conclusions and suboptimal decisions. Missing data arises when key information is unavailable or has not been recorded, such as missing test results or patient information. This absence of critical details can hinder accurate diagnosis and treatment planning.

Incomplete data refers to records that lack certain values, such as incomplete medical histories or missing medical records. These gaps can limit the ability to understand a patient's condition fully or make informed clinical decisions. Noisy data, on the other hand, includes irrelevant, inconsistent, or erroneous data points that interfere with accurate analysis. This could result from input errors, equipment malfunctions, or other inconsistencies in data collection.

Several techniques can be employed to address issues related to missing, incomplete, or noisy data. One such technique is data imputation, which involves estimating missing values based on available data. However, this approach must be applied carefully to avoid introducing bias or distorting the dataset.

Another effective strategy is data cleaning, which focuses on identifying and correcting errors in the data. This includes removing duplicates, resolving inconsistencies, and ensuring that the data is accurate and relevant for analysis. Additionally, robust algorithms can be utilized. These algorithms are designed to be resistant to noise and can handle missing data without significantly compromising the accuracy of results.

While these solutions can enhance data quality, their implementation requires careful consideration to avoid inadvertently affecting the integrity of the analysis. Ensuring that these techniques are applied appropriately is essential for maintaining the reliability and validity of healthcare data.

Regulatory issues also extend to the ethical use of patient data for research. Data sharing between healthcare organizations, researchers, and pharmaceutical companies has the potential to drive advancements in medicine, but it also raises concerns about privacy and informed consent. Stringent data-sharing agreements and ethical guidelines must be in place to ensure that data is used responsibly. Federated machine learning techniques and privacy-preserving machine learning can be used to overcome some of these issues.

1.9 Conclusion

The anatomy of medical data is both complex and multifaceted, yet it holds immense promise for advancing healthcare delivery and research. As we have seen throughout this chapter, different types of medical data—ranging from imaging and genomics to electronic health records—present unique opportunities and challenges. By developing robust methods for analysing and visualizing these data, clinicians can make better-informed decisions, while researchers can uncover new insights that may revolutionize our understanding of health and disease.

The integration of machine learning, AI, and advanced analytics has the potential to transform medical data from a passive archive into an active tool that drives clinical innovation. However, realizing this potential requires overcoming technical, ethical, and regulatory hurdles, as well as fostering a deep understanding of the data's nuances and limitations.

As medical data continues to grow in volume and complexity, its effective utilization will rely heavily on interdisciplinary collaboration between clinicians, data scientists, bioinformaticians, and policymakers. The future of healthcare will not only be shaped by the data we collect but by how we understand, interpret, and apply that data to improve patient outcomes, drive innovation, and address global health challenges.

References

Ahmed A, Aziz S, Toro CT, Alzubaidi M, Irshaidat S, Serhan HA et al (2022) Machine learning models to detect anxiety and depression through

social media: a scoping review. Comput Methods Progr Biomed Update 2. https://doi.org/10.1016/j.cmpbup.2022.100066
Auslander N, Gussow AB, Koonin EV (2021) Incorporating machine learning into established bioinformatics frameworks. Int J Mol Sci 22(6). https://doi.org/10.3390/ijms22062903
Avram R, Olgin JE, Kuhar P, Hughes JW, Marcus GM, Pletcher MJ et al (2020) A digital biomarker of diabetes from smartphone-based vascular signals. Nat Med 26(10). https://doi.org/10.1038/s41591-020-1010-5
Bachtiger P, Petri CF, Scott FE, Park SR, Kelshiker MA, Sahemey HK et al (2022) Point-of-care screening for heart failure with reduced ejection fraction using artificial intelligence during ECG-enabled stethoscope examination in London, UK: a prospective, observational, multicentre study. Lancet Digit Health 4(2). https://doi.org/10.1016/S2589-7500(21)00256-9
Balagué-Dobón L, Cáceres A, González JR (2022) Fully exploiting SNP arrays: a systematic review on the tools to extract underlying genomic structure. Brief Bioinform 23(2). https://doi.org/10.1093/bib/bbac043
Bar-Lev S, Reichman S, Barnett-Itzhaki Z, Bar-Lev S, Reichman S, Barnett-Itzhaki Z (2021) Prediction of vaccine hesitancy based on social media traffic among Israeli parents using machine learning strategies. Israel J Health Pol Res 10(1). https://doi.org/10.1186/s13584-021-00486-6
Bellens S, Guerrero P, Vandewalle P, Dewulf W (2024) Machine learning in industrial X-ray computed tomography—a review. CIRP J Manuf Sci Technol 51. https://doi.org/10.1016/j.cirpj.2024.05.004
Ben Moshe T, Ziv I, Dershowitz N, Bar K, Ben Moshe T, Ziv I et al (2024) The contribution of prosody to machine classification of schizophrenia. Schizophrenia 10(s). https://doi.org/10.1038/s41537-024-00463-3
Bohlmann A, Mostafa J, Kumar M (2021) Machine learning and medication adherence: scoping review. JMIRx Med 2(4). https://doi.org/10.2196/26993
Chan S, Reddy V, Myers B, Thibodeaux Q, Brownstone N, Liao W (2020) Machine learning in dermatology: current applications, opportunities, and limitations. Dermatol Ther 10(3). https://doi.org/10.1007/s13555-020-00372-0
Chen F, Zhang W, Mfarrej MFB, Saleem MH, Khan KA, Ma J et al (2024) Breathing in danger: understanding the multifaceted impact of air pollution on health impacts. Ecotoxicol Environ Saf 280. https://doi.org/10.1016/j.ecoenv.2024.116532
Dall'Olio L, Curti N, Remondini D, Safi Harb Y, Asselbergs FW, Castellani G et al (2020) Prediction of vascular aging based on smartphone acquired PPG signals. Sci Reports 10(1). https://doi.org/10.1038/s41598-020-76816-6
Fallahpoor M, Chakraborty S, Pradhan B, Faust O, Barua PD, Chegeni H, Acharya R (2024) Deep learning techniques in PET/CT imaging: a comprehensive review from sinogram to image space. Comput Methods Prog Biomed 243. https://doi.org/10.1016/j.cmpb.2023.107880
Gao C, Goswami M, Chen J, Dubrawski A (2022) Classifying unstructured clinical notes via automatic weak supervision. https://doi.org/10.48550/arXiv.2206.12088
Ghassemi M, Naumann T, Schulam P, Beam AL, Chen IY, Ranganath R (2020) A review of challenges and opportunities in machine learning for health. AMIA Jt Summits Transl Sci Proc 2020:191–200
Gianfrancesco MA, Tamang S, Yazdany J, Schmajuk G (2018) Potential biases in machine learning algorithms using electronic health record data. JAMA Intern Med 178(11). https://doi.org/10.1001/jamainternmed.2018.3763
Gogishvili D, Vromen EM, Koppes-den Hertog S, Lemstra AW, Pijnenburg YAL, Visser PJ et al (2023) Discovery of novel CSF biomarkers to predict progression in dementia using machine learning. Sci Reports 13(1). https://doi.org/10.1038/s41598-023-33045-x
Gudigar A, R U, Samanth J, Vasudeva A, Nayak K, Tan RS, Ciaccio EJ, Ooi CP, Barua PD, Molinari F, Acharya UR (2022) Role of four-chamber heart ultrasound images in automatic assessment of fetal heart: a systematic understanding. Informatics 9(2):34. https://doi.org/10.3390/informatics9020034
Hsu BW, Chen YM, Yang YH, Tseng VS (2024) Predicting fine-grained behavioral and psychological symptoms of dementia based on machine learning and smart wearable devices. https://doi.org/10.48550/arXiv.2410.18091
Huang D-M, Huang J, Qiao K, Zhong N-S, Lu H-Z, Wang W-J et al (2023) Deep learning-based lung sound analysis for intelligent stethoscope. Mil Med Res 10(1). https://doi.org/10.1186/s40779-023-00479-3
Iaboni A, Spasojevic S, Newman K, Martin LS, Wang A, Ye B et al (2022) Wearable multimodal sensors for the detection of behavioral and psychological symptoms of dementia using personalized machine learning models. Alzheimer's Dement 14(1). https://doi.org/10.1002/dad2.12305
Jeong HK, Park C, Henao R, Kheterpal M (2023) Deep learning in dermatology: a systematic review of current approaches, outcomes, and limitations. JID Innov 3(1). https://doi.org/10.1016/j.xjidi.2022.100150
Johnson A, Bulgarelli L, Shen L, Gayles A, Shammout A, Horng S et al (2023) MIMIC-IV, a freely accessible electronic health record dataset - PubMed. Sci Data 10(1). https://doi.org/10.1038/s41597-022-01899-x
Kulyabin M, Zhdanov A, Nikiforova A, Stepichev A, Kuznetsova A, Ronkin M et al (2024) OCTDL: optical coherence tomography dataset for image-based deep learning methods. Sci Data 11(1). https://doi.org/10.1038/s41597-024-03182-7
Leandro I, Lorenzo B, Aleksandar M, Dario M, Rosa G, Agostino A et al (2023) OCT-based deep-learning models for the identification of retinal key signs. Sci Reports 13(1). https://doi.org/10.1038/s41598-023-41362-4
Lee S, Ku H, Hyun C, Lee M (2022) Machine learning-based analyses of the effects of various types of air

pollutants on hospital visits by asthma patients. Toxics 10(11). https://doi.org/10.3390/toxics10110644
Leipzig J (2017) A review of bioinformatic pipeline frameworks. Brief Bioinform 18(3). https://doi.org/10.1093/bib/bbw020
Liu T, Krentz A, Lu L, Curcin V (2025) Machine learning based prediction models for cardiovascular disease risk using electronic health records data: systematic review and meta-analysis. Eur Heart J 6(1). https://doi.org/10.1093/ehjdh/ztae080
Lu C, Tzovaras BG, Gough J (2021) A survey of direct-to-consumer genotype data, and quality control tool (GenomePrep) for research. Comput Struct Biotechnol J 19. https://doi.org/10.1016/j.csbj.2021.06.040
Momtazmanesh S, Nowroozi A, Rezaei N (2022) Artificial intelligence in rheumatoid arthritis: current status and future perspectives: a state-of-the-art review. Rheumatol Ther 9(5). https://doi.org/10.1007/s40744-022-00475-4
Najjar R, Najjar R (2023) Redefining radiology: a review of artificial intelligence integration in medical imaging. Diagnostics 13(17):2760. https://doi.org/10.3390/diagnostics13172760
National Human Genome Research Institute (2023) DNA sequencing costs: Data. Retrieved from https://www.genome.gov/about-genomics/fact-sheets/DNA-Sequencing-Costs-Data
Noaeen M, Amini S, Bhasker S, Ghezelsefli Z, Ahmed A, Jafarinezhad O, Abad ZS (2023) Unlocking the power of EHRs: harnessing unstructured data for machine learning-based outcome predictions - PubMed. In: Annual International Conference of the IEEE Engineering in Medicine and Biology Society. IEEE Engineering in Medicine and Biology Society. Annual International Conference. IEEE. https://doi.org/10.1109/EMBC40787.2023.10340232
Ouyang D, He B, Ghorbani A, Yuan N, Ebinger J, Langlotz CP et al (2020) Video-based AI for beat-to-beat assessment of cardiac function. Nature 580(7802). https://doi.org/10.1038/s41586-020-2145-8
Rigas ES, Lagakis P, Karadimas M, Logaras E, Latsou D, Hatzikou M et al (2024) Semantic interoperability for an AI-based applications platform for smart hospitals using HL7 FHIR. J Syst Softw 215. https://doi.org/10.1016/j.jss.2024.112093
Sabry F, Eltaras T, Labda W, Alzoubi K, Malluhi Q (2022) Machine learning for healthcare wearable devices: the big picture. J Healthc Eng 2022. https://doi.org/10.1155/2022/4653923
Santos-Silva MA, Sousa N, Sousa JC (2024) Frontiers | Artificial intelligence in routine blood tests. Front Med Eng 2. https://doi.org/10.3389/fmede.2024.1369265
Segar MW, Hall JL, Jhund PS, Powell-Wiley TM, Morris AA, Kao D et al (2022) Machine learning–based models incorporating social determinants of health vs traditional models for predicting in-hospital mortality in patients with heart failure. JAMA Cardiol 7(8). https://doi.org/10.1001/jamacardio.2022.1900
Shah S, Shah M (2024) The effects of machine learning algorithms in magnetic resonance imaging (MRI), and biomarkers on early detection of Alzheimer's disease. Adv Biomarker Sci Technol 6. https://doi.org/10.1016/j.abst.2024.08.004
Slatko BE, Gardner AF, Ausubel FM (2018) Overview of next generation sequencing technologies. Curr Protoc Mol Biol 122(1). https://doi.org/10.1002/cpmb.59
Sullivan R, Williams J, Robinson J, Thompson I, McNicoll I, Nichols T (2023) Pathways to interoperable electronic patient records for health and social care: part 1: for those involved directly in care - PubMed. Future Healthc J 10(3). https://doi.org/10.7861/fhj.2023-0071
Trerotola M, Relli V, Simeone P, Alberti S, Trerotola M, Relli V et al (2015) Epigenetic inheritance and the missing heritability. Hum Genom 9(1). https://doi.org/10.1186/s40246-015-0041-3
Varghese J, Brenner A, Fujarski M, van Alen CM, Plagwitz L, Warnecke T et al (2024) Machine learning in the Parkinson's disease smartwatch (PADS) dataset. npj Parkinson's Dis 10(1). https://doi.org/10.1038/s41531-023-00625-7
Wabl MR, Brun RB, Pasquier LD (1975) Lymphocytes of the toad Xenopus laevis have the gene set for promoting tadpole development. Science. https://doi.org/10.1126/science.1198115
Wasserzug Y, Degani Y, Bar-Shaked M, Binyamin M, Klein A, Hershko S, Levkovitch Y (2023) Development and validation of a machine learning-based vocal predictive model for major depressive disorder - PubMed. J Affect Disord 325. https://doi.org/10.1016/j.jad.2022.12.117
Wei L, Naqa IE (2020) AI for response evaluation with PET/CT. Semin Nucl Med 51(2). https://doi.org/10.1053/j.semnuclmed.2020.10.003
Weng W-H, Baur S, Daswani M, Chen C, Harrell L, Kakarmath S et al (2024) Predicting cardiovascular disease risk using photoplethysmography and deep learning. PLOS Glob Public Health 4(6). https://doi.org/10.1371/journal.pgph.0003204

Machine Learning Algorithms for Medical Imaging

2

Viraj Shah and Hariharan Subbiah Ponniah

Abstract

This chapter highlights the profound impact of machine learning (ML) on the field of medical imaging. Medical imaging is vital to modern healthcare, providing clinicians with vital visual insights for diagnosis and treatment planning without invasive procedures. The integration of ML algorithms, such as convolutional neural networks (CNNs), recurrent neural networks (RNNs), support vector machines (SVMs), and decision trees/random forests, is fundamentally transforming how imaging data is analysed and utilized. ML enhances diagnostic accuracy, enables personalized treatment strategies, and streamlines workflow efficiency in medical imaging applications. Despite significant progress, challenges including data requirements, interpretability, and ethical considerations must be addressed through interdisciplinary collaboration. Future efforts focusing on data acquisition, privacy preservation, and regulatory standards will drive transformative advancements in ML-driven medical imaging, ultimately enhancing healthcare delivery and improving patient outcomes across mortality, safety, patient experience, effectiveness, and patient satisfaction.

Keywords

Machine learning · Medical imaging · Diagnostic imaging · Diagnostic accuracy

2.1 Introduction to Medical Imaging

Medical imaging continues to form a cornerstone pillar of twenty-first century healthcare. It provides clinicians with non-invasive methods to visualize internal structures to assess a patient's pathological state. Over the last 100 years, advancements in imaging have been the catalyst for enormous improvements in medical diagnosis and treatment planning, leading to improved patient outcomes and care.

2.2 Overview of Medical Imaging Techniques

2.2.1 Magnetic Resonance Imaging (MRI)

MRI is a powerful imaging modality that employs magnetic fields and radio waves to produce detailed images of internal organs, tissues, and

V. Shah (✉) · H. Subbiah Ponniah
Department of Medicine, Faculty of Medicine, Imperial College London, London, UK
e-mail: viraj.shah19@imperial.ac.uk

J. Malawana et al. (eds.), *Artificial Intelligence in Healthcare and Biomedical Visualization*, Biomedical Visualization 10, https://doi.org/10.1007/978-3-032-06520-9_2

structures within the body. By detecting signals emitted by hydrogen atoms in water, MRI-produced images play useful roles in visualizing soft tissue. As such, MRI is commonly used in diagnosis and condition monitoring of a range of pathology—such as brain tumours, spinal cord injuries, musculoskeletal disorders, and cardiovascular diseases.

2.2.2 Computed Tomography (CT) Scan

CT scan, known in long-form as a computerized axial tomography (CAT) scan, utilizes X-rays and computer processing to generate cross-sectional images of the body. CT imaging provides detailed anatomical information and is therefore valuable for detecting abnormalities in the chest, abdomen, and pelvis. CT scans are widely used in the diagnosis of conditions such as cancer, trauma, vascular diseases, and pulmonary embolism.

2.2.3 X-Ray Imaging

X-rays are one of the oldest and most commonly used imaging formats. They involve exposing the body to a small dose of ionizing radiation—this subsequently leads to the creation of images of bones, tissues, and organs. X-rays are so widely used largely because they are quick and effective for detecting fractures, lung conditions, and gastrointestinal pathology. Additionally, fluoroscopy, a type of real-time X-ray imaging, is used for procedures such as angiography and barium-led studies.

2.3 Accurate Diagnostics in Medical Imaging

Accurate diagnostic interpretation underpins the clinical utility of medical imaging. It forms the basis for high-quality decision-making across the patient care continuum: from initial assessment and diagnosis to treatment selection, monitoring, and prognostication. Imaging is no longer a supplementary tool, but a central pillar of modern evidence-based medicine.

2.3.1 Early Detection of Disease

One of the principal contributions of imaging is its role in facilitating the early identification of pathological changes, often prior to the manifestation of clinical symptoms. This pre-symptomatic detection is critical in diseases where prognosis is closely linked to the stage at diagnosis. In breast cancer, for example, mammographic screening enables visualization of microcalcifications and non-palpable masses, contributing to a stage shift towards earlier diagnosis and improved survival outcomes. The identification of such radiological signs prompts further investigation and biopsy, often years before a clinical presentation would otherwise occur.

2.3.2 Refinement of Differential Diagnosis

Imaging contributes to diagnostic precision by allowing visual differentiation between a spectrum of disease entities that may present with overlapping clinical features. For example, in patients with non-specific abdominal pain, CT imaging can discriminate between inflammatory, obstructive, ischaemic, or neoplastic aetiologies. This granularity is critical in tailoring management: distinguishing between Crohn's disease and colorectal malignancy, for instance, leads to fundamentally different therapeutic approaches. Similarly, chest imaging plays a pivotal role in differentiating pulmonary embolism, pneumonia, and malignancy in patients presenting with dyspnoea or chest pain, guiding urgent and appropriate treatment.

2.3.3 Treatment Planning and Therapeutic Monitoring

Beyond its diagnostic function, medical imaging is essential in formulating and refining treatment strategies. In radiotherapy planning, high-resolution CT is used to delineate tumour margins with millimetric precision, enabling conformal radiation delivery while preserving adjacent normal structures—thereby reducing adverse effects. MRI, with its superior soft tissue contrast, is particularly valuable in neuro-oncology and musculoskeletal malignancies, facilitating accurate assessment of tumour response to chemotherapy or radiotherapy over time. In chronic neurological conditions such as multiple sclerosis, imaging biomarkers such as T2 lesion load and gadolinium enhancement status are incorporated into clinical decision-making frameworks to assess disease activity and escalate or de-escalate therapy accordingly.

2.3.4 Clinical Illustrations and Supporting Evidence

The clinical implications of imaging accuracy are well exemplified in multiple disease contexts. In the management of multiple sclerosis, Filippi et al. (2019) demonstrate the indispensable role of MRI in identifying demyelinating lesions within both the brain and spinal cord. Imaging informs diagnosis under the McDonald criteria, guides treatment decisions, and enables longitudinal monitoring of disease progression—thereby influencing patient outcomes across the disease course.

In the context of acute surgical emergencies, CT imaging provides timely and high-yield diagnostic information. This has been evidenced before across the literature including in suspected appendicitis, where early imaging has facilitated rapid surgical referral, avoided diagnostic delay, and reduced the risk of perforation or abscess formation.

Systematic evidence also supports the diagnostic accuracy of specific modalities. Previous evidence reports consistently high sensitivity and specificity for MRI in the detection of breast cancer, reinforcing its role not only in screening high-risk populations but also in problem-solving cases with equivocal mammography or ultrasound findings. Meanwhile, other examples highlight the diagnostic value of CT pulmonary angiography in suspected pulmonary embolism, demonstrating high performance in identifying embolic burden and directly contributing to timely anticoagulation initiation and improved patient survival.

2.4 Role of Machine Learning in Medical Imaging

Machine learning is increasingly fundamental in medical imaging due to its ability to revolutionize the way we interpret and utilize imaging data in healthcare. Machine learning (ML), a subset of artificial intelligence, harnesses algorithms to analyse data, recognize patterns, and make predictions. This has profound implications in enhancing diagnostic accuracy, improving workflow efficiency, and enabling personalized treatment strategies.

A fundamental advantage of ML in medical imaging is the ability to handle large and complex datasets more efficiently than traditional methods. Medical images inherently produce enormous volumes of data that require precise analysis for accurate diagnosis. ML algorithms excel in processing this wealth of information, extracting meaningful features and patterns from images that contribute to the early detection of diseases and abnormalities, enabling a shift from qualitative to quantitative analysis of medical imaging.

ML algorithms can be trained using supervised or unsupervised learning methods, each offering unique advantages in medical imaging. In supervised learning, algorithms are trained on labelled datasets to recognize specific patterns and make predictions, such as identifying and segmenting anatomical structures or classifying diseases based on imaging features. This approach enhances the precision and accuracy of diagnostic processes, facilitating more informed decision-making by healthcare providers. On the other hand, unsupervised learning explores datasets without predefined labels, allowing algorithms to uncover hidden insights and patterns that may not be apparent through manual analysis. This exploratory analysis can lead to novel discoveries and a deeper understanding of complex medical conditions through various imaging modalities.

Integration of ML into medical imaging workflows addresses critical challenges encountered in healthcare. First, ML enhances diagnostic accuracy and consistency by minimizing human error and variability in image interpretation. Algorithms trained on extensive datasets can detect subtle changes or abnormalities within images that might otherwise go unnoticed, thus leading to improved diagnosis and prognosis of underlying medical conditions, enabling timely interventions and ultimately improving patient outcomes.

A key aspect contributing to this increased accuracy is image processing and segmentation. ML algorithms automate and enhance the process of partitioning digital images into meaningful segments. ML algorithms, particularly deep learning models like convolutional neural networks (CNNs), automate and enhance this process traditionally done manually, leading to more accurate and reliable results (Hesamian et al. 2019). By leveraging ML for segmentation, clinicians benefit from detailed insights into anatomical structures and pathological features, such as delineating tumour boundaries or extracting quantitative imaging biomarkers (Koh et al. 2022; Hajjo et al. 2021). This automation not only saves time and reduces human error but also enables the extraction of rich data from specific regions within images, facilitating more informed clinical judgments and enhancing diagnostic and therapeutic decision-making across various medical specialties.

Secondly, ML optimization of resource allocation and workflow processes streamlines the efficiency of delivering care. By automating routine tasks such as image triage and preliminary analysis, ML algorithms enable clinicians to focus more on complex cases and provide more personalised patient care (Yala et al. 2019). This workflow optimization is particularly impactful in environments where there is a shortage of skilled healthcare professionals or where rapid turnaround times are essential for patient outcomes. ML-driven optimization not only expedites routine tasks but also facilitates opportunistic screening for serious underlying conditions (Bendifallah et al. 2022; Hickman et al. 2021; Sebro and De la Garza-Ramos 2022). By swiftly identifying potential issues through automated analysis, ML helps prevent long-term sequelae and ensures appropriate pathways for timely intervention. This proactive approach underscores ML's capacity to augment healthcare delivery, enhancing both efficiency and quality of care.

Moreover, ML facilitates the advancement of personalized medicine by integrating imaging data with other patient-specific information such as genetic profiles, clinical histories, and biomarkers (Libbrecht and Noble 2015; Quazi 2022). By analysing this comprehensive dataset, ML algorithms can recommend tailored treatment plans tailored to individual patient characteristics and preferences thus optimizing therapeutic interventions, minimizing adverse effects, and enhancing patient recovery.

2.5 Common Machine Learning Algorithms Used in Medical Imaging

A wide variety of machine learning algorithms have been employed across the spectra of medical imaging, from disease identification and detection to image data throughput. Electing the optimal algorithm for a particular imaging use case requires high specificity for the case in hand, requiring a deep knowledge of an algorithm's architecture. In this section, we delve into four common machine learning algorithms used in medical imaging: convolutional neural networks (CNNs), recurrent neural networks (RNNs), support vector machines (SVMs), and decision trees/random forest models.

2.5.1 Convolutional Neural Networks (CNNs)

CNNs have emerged as a critical mass in medical imaging, foremost for their ability to automatically process hierarchical representations from raw pixel data. An example of deep learning, CNN architecture finds itself suited to image classification, segmentation, and object detection—underscoring their extensive deployment across tumour detection, organ segmentation, and disease classification.

A CNN comprises 3 core components: a convolutional layer, a pooling layer, and a fully connected layer. Through the convolutional layer, a CNN is able to capture spatial maps within inputted images through the application of filters in the layer. This characteristic makes them highly effective for tasks where analysing the depth of local patterns is crucial for accurate classification, such as picking up an abnormality in a radiograph. Contrastingly, the fully connected layer serves an important role in making the ultimate prediction based on this analysis. With the rise of one of the first widely used CNN architectures, U-Net, CNN performance has accelerated in tasks where this precise segmentation is paramount, such as delineating tumour boundaries in an MRI or CT scan.

One of the earliest successful use cases of CNNs was identified in the work of Esteva et al. (2017), who created a CNN-based algorithm capable of classifying skin cancer with an accuracy comparable to dermatologists. The algorithm was trained on a dataset of approximately 130,000 clinical images, and showed significant signs of success in skin cancer detection—for example, the CNN distinguished malignant melanomas from benign nevi, with an area under the curve (AUC) exceeding 91%, outperforming the average of 21 board-certified dermatologists.

2.5.2 Recurrent Neural Networks (RNNs)

While CNNs play a crucial role in spatial analysis, RNNs hold greater utility in the analysis of sequential data, such as that of a time series. Such information is critical in the context of medical imaging, and so RNN applications remain equally diverse—spanning use cases in dynamic imaging modalities like functional MRI (fMRI) or the tracking of disease course over time.

The ability of RNNs to inherently retain ‘knowledge’ of past states enables their use in the modelling of temporal dependencies within varying medical image sequences. This proves important in situations where longitudinal data is necessary for predicting outcomes, or there is a necessity to remain alert to the small delta—a subtle change that may indicate potential progression of disease. Additionally, tailored variants of RNNs, including long short-term memory (LSTM) networks, have already demonstrated success in capturing long-range dependencies. The ‘vanishing gradient’ problem has historically been a key risk factor for RNNs. In an RNN, which is essentially trying to learn from sequences of data over time, information from earlier in the sequence may be ‘forgotten’ or too intrinsically small to remember as later parts are processed. This happens due to the fact that gradients (which enable the network to develop by adjusting interneuron connections) may become increasingly smaller as they’re passed back through time, limiting how hard it is for an RNN to pick out patterns in the data. The recent rise of LSTM networks effectively mitigates this, further enhancing their utility and reliability in medical imaging.

An early proposition of this is the RNN-based framework for predicting Alzheimer’s disease progression using longitudinal MRI image data. By capturing temporal patterns in the scans, Liang et al.’s 2021 model leveraged high accuracy in predicting disease progression, allowing for rapid intervention and tailored care planning, specifically achieving up to 11.8% improvement over baselines.

2.5.3 Support Vector Machines (SVMs)

SVMs form a class of supervised algorithms that perform optimally in binary classification tasks. They are able to identify the optimal hyperplane—that is, the separating boundary for data points belonging to different classes, to discrete grouped output classes for ease of classification. A more traditional algorithm, SVMs are able to handle high-dimensional data well, of which there is much in medical imaging. Moreover, their ability to classify unknown data into categories is a vital solution in imaging. Thus, they continue to find use cases due to their performance track record.

In medical imaging, SVMs are utilized extensively for tumour classification, disease diagnosis, and outcome prediction. Their ability to effectively handle markedly non-linear data via the use of kernel functions makes them useful in cases where finding the decision boundary itself is complex and non-linear—notably seen when distinguishing between different tissue types in MRI scans. Moreover, SVMs are known for their ability to handle small sample sizes and high-dimensional feature spaces, making them highly specialized to medical image datasets which share similar characteristics on the fronts of limited availability and high data dimensionality.

2.5.4 Decision Trees and Random Forests for Decision-Making

Decision trees and random forest models are entry-level algorithms that have become well-known within medical imaging and beyond, with their high accessibility making them ideal for early-stage programmers. These popular algorithms are noted for their simplicity, high interpretability and explainability. Explainability remains a cornerstone issue for the clinical utility of many ML algorithms, where algorithms' black-box characteristics represent an ever-increasing problem. This track record on performance spans both classification and regression. In medical imaging, these algorithms are perhaps most useful in decision-making processes such as disease diagnosis, treatment planning, and risk stratification.

Decision trees operate by repeatedly partitioning the feature space of a dataset (the dimensions inhabited by the variables) into smaller subsets based on increasing discrimination and categorization. This creates a tree-like structure where each internal node represents a decision based on a feature value. Each decision tree, in this way, may form a specific cluster of decisions. Random Forests, on the other hand, aggregate the predictions of multiple decision trees, thereby reducing overfitting and improving generalization performance.

In medical imaging, decision trees and random forests have been used for tasks such as identifying anatomical structures, classifying pathological states, and predicting outcomes. Their ability to handle a mix of numerical and categorical data, combined with their advanced feature selection capacities, suits them to analysing diverse types of medical imaging data.

One of the earliest demonstrations of machine learning in oncology came from Daemen et al. (2013), who used random forests and to predict breast cancer therapy response across 70 cell lines treated with 90 drugs. By integrating multi-omic data, such as gene expression, mutations, and protein levels, they showed that combining data types improved predictive performance for 65% of agents, while transcriptional subtype alone predicted response for 25%. These models, validated on patient data, highlighted the promise of interpretable ensemble models for guiding precision treatment strategies.

2.6 Applications of Machine Learning in Medical Imaging

The application of machine learning (ML) in medical imaging has profound implications across various medical specialties, particularly in oncology and pathology.

In the field of oncology, ML has become an essential asset, profoundly influencing all aspects of cancer care by transforming the landscape for cancer detection, characterization, and treatment (Suzuki 2022). ML has proven to be pivotal in the domain of early detection, pertaining to the aforementioned point of pinpointing subtle abnormalities that might otherwise elude human observation. An example of this is the ML-powered computer-aided detection (CADe) systems, which excel at pinpointing subtle abnormalities in mammograms, low-dose CT scans, and other modalities for breast and lung cancer (Arun Kumar and Sasikala 2023; El-Baz et al. 2013). This may hypothetically translate to earlier diagnoses, a critical factor in enhancing cancer survival rates. Furthermore, ML can leverage this information alongside other risk factors like family history and genomic data to facilitate targeted screening programs and implement preventive measures aimed at cancer prevention.

Beyond detection, machine learning plays a critical role in tumour characterization and staging. Advanced algorithms can analyse tumour features on MRI, CT scans, and PET scans to differentiate between benign and malignant lesions and assist in staging (Wang et al. 2022). This not only reduces the necessity for unnecessary biopsies but also informs treatment decisions by providing vital insights into the tumour's aggressiveness, determined by ML models analysing its characteristics from imaging data. This information is crucial for selecting the most appropriate treatment modality, whether surgery, radiation, or chemotherapy (Suzuki 2022).

ML-driven segmentation is also particularly beneficial for identifying organs at risk (OARs) and tumour volumes in radiotherapy planning, optimizing radiation dose delivery while minimizing harm to healthy tissues. This facilitates the use of adaptive radiotherapy techniques, which are guided by real-time imaging, can improve treatment precision and efficacy, as demonstrated by Erdur et al. (2025).

The impact of ML extends further into personalized treatment planning. By analysing a patient's unique tumour characteristics and genetic profile, ML algorithms can forecast their potential response to different treatment options (Kourou et al. 2015). This empowers clinicians to customize treatment plans for each individual, potentially resulting in therapies that are more effective with fewer side effects. Additionally, ML models optimize radiation therapy by analysing tumour location and surrounding healthy tissues, facilitating the creation of precise radiation plans that minimize the risk of damage to nearby organs, as exhibited in Ger et al. (2022).

Machine learning (ML) is also demonstrably transforming the landscape of pathology, leveraging advancements in digital pathology and data analysis to propel diagnostic accuracy and refine treatment strategies. Histopathology, traditionally reliant on microscopic tissue examination, has witnessed a paradigm shift with the utilization of vast libraries of digitized slides for training sophisticated ML algorithms. Convolutional neural networks (CNNs) have emerged as adept assistants, achieving impressive accuracy in the identification of a wide range of tissue abnormalities, including cancerous lesions and infectious diseases. Their ability to recognize complex patterns within digital slides allows them to distinguish pathologies with high sensitivity and specificity (Cui and Zhang 2021).

The impact of ML extends far beyond mere disease detection. It has the potential to revolutionize patient care by predicting disease progression and tailoring treatment plans to individual needs. By meticulously analysing the digitized features extracted from tissue samples, ML-driven prognostic models can forecast patient outcomes, with a qualitative 'high precision' (Madabhushi and Lee 2016). This empowers pathologists to craft personalized treatment strategies, ensuring that patients receive therapies that are most effective for their specific condition, improving patient care by optimizing treatment efficacy while minimizing unnecessary interventions.

2.7 Challenges and Limitations

2.7.1 Ethical Dilemmas

Implementing ML models in medical imaging introduces complex ethical dilemmas, particularly when considering potential conflicts of interest between clinicians and ML developers. Such conflicts may revolve around autonomy and such tensions necessitate a careful, transparent, and multidisciplinary approach to development and implementation, in which all stakeholders, including patients, are meaningfully involved in shaping the ethical boundaries and practical applications of these technologies (Rigby 2019).

It is imperative that stakeholders and researchers actively mitigate the risk of algorithmic bias, both in training datasets and in institutional pressures, by promoting open dialogue, diverse data representation, and clinical validation across settings. ML systems should be framed as decision-support tools designed to augment rather than replace imaging professionals. Indeed, numerous studies have shown that when used synergistically, ML and radiologists may theoretically outperform either alone in terms of diagnostic accuracy, efficiency, and consistency, particularly in tasks such as detecting pulmonary embolism or breast cancer on imaging (McKinney et al. 2020).

Prioritizing patient care over professional rivalry or economic gain must remain the guiding principle. Ethical integration of ML in radiology requires ongoing oversight, interdisciplinary collaboration, and a shared commitment to equity, safety, and clinical efficacy. Only by fostering mutual trust and transparency can these technologies fulfil their promise of enhancing, not undermining, human expertise in healthcare.

2.7.2 Data Requirements and Clinical Implementation

The substantial data requirements for training high-quality ML algorithms pose a grave future challenge in medical imaging. Clinical research has already generated vast amounts of data, presenting an opportunity for ML to bridge the gap between existing complex datasets and clinical decision-making. However, the dynamic nature of medical practice and limitations of sourcing retrospective data may complicate ML's future growth. With ML growth far outpacing the generation of novel data, concerns around a plateau point of data availability require careful consideration to prevent ML applications from stagnating. Infamous theories such as the idea of feeding the output generation of ML models back as input material have recently arisen, underscoring the importance of ethical data handling. Intrinsically linked to this, the generally established limitations of ML, including the capacity for models to repropagate the inherent inaccuracies of datasets (the 'rubbish in, rubbish out' phenomenon), remain valid concerns. These concerns arise from poor representation of diverse demographic groups in training datasets, renewing the conversation around data diversity, sample optimization, and research equity.

Nevertheless, ML advancements continue to adapt. ANNs (artificial neural networks) have demonstrated high prediction performance in breast cancer surgery outcomes, showcasing their adaptability to diverse and noisy datasets. Lou et al. showed that these networks yield the highest prediction performance index, providing robust predictions even with non-normally distributed data such as that found in imaging.

2.7.3 Interpretability and Explainability

The lack of interpretability and explainability in ML algorithms presents a considerable obstacle in medical imaging. For example, a radiologist may rely on understanding the rationale behind diagnostic decisions, which is often obscured in black-box models. This sense of 'opacity' undermines trust and may lead to discrepancies between ML output and academic consensus. Addressing this challenge requires the development of interpretable and explainable AI models that provide insights into the model's decision-making processes, enhancing clinician confidence in ML diagnostics and overcoming the key challenge to ML's practical application in imaging—namely, the distrust presented by clinician laggards.

Moreover, explainable machine learning approaches offer potential solutions by providing clinicians with transparent justifications for an ML model's prediction, allowing them to weigh up their opinion versus that of an algorithm, with sufficient depth of information—akin to the way clinicians view their patients when gaining consent for a clinical plan. Interestingly, the rise of attention mechanisms and saliency maps can highlight the regions of interest in medical images, enabling individuals to understand the basis for AI predictions.

2.7.4 Looking Beyond

It is clear that clinicians must remain cautious about the limitations and risks of AI technology, including data biases, algorithmic complexity, and ethical dilemmas. Collaborative efforts between healthcare professionals, AI experts, and patients are essential to navigate these challenges and ensure the responsible implementation of ML in medical imaging. While ML holds tremendous promise for enhancing medical imaging and improving patient care, its integration into clinical practice presents a challenge. By addressing ethical concerns, including data diversity alongside interpretability, and by fostering collaborative approaches, clinicians can harness the full potential of ML in imaging. Interdisciplinary collaboration and ongoing research are crucial to overcome these challenges.

2.8 Future Perspectives and Opportunities

Machine learning has emerged as a powerful tool in the realm of medical imaging, offering the potential to transform diagnostics and patient care. However, the integration of machine learning (ML) algorithms into clinical practice presents several notable challenges along with promising opportunities for future development.

One of the primary challenges lies in data acquisition and diversity. High-quality, diverse datasets are essential for training robust ML models, yet obtaining such data is hindered by privacy regulations, data silos across healthcare institutions, and complexities in data sharing agreements. Future efforts must focus on developing secure, collaborative platforms for data sharing while ensuring compliance with ethical and legal standards.

Privacy and data security are critical considerations in healthcare applications of ML. Protecting patient privacy and ensuring data security requires the implementation of robust security measures and privacy-preserving techniques, such as federated learning and differential privacy. These efforts are crucial for fostering trust and facilitating data sharing among healthcare stakeholders.

Integrating ML models into existing healthcare systems presents another significant challenge. This process requires seamless collaboration between data scientists, clinicians, and IT professionals to overcome technical and cultural barriers. Developing interoperable systems and tools tailored to the needs of healthcare providers is essential for successful integration.

Standardization, validation, and regulation are imperative as ML algorithms become more prevalent in medical imaging. Establishing rigorous validation protocols and ethical guidelines is essential to ensure the safety, efficacy, and fairness of ML-driven diagnostics. Collaboration with regulatory bodies, industry experts, and policymakers is necessary to navigate these regulatory challenges effectively.

The interpretability of ML models in medical imaging is crucial for gaining acceptance and trust from clinicians and patients. Advancements in explainable AI techniques, such as attention mechanisms and model-agnostic approaches, will enhance transparency and facilitate clinical adoption of ML-driven diagnostics.

Looking ahead, future developments in ML for medical imaging will require collaborative data initiatives to create large-scale, diverse datasets through multi-institutional partnerships and data sharing agreements. Additionally, investing in research and development of privacy-preserving ML techniques, developing interoperable healthcare systems, establishing regulatory standards, and advancing explainable AI methods specific to medical imaging are key priorities.

In conclusion, while challenges exist in integrating ML into medical imaging, concerted efforts from researchers, clinicians, policymakers, and industry stakeholders can pave the way for transformative advancements. By fostering interdisciplinary collaboration, investing in innovative technologies, and upholding ethical standards, the field of ML in medical imaging can realize its full potential and positively impact healthcare delivery and patient outcomes.

2.9 Conclusion

Machine learning algorithms certainly present promising avenues for enhancing diagnostic accuracy and efficiency in medical imaging, offering the ability to understand and extract meaningful patterns from complex data, with the goal of improving patient outcomes. However, challenges such as ethical dilemmas, data requirements, and interpretability must be addressed via interdisciplinary collaboration and multicentre research. The integration of machine learning into medical imaging holds real potential to catalyse diagnostics and treatment planning if correctly executed in this critical growth period.

References

Arun Kumar S, Sasikala S (2023) Review on deep learning-based CAD systems for breast cancer diagnosis. Technol Cancer Res Treat 22:15330338231177977

Bendifallah S, Puchar A, Suisse S, Delbos L, Poilblanc M, Descamps P, Golfier F, Touboul C, Dabi Y, Daraï E (2022) Machine learning algorithms as new screening approach for patients with endometriosis. Sci Rep 12:639

Cui M, Zhang DY (2021) Artificial intelligence and computational pathology. Lab Investig 101:412–422

Daemen A, Griffith OL, Heiser LM, Wang NJ, Enache OM, Sanborn Z, Pepin F, Durinck S, Korkola JE, Griffith M et al (2013) Modeling precision treatment of breast cancer. Genome Biol 14:R110

El-Baz A, Beache GM, Gimel'farb G, Suzuki K, Okada K, Elnakib A, Soliman A, Abdollahi B (2013) Computer-aided diagnosis systems for lung cancer: challenges and methodologies. Int J Biomed Imaging 2013:942353

Erdur AC, Rusche D, Scholz D, Kiechle J, Fischer S, Llorián-Salvador Ó, Buchner JA, Nguyen MQ, Etzel L, Weidner J, Metz M-C, Wiestler B, Schnabel J, Rueckert D, Combs SE, Peeken JC (2025) Deep learning for autosegmentation for radiotherapy treatment planning: State-of-the-art and novel perspectives. Strahlenther Onkol 201:236–254

Esteva A, Kuprel B, Novoa RA, Ko J, Swetter SM, Blau HM, Thrun S (2017) Dermatologist-level classification of skin cancer with deep neural networks. Nature 542(7639):115–118

Filippi M, Brück W, Chard D et al (2019) Association between pathological and MRI findings in multiple sclerosis. Lancet Neurol 18(2):198–210

Ger RB, Netherton TJ, Rhee DJ, Court LE, Yang J, Cardenas CE (2022) Auto-contouring for image-guidance and treatment planning. In: El Naqa I, Murphy MJ (eds) Machine and deep learning in oncology, medical physics and radiology. Springer International Publishing, Cham

Hajjo R, Sabbah DA, Bardaweel SK, Tropsha A (2021) Identification of tumor-specific MRI biomarkers using machine learning (ML). Diagnostics [Online], 11

Hesamian MH, Jia W, He X, Kennedy P (2019) Deep learning techniques for medical image segmentation: achievements and challenges. J Digit Imaging 32:582–596

Hickman SE, Woitek R, Le EPV, Im YR, Mouritsen Luxhøj C, Aviles-Rivero AI, Baxter GC, Mackay JW, Gilbert FJ (2021) Machine learning for workflow applications in screening mammography: systematic review and meta-analysis. Radiology 302:88–104

Koh D-M, Papanikolaou N, Bick U, Illing R, Kahn CE, Kalpathi-Cramer J, Matos C, Martí-Bonmatí L, Miles A, Mun SK, Napel S, Rockall A, Sala E, Strickland N, Prior F (2022) Artificial intelligence and machine learning in cancer imaging. Commun Med 2:133

Kourou K, Exarchos TP, Exarchos KP, Karamouzis MV, Fotiadis DI (2015) Machine learning applications in cancer prognosis and prediction. Comput Struct Biotechnol J 13:8–17

Liang W, Zhang K, Cao P, Liu X, Yang J, Zaiane O (2021) Rethinking modeling Alzheimer's disease progression from a multi-task learning perspective with deep recurrent neural network. Comput Biol Med 138:104935. Available at: https://doi.org/10.1016/j.compbiomed.2021.104935

Libbrecht MW, Noble WS (2015) Machine learning applications in genetics and genomics. Nat Rev Genet 16:321–332

Madabhushi A, Lee G (2016) Image analysis and machine learning in digital pathology: challenges and opportunities. Med Image Anal 33:170–175

Mckinney SM, Sieniek M, Godbole V et al (2020) International evaluation of an AI system for breast cancer screening. Nature 577:89–94

Quazi S (2022) Artificial intelligence and machine learning in precision and genomic medicine. Med Oncol 39:120

Rigby MJ (2019) Ethical dimensions of using artificial intelligence in health care. AMA J Ethics 21:E121–E124

Sebro R, De La Garza-Ramos C (2022) Machine learning for opportunistic screening for osteoporosis from CT scans of the wrist and forearm. Diagnostics [Online], 12

Suzuki K (2022) Computerized detection of lesions in diagnostic images with early deep learning models. In: El Naqa I, Murphy MJ (eds) Machine and deep learning in oncology, medical physics and radiology. Springer International Publishing, Cham

Wang J, El Naqa I, Yang Y (2022) Classification of malignant and benign tumors. In: El Naqa I, Murphy MJ (eds) Machine and deep learning in oncology, medical physics and radiology. Springer International Publishing, Cham

Yala A, Schuster T, Miles R, Barzilay R, Lehman C (2019) A deep learning model to triage screening mammograms: a simulation study. Radiology 293:38–46

3 Virtual Reality in Medical Training

Leila Ellis

Abstract

The integration of technology into the continually evolving landscape of medical education and training has become pivotal to enhancing learning experiences. Among the array of innovative tools, virtual reality stands out as a transformative force, offering immersive and interactive simulations that bridge the gap between theoretical knowledge and practical application. This chapter covers the current capabilities as well as potential future applications of virtual reality simulations for surgical training, anatomy education, and patient-care scenarios, along with its benefits and challenges.

Keywords

Virtual reality · Medical education and training

L. Ellis (✉)
University of Bristol, Bristol, UK
e-mail: leila.ellis@bristol.ac.uk

3.1 Transformative Impact of Virtual Reality

3.1.1 The Paradigm Shift in Medical Education Due to Immersive Technology

The integration of technology into the continually evolving landscape of medical education and training has become pivotal to enhancing learning experiences. There is a wide array of digital education tools available, from the simple conversion of a book into PDF format to complex modalities such as mobile learning, virtual patients, gamification, large open online courses, and digital psychomotor skills trainers. Extended reality (XR) refers to the various types of immersive technologies that create a three-dimensional image that can be interacted with in real-time. Fully immersive virtual reality (VR) provides users with a complete sense of presence in an entirely artificial computer-simulated environment through head-mounted displays and motion tracking systems. It offers the highest level of immersion, making it ideal for simulations requiring full sensory engagement, such as surgical training. Augmented reality (AR), on the other hand, overlays virtual elements onto the real world, enhancing the user's perception of their surroundings. AR is valuable for contextualising information in real-world settings, such as anatomical visualisation during medical proce-

J. Malawana et al. (eds.), *Artificial Intelligence in Healthcare and Biomedical Visualization*, Biomedical Visualization 10, https://doi.org/10.1007/978-3-032-06520-9_3

dures. For example, AccuVein superimposes a map of vasculature on the surface of a patient's skin to help medical professionals find veins for phlebotomy (Sakakibara et al. 2025). Mixed reality (MR) combines elements of both VR and AR, allowing virtual objects to interact with the physical environment and vice versa. MR offers versatility, enabling users to engage with virtual content while maintaining awareness of their surroundings, making it suitable for scenarios requiring physical interaction, such as patient examinations. Each type of XR technology has its strengths and limitations, and the choice depends on the specific educational objectives and requirements of training programs. This chapter aims to explore the multifaceted role of VR in bridging the gap between theoretical knowledge and practical application in medical education.

Medical education today comprises both classroom learning as well as hospital-based learning, where students are able to gain clinical experience. However, the hospital model has been criticised for being costly and restricted by insufficient resources. One of the fundamental challenges is the limited exposure to diverse clinical cases and procedures, often resulting in a gap between theoretical learning and real-world practice. VR addresses this challenge by offering students an opportunity to engage in a broad spectrum of realistic clinical scenarios, ranging from routine consultations to rare emergencies, with real-time feedback. VR programs place learners in a key role through the exercise of their complex cognitive thinking skills, psychomotor control, and communication skills. It empowers learners to develop critical decision-making, refine procedural techniques, and cultivate confidence in a safe and controlled environment. Moreover, VR offers a platform for shared learning, enabling students to engage in group exercises, interprofessional consultations, and peer-to-peer debrief sessions (Pottle 2019). Through the development of teamwork, situational awareness, and empathy, VR supports a collaborative learning environment reflective of real clinical settings, where collective performance is paramount to patient outcomes.

3.1.2 Understanding the Evidence for Virtual Reality as an Education Tool

There is significant cost and effort involved in designing VR programs in the early stage, as well as in the training of educators. As such, research is needed to provide reliable evidence of its effectiveness by comparing it with existing education methods. VR simulations in surgical programs and medical curricula have shown promise in enhancing operative efficiency, minimising errors, and improving patient safety. Immersive interactive VR has demonstrated superior knowledge acquisition compared to screen-based learning, making it a standard in clinical skills development.

A scoping review by Jiang et al. (2022) delineated existing research on the role of VR in undergraduate medical education. Searches of four databases yielded 114 relevant studies. Findings showed that most studies reported the use of commercially available surgical VR simulators. Other VR modalities included three-dimensional (3D) models and virtual worlds, which were mainly used for anatomy education. Most VR modalities were semi-immersive and highly interactive. Notably, few studies reported using theoretical or conceptual frameworks to guide VR design. This highlights a need to explore the potential of VR beyond surgery and anatomy, with particular focus on emerging VR modalities, including mobile VR, haptic-enabled systems, 360° video simulations, artificial intelligence (AI) driven adaptive platforms, and multi-user or group-based learning environments.

VR offers a multitude of benefits in enhancing long-term retention of medical knowledge and skills. By immersing learners in realistic and interactive environments, VR engages multiple senses, thereby enhancing cognitive processing and memory retention. Studies have shown that experiential learning through VR leads to deeper encoding of information, making it more likely to be retained over time (Essoe et al. 2022). VR enables learners to contextualise their knowledge by applying it to real-world scenarios, which strengthens neural connections and facilitates transfer of learning to clinical practice. The ability to repeat simulations and practice procedures in VR allows for spaced repetition, a proven method for long-term retention. Furthermore, the emotional engagement elicited by VR experiences can enhance memory consolidation, ensuring that learners remember key concepts and procedures well beyond the initial training sessions.

In a one-year follow-up study, Gan et al. (2023) examined the impact of VR tendon suturing training compared to traditional methods on 117 participants from an initial randomised controlled study. Of these, 108 completed the follow-up. Participants were divided into VR and control groups and assessed using questionnaires, surgical internship scores, and OSCE graduation scores. Results showed that the VR group exhibited more positive career choices and study habits, alongside better clinical practice scores and OSCE performance in physical examination, suturing and knotting, and image reading. This suggests VR teaching enhances career determination, learning willingness, and clinical proficiency among medical students.

Furthermore, a recent systematic review (Foronda et al. 2024) aimed to compare VR to traditional simulation in terms of learning outcomes. Searching eight databases yielded 15 studies, including 11 randomised controlled trials. Data were evaluated against Kirkpatrick and Kirkpatrick's (2006) Four Levels of Training Evaluation. All studies included level one outcomes of learner reactions and level two outcomes evaluating knowledge or learning. No studies reported level three outcomes considering behaviour changes. Only one study (Katz et al. 2020) evaluated level four outcomes of system-level impact, which suggested that VR sessions were more efficient and less expensive. More evidence is needed to improve understanding of the longitudinal impact of VR learning experiences, including costs, patient outcomes, and other performance indicators.

3.1.3 Integration of Virtual Reality in Medical Education and Training Programs

In recent years, the integration of VR technology into medical education has transformed the way students learn and prepare for clinical practice. Medical schools in the United Kingdom (UK) have been at the forefront of adopting VR solutions to enhance learning experiences and better prepare future healthcare professionals.

Introducing VR into medical school curricula poses several significant challenges that require careful consideration and strategic planning. Among these challenges is the issue of cost and accessibility, as high-quality VR equipment and software can be prohibitively expensive for some institutions, potentially widening the gap in learning opportunities between students. One of the primary avenues through which VR has been introduced is through collaborations and partnerships with technology companies specialising in medical simulation. These collaborations often involve joint research projects, software development, and customisation of VR solutions to align with curricula requirements and educational objectives of medical schools. Logistical hurdles include ensuring that medical schools have the necessary technical infrastructure to support VR integration, including reliable internet connections and adequate space for VR simulations. Furthermore, faculty members may require training and support to effectively incorporate VR technology into their teaching practices, highlighting the importance of ongoing professional development initiatives. Many UK medical schools have established dedicated simulation centres equipped with VR technology, providing students with access to a wide range of VR simulations and scenarios. The University of Leeds School of Medicine established the Medical Simulation Centre in the late 1990s, pioneering the integration of VR into medical education in the UK. These simulation centres offer students the opportunity to engage in realistic patient encounters within a standardised and repeatable environment. Finally, validating the educational value of VR simulations and addressing ethical and legal considerations related to patient privacy and data security are essential steps in the successful integration of VR into medical education. By addressing these challenges proactively, medical schools can maximise the potential of VR technology to enhance learning experiences.

Beyond the realm of medical schools, VR has also emerged as a valuable tool for continuing medical education and professional development. With the rapid advancements in medical technology and procedures, healthcare professionals must continually update their knowledge and skills to deliver optimal patient care. VR-based training programs offer clinicians an avenue to explore new techniques, refine existing skills, and stay abreast of emerging trends in their respective fields, ultimately enhancing the quality and safety of healthcare delivery.

3.1.4 Global Market for Virtual Reality in Healthcare

The global healthcare market for VR in healthcare is projected to grow from USD 4.18 billion in 2024 to USD 38.46 billion by 2032, at a Compound Annual Growth Rate of 32.0% (Fortune Business Insights 2024). The VR in medical education market is highly competitive, marked by its dynamic nature and diverse range of players, from industry giants to start-ups. This competition drives continuous innovation and excellence, as companies differentiate themselves through product quality, pricing, and customer service. Market dynamics are influenced by technological advancements, environmental impact, regulations, and consumer preferences, presenting challenges and opportunities for participants. This environment leads to strategic partnerships, mergers, and acquisitions as companies strive to maintain their competitive edge.

3.2 Virtual Reality for Surgical Training

3.2.1 Evolution of Surgical Training Methods

Historical surgical training often involved apprenticeships, where aspiring surgeons learned through direct observation and hands-on experience under the guidance of a senior. During the Renaissance, formalised apprenticeships became more structured, with some institutions offering more systematic training. Dissection of cadavers became a key component of surgical education, contributing to a deeper understanding of anatomy. The nineteenth century saw the establishment of anatomy lectures and the widespread use of cadavers in medical education. The Flexner Report (1910) in the United States led to the restructuring of medical education, emphasising scientific principles and standardising curricula. Surgical training became more formalised within medical schools, incorporating didactic lectures and hands-on experiences. Simulated training methods, such as using rubber models and animal tissues, gained popularity in the mid-twentieth century. These methods allowed for controlled practice of specific skills before applying them in real surgical settings. The advent of laparoscopic surgery brought about a shift in training methods. Simulators for laparoscopic procedures were introduced, providing surgeons-in-training with a virtual platform to practice minimally invasive techniques. Most modern surgical training programmes are evolving from time-related models towards a competency-based framework. Trainees are now expected to demonstrate achievement of defined procedural milestones before completing specialisation. This underscores the importance of providing trainees with efficient and effective tools for skill development.

3.2.2 Introduction of Virtual Reality Simulations for Surgical Procedures

VR emerged as a transformative tool for surgical training. VR simulations offer opportunities for practicing various surgical procedures, providing a safe and controlled environment for skill development. The emphasis is on creating highly realistic simulations that closely mimic the complexity of surgical procedures. VR incorporation into surgical training programs is supported by high-quality, albeit heterogeneous, studies demonstrating improved task completion, procedural times, accuracy, positive user ratings, and cost-effectiveness (Bielsa 2021; Mao et al. 2021; McKinney et al. 2022; Vrillon et al. 2022). However, the extent of these benefits across different surgical skills is not well characterised. A Cochrane meta-analysis (Khan et al. 2019) of 18 trials with 3817 endoscopic procedures suggested that VR simulation training was advantageous over no training, but that there was insufficient evidence of benefit when compared to conventional training. As such, adaptation into surgical curricula is often in conjunction with other forms of surgical education (Feeley et al. 2021).

3.2.3 Benefits of Using Virtual Reality in Surgical Training

3.2.3.1 Enhanced Realism and Controlled Environment

VR fosters active learning by allowing students to engage with content rather than passively receiving information. Hands-on experiences and interactive simulations enhance understanding and retention of medical concepts. VR simulators allow for 3D visualisation of anatomical structures, offering a more comprehensive understanding of spatial relationships. Trainees can explore and manipulate virtual anatomy, leading to improved surgical planning and decision-making. Moreover, VR platforms can give prompt feedback to learners from multisensory and multiangle viewpoints. Haptic feedback allows users to feel resistance and pressure akin to real surgical scenarios.

Trainees can practice procedures repeatedly in a controlled, risk-free virtual environment. This repetitive practice helps build muscle memory and fine-tune techniques without the potential consequences associated with real-life surgeries. VR simulations can be customised to different skill levels, allowing trainees to progress at their own pace while receiving personalised feedback to enhance learning outcomes. Subsequently, surgeons enter real-life scenarios with increased confidence and competence, minimising the risk of errors.

3.2.3.2 Objective Performance Assessment

VR enables assessment of medical skills through data-driven analytics. VR platforms provide objective data on trainee performance, including metrics related to precision, speed, and accuracy. Immediate feedback on performance allows for continuous improvement through targeted skill development and progress tracking. Real-time kinetic data and physiological measures from the user can provide adaptations to controlled elements in the simulation. Similarly, reinforcement learning algorithms can be used to adjust feedback content, type, and timing to improve the perceived feedback value (Zahabi and Abdul Razak 2020). Moreover, objective performance assessment in VR allows for standardised evaluation across trainees, ensuring consistency and reliability in measuring proficiency levels.

3.2.4 Addressing Challenges in Developing Effective Virtual Reality Surgical Simulations

3.2.4.1 Technological Limitations

Technological limitations pose significant challenges when using VR for surgical training, impacting the effectiveness and accessibility of training programs. The fidelity of VR simulations may not accurately replicate the tactile feedback and haptic sensations experienced during real surgical procedures. Any lack of realism can hinder trainees' ability to develop precise motor skills and may diminish the overall learning experience. Additionally, VR hardware and software may have technical constraints, such as low-quality graphical rendering or latency issues, which can detract from the immersive nature of simulations. Prioritising compatibility with a wide range of VR devices is essential to maximise accessibility, ensuring that trainees can access training programs regardless of the VR hardware they use. Overcoming these technological limitations requires ongoing advancements in VR technology, including the development of more sophisticated haptic feedback systems and improvements in hardware performance. There is increasing interest in the integration of AI algorithms to enhance effectiveness. AI can contribute to dynamic responses within simulations, creating more realistic and personalised learning experiences. Furthermore, adopting a modular development approach allows for incremental updates and improvements, breaking down the simulation into manageable components and facilitating easier integration of new technologies as they become available.

3.2.4.2 Cost Implications

While the initial investment associated with implementing VR technology, including purchasing hardware, software, and training personnel, can be significant, they are often offset by the potential savings in traditional educational methods. VR platforms offer the advantage of reusable simulations, allowing trainees to practice procedures repeatedly without the need for additional resources. VR reduces the reliance on costly materials, such as cadavers or medical supplies, and minimises the risks associated with practicing on live patients. However, ongoing maintenance and updates to VR systems can incur additional expenses over time.

3.2.4.3 Integration with Existing Curricula

Integrating VR into both undergraduate and postgraduate surgical curricula offers a promising avenue to enhance learning experiences and skill development. For undergraduate students, VR can supplement traditional anatomy courses by providing immersive, interactive experiences that allow them to explore anatomical structures in depth. VR simulations can be developed to cater to various skill levels to ensure that trainees receive tailored training experiences that align with their proficiency levels. Similarly, for postgraduate training, VR offers advanced simulation for procedural skills such as laparoscopic surgery, endoscopy, interventional radiology, echocardiography, and lumbar puncture (Duarte et al. 2021; O'Sullivan et al. 2021; Vrillon et al. 2022). For example, the Royal College of Surgeons of England (Lam 2022) has developed VR modules for laparoscopic training, allowing trainees to practice surgical techniques. Challenges in integration may include the need for specialised VR content and interoperability with existing training programs. While repeated practice enhances skills up to a certain extent, deliberate practice, rather than mere repetition, is essential for continual improvement and optimal outcomes. The combination of simulation and deliberate practice is considered superior to the traditional Halstedian "see one, do one, teach one" approach regarding the acquisition of skills (McGaghie et al. 2011). Thus, it is necessary to align VR with existing curricula using the principles of Kolb's Experiential Learning Cycle (2014), whereby trainees engage in hands-on virtual simulations to gain experience, during which outcomes are observed and reflected on with the subsequent application of insights gained from the virtual experience to real-world surgical practice.

3.3 Virtual Reality for Anatomy Education

3.3.1 Traditional Methods of Anatomy Education in Medical Schools

Anatomy education in medical schools has historically relied on a combination of traditional methods to impart knowledge of the human body's intricate structures. Didactic teaching serves as the foundation, with instructors delivering lectures in a classroom setting to cover the theoretical aspects of anatomy. These lectures provide students with essential conceptual frameworks and a strong theoretical foundation in anatomy. Anatomical atlases and textbooks play a crucial role as essential references, allowing students to study and review anatomical structures in detail, reinforcing their learning from lectures. Cadaveric dissection stands as a hallmark of anatomy education, offering students a hands-on approach to studying the structural relationships between different body parts. The practice involves students meticulously dissecting human cadavers under the guidance of experienced anatomists. Through dissection, students gain a profound understanding of anatomical variations, spatial relationships, and the three-dimensional complexity of the human body. Additionally, pre-prepared prosected specimens may be used for instructional purposes, providing students with opportunities to observe specific anatomical structures in isolation and enhance their understanding. The integration of medical imaging techniques such as X-rays, Computed Tomography scans, and Magnetic Resonance Imaging has become increasingly prevalent in anatomy education. These imaging modalities allow students to correlate anatomical structures with real-life clinical images, bridging the gap between theoretical knowledge and clinical practice.

3.3.2 Benefits of Using Virtual Reality in Anatomy Education

3.3.2.1 Three-Dimensional Visualisation and Spatial Understanding

VR allows students to move beyond static two-dimensional images and experience anatomy in a dynamic, three-dimensional space. VR simulations replicate realistic anatomical environments, offering a level of detail and realism comparable to traditional cadaveric dissection. Virtual anatomy models can be manipulated in real-time, allowing students to rotate, zoom, and explore structures from various angles. Virtual dissection tools allow for the exploration of structures layer by layer, enhancing the understanding of complex anatomical relationships. This level of immersion enhances engagement and retention, as users can explore anatomy from multiple perspectives without real-world distractions (Miltykh et al. 2023).

3.3.2.2 Personalised Learning Experiences

VR platforms can be leveraged for self-directed anatomy learning as they allow students to interact with models at their own pace and focus on areas requiring additional practice (Fairén et al. 2020). A recent scoping review (Sinha et al. 2023) identified determinants of learning within immersive VR environments, noting their capacity to facilitate personalised learning trajectories, whereby learners can revisit challenging content and progress to more complex structures. The review also recommended further development of customisation features and integrated analytics to provide adaptive data-driven feedback.

3.3.3 Addressing Challenges in Implementing Virtual Reality for Anatomy Education

3.3.3.1 Content Development and Accuracy

The educational value of VR anatomy depends on model fidelity. Advances in photogrammetry and high-resolution 3D scanning now enable the creation of highly accurate, photorealistic models derived directly from cadaveric dissections (Krause et al. 2023). Iterative refinement processes, carried out in collaboration with anatomists, clinicians, and educators, are essential to validate virtual content across physiological and pathological variations (Esmaeeli et al. 2025).

3.3.3.2 Accessibility for all Students

Universal access demands VR solutions compatible with a broad spectrum of hardware. Cloud-based VR streaming interfaces support remote participation without high-end headsets (Zhang 2024). Embedding VR modules within existing learning management systems (e.g. Moodle, Canvas) promotes seamless curriculum integration. For example, 3D-VR tools have been successfully deployed alongside traditional learning management systems to complement cadaver labs (Stepan et al. 2017). Inclusive design that integrates voice commands, gesture controls and audio descriptions improves usability for students with visual or motor impairments (Vargas and González 2018). Finally, motion sickness remains a barrier, with mitigating strategies including reduced latency, optimised frame rates, and comfort settings such as adjustable field of view (Alexander et al. 2023; O'Hara et al. 2021).

3.3.3.3 Faculty Training and Acceptance

Faculty buy-in is essential for consistent VR adoption. Early reviews have emphasised the need for comprehensive training programmes to address educators' concerns and demonstrate VR's pedagogical advantages, thereby fostering a culture of innovation (Vargas and González 2018). One-on-one tutoring systems that connect instructors and students in shared VR spaces also show promise for building faculty confidence. Saalfeld et al. (2020) developed a networked VR tutoring platform where instructors guide student exploration and provide in situ annotations, enhancing educator control and acceptance.

3.4 Virtual Reality for Patient-Care Scenarios

3.4.1 Importance of Practical Patient-Care Experience in Medical Training

Practical patient-care experience is essential in medical education as it bridges the gap between theoretical knowledge and clinical application, equipping medical students with essential skills and competencies for effective healthcare delivery. Through direct interaction with patients, students learn to conduct thorough medical histories, perform physical examinations, and formulate accurate diagnoses under the supervision of experienced clinicians. Practical experience also cultivates empathy, communication, and professionalism, essential qualities for establishing trusting relationships with patients and delivering compassionate care. Moreover, exposure to diverse patient cases enhances students' clinical reasoning and problem-solving abilities, preparing them to navigate complex healthcare scenarios encountered in real-world practice. In addition to technical competence, experiential patient care promotes understanding of the social, cultural, and ethical contexts of medicine, contributing to the development of patient-centred practitioners.

3.4.2 Utilising Virtual Reality for Immersive Patient-Care Simulations

High-fidelity simulation-based medical education (SBME) with deliberate practice is well supported by meta-analytic evidence but remains logistically demanding, resource-intensive, and costly to implement at scale (McGaghie et al. 2011). In contrast, VR offers a more economical, space-efficient alternative that can be deployed without extensive supervisor oversight or physical infrastructure (Kyaw et al. 2019; Moro et al. 2017). VR simulations prioritise safety by allowing learners to practise high-risk scenarios without endangering patients (Padilha et al. 2019) and support experiential learning in realistic, interactive environments (Kyaw et al. 2019). The capacity to recreate authentic clinical situations enhances preparedness for real-world practice, and immersive scenarios reinforce patient-centred care by focusing on understanding patients' perspectives and honing communication skills (Padilha et al. 2019; Kyaw et al. 2019).

3.4.3 Benefits of Virtual Reality in Patient-Care Training

3.4.3.1 Exposure to Diverse Medical Scenarios

VR allows learners to encounter a broad spectrum of patient presentations across age, gender, ethnicity, and socio-economic backgrounds in a controlled setting (Rothlind et al. 2021). This diversity not only ensures exposure to conditions that may be uncommon in clinical rotations but also helps students develop cultural competence and sensitivity to social determinants of health. Furthermore, VR enables repeated practice and mastery learning, allowing learners to revisit challenging scenarios, refine their skills, and consolidate clinical reasoning and communication skills.

3.4.3.2 Developing Critical Decision-Making Skills

VR training can provide students with exposure to high-pressure and uncertain scenarios to improve clinical decision-making, prioritisation, and situational awareness without compromising patient safety. One study found that paramedic science students using a bespoke VR mass-casualty simulation achieved equivalent triage accuracy to live drills but allocated patients more quickly and at ~1/13th the cost of traditional exercises (Mills et al. 2020). Similarly, VR obstetrics modules for shoulder dystocia management have been shown to improve adherence to emergency algorithms and reduce diagnosis-to-delivery intervals (Farr et al. 2024). Moreover, VR enables exposure to complex or rare conditions, including psychiatric emergencies, infectious diseases, and genetic disorders. This allows learners to practise rapid assessment, prioritisation, and evidence-based decision-making in situations that may be difficult to encounter in clinical rotations and challenging to reproduce in traditional simulations.

3.4.3.3 Improving Communication and Empathy

VR simulations immerse students in scenarios that simulate diverse patient encounters, enabling them to practice effective communication techniques and empathetic responses. VR platforms, namely Embodied Labs, SimX, Health Scholars, and Virti, offer simulations where students embody the perspective of patients with chronic conditions, such as sensory impairments, Alzheimer's disease or Parkinson's disease, fostering empathy and a deeper understanding of lived experiences. These insights enable students to develop rapport, active listening skills, and nonverbal communication techniques essential for building trusting relationships with patients.

The University of New England (Dyer et al. 2018) successfully introduced VR software to the medical, physician assistant, physical therapy, and nursing curricula to teach empathy. They encouraged students to simulate being a patient with age-related conditions, such as macular degeneration and high-frequency hearing loss. The programme was met with positive feedback from students, with assessment results indicating increased understanding of and empathy towards those with age-related conditions.

Other examples include mental health simulations where students can engage with virtual patients experiencing symptoms of anxiety or depression, learning to communicate effectively and de-escalate emotional distress. Similarly, VR simulations can simulate challenging conversations, such as delivering bad news or discussing end-of-life care, allowing students to practice empathy and compassionate communication in emotionally charged situations.

3.4.4 Addressing Challenges in Implementing Virtual Reality for Patient-Care Training

3.4.4.1 Ethical Considerations

When implementing VR for patient-care training, it is imperative to consider ethical implications using established frameworks, such as the principlist approach (Beauchamp and Childress 1979). Grounded in the principles of beneficence, non-maleficence, respect for autonomy, and justice, this framework provides a structured guide for ethical decision-making in healthcare contexts.

Beneficence in VR-based training entails actively promoting the wellbeing of both trainees and simulated patients by designing scenarios that maximise educational value. This includes ensuring that learning objectives are achievable, feedback is constructive, and the simulation environment does not inadvertently cause stress, anxiety, or confusion that could undermine the learning experience.

Non-maleficence obligates educators to prevent harm to both trainees and simulated patients by carefully considering and minimising physical, psychological, and cognitive risks associated with VR simulations. This includes anticipating potential stressors, monitoring for signs of discomfort, and preventing overreliance by ensuring learners appropriately contextualise simulation experiences within real-world patient care.

Autonomy emphasises the need to represent virtual patients with dignity and respect while ensuring that trainees are fully informed about the capabilities and limitations of the technology, including data collection and performance monitoring. Learners should provide informed consent before engaging with simulations, recognising how their interactions may be recorded or assessed.

Finally, justice demands equitable access to VR training opportunities, ensuring that all trainees, regardless of background or resources, have equal access. This includes addressing disparities in access to technology and internet connectivity, which may disproportionately affect certain groups. A large cohort implementation study in Germany (Mahling et al. 2023) showed that following a VR-based emergency medicine teaching session, test scores were not influenced by gender, age, or prior experience in emergency medicine or with VR. However, the reported positive attitude regarding learning experience was comparatively lower among female students, indicating that gender differences need to be considered. Additionally, considerations of justice extend to the selection of content for VR simulations, ensuring that scenarios are inclusive and representative of diverse patient populations.

By applying the principlist approach, educators can navigate complex ethical considerations to ensure that VR-enhanced patient-care training upholds ethical standards while promoting learning and professional development.

3.4.4.2 Realism and Emotional Engagement

Advances in VR technology have increasingly focused on enhancing emotional realism to support immersive and effective learning experiences. Dechsling et al. (2023) evaluated the feasibility of embedding dynamic facial expressions into avatars generated from real person photos, demonstrating that tailored emotion expressions can be rendered in VR but require further refinement to ensure accurate perception of subtle emotional cues. Similarly, Mavrogiorgou et al. (2024) reported on the Bochum Avatar Exploration Project (AVEX), in which medical students conducted psychiatric history interviews with virtual avatars. While students felt the experience enhanced their understanding of psychiatric assessment and interview stills, their feedback highlighted limitations in the naturalness of dialogue and the need for more nuanced emotional response systems. Furthermore, preparing learners for the emotional demands of immersive scenarios is key to safe and effective engagement with VR. Cieslowski et al. (2024) conducted an integrative review of VR/AR simulations in nursing education and stressed that comprehensive, standardised pre-training briefings are essential to mitigate potential stress or discomfort.

3.4.4.3 Integration into Clinical Rotations

Medical curricula undergo rigorous review processes to ensure that content aligns with accreditation standards and clinical competencies. As a result, introducing new educational technologies like VR requires careful consideration and validation to demonstrate their effectiveness and relevance. Institutions need to identify specific learning objectives and competencies that can be enhanced through VR experiences, ensuring alignment with the clinical topics covered during each training stage.

In 2020, more than 30 medical schools from across the UK and Ireland combined forces to create Virtual Primary Care, a digital learning resource that makes complete and authentic primary care consultations available for use in UK undergraduate medical education. The material provided is adaptable to individual medical school curricula and has been mapped to the General Medical Council's *Outcomes for Graduates* (2018). Each consultation is tagged for clinical and educational content and is accompanied by associated learning and discussion points as well as additional learning resources.

3.5 Conclusion

3.5.1 Transformative Impact of Virtual Reality in Medical Education and Training

VR holds immense potential to revolutionise medical education by providing cost-effective solutions that offer high-fidelity graphics and realism. Through VR, students can engage in immersive learning experiences that simulate real-world medical scenarios, enhancing their understanding of complex concepts and procedures. User training and support play a pivotal role in the successful implementation of VR in medical education. Faculty training programs should be provided to familiarise educators with the use of VR simulations in teaching, empowering them to effectively leverage these tools to enhance student learning. Scalability is another key consideration, as institutions seek to expand the use of VR across various disciplines and educational levels.

Use of open-source platforms and partnerships with technology companies can reduce licensing and development costs, ensuring affordability for educational institutions with limited budgets. However, challenges such as data security and privacy must be addressed to safeguard sensitive patient information stored within VR software. Moreover, ensuring device compatibility and accessibility remains crucial to enable seamless integration into existing educational infrastructure and accommodate diverse learning needs.

In harnessing the full potential of VR technology, medical education can undergo a transformative shift towards more immersive, engaging, and effective learning experiences. Through collaborative initiatives, VR can expand access to high-quality medical education, equipping healthcare professional with the skills and knowledge required to provide safe, effective, and patient-centred care.

3.5.2 Future Prospects and Advancements in Virtual Reality Technology for Medical Education

Whilst digital simulations have been available for decades, the current landscape suggests a pivotal moment for immersive simulation technologies due to substantial investments and notable advancements in affordable computing and artificial intelligence. However, the potential for future progress may be undermined by inadequate implementation and unstructured evaluation processes. Mathew et al. (2021) consulted clinicians, researchers, and industry to develop three guiding principles to maximise the utility of these technologies for educational purposes. These include: (1) design and development should be driven by learning needs; (2) implementation must be supported by rigorous evaluation; (3) collaboration should be fostered to ensure efficient and effective use. Continued advancement will require the alignment of innovation with evidence-based practice to realise the full potential of VR in medical education and training.

References

Beauchamp TL, Childress JF (1979) Principles of biomedical ethics. Oxford University Press, Oxford, p 314. ISBN: 0195024885

Bielsa VF (2021) Virtual reality simulation in plastic surgery training. Literature review. J Plast Reconstr Aesthet Surg 74(9):2372–2378

Cieslowski BJ, Craig S, Gummadi SD, Butler K (2024) Prebrief time for immersive virtual and augmented reality simulation: an integrative review. Nurse Educ 49(1):E7–E11. https://doi.org/10.1097/NNE.0000000000001477. PMID:37467148

Dechsling A, Cogo-Moreira H, Spydevold Gangestad J, Johannessen SN, Nordahl-Hansen A (2023) Evaluating the feasibility of emotion expressions in avatars created from real person photos: pilot web-based survey of virtual reality software. JMIR Format Res 7:e44632. https://doi.org/10.2196/44632. PMID:37166970

Duarte ML, Assis AM, Guimarães Junior JB, Carnevale FC (2021) Virtual reality in interventional radiology education: a systematic review. Radiol Bras 54:254–260

Dyer E, Swartzlander BJ, Gugliucci MR (2018) Using virtual reality in medical education to teach empathy. J Med Libr Assoc 106(4):498–500. https://doi.org/10.5195/jmla.2018.518

Esmaeeli E, Soleimani A, Sadat Khorashadizadeh M, Shahmoradi L, Nekoonam S (2025) A practical framework for developing a virtual reality-based anatomy education application: key content and technical requirements. Sci Rep 15:12536. https://doi.org/10.1038/s41598-025-96074-8

Essoe JK, Reggente N, Ohno AA, Baek YH, Dell'Italia J, Rissman J (2022) Enhancing learning and retention with distinctive virtual reality environments and mental context reinstatement. NPJ Sci Learn 7(1):31

Fairén M, Ramírez-Serrano A, Casas R (2020) VR4Health: personalized teaching and learning anatomy using virtual reality. Int J Adv Life Sci 12(1):1–10. PMID:32193612

Farr A, Farr F et al (2024) Impact of a virtual reality-based simulation training for shoulder dystocia management. Sci Rep. https://doi.org/10.1038/s41598-024-57785-6

Feeley A, Feeley I, Merghani K, Sheehan E (2021) Use of virtual reality simulation in surgical training: a systematic review on predictive validity and current use in surgical curricula. J Surg Simul 8:1–13

Flexner A (1910) Medical education in the United States and Canada. Science 32(810):41–50

Foronda CL, Gonzalez L, Meese MM, Slamon N, Baluyot M, Lee J, Aebersold M (2024) A comparison of virtual reality to traditional simulation in health professions education: a systematic review. Simul Healthc 19(1S):S90–S97

Fortune Business Insights (2024) Virtual Reality (VR) in healthcare market size, share & industry analysis, by component (Hardware, software, and content), by application (pain management, education & training, surgery, patient care management, rehabilitation & therapy procedures, and Post-Traumatic Stress Disorder (PTSD)), and regional forecast, 2024–2032

Gan W, Mok TN, Chen J, She G, Zha Z, Wang H, Li H, Li J, Zheng X (2023) Researching the application of virtual reality in medical education: one-year follow-up of a randomized trial. BMC Med Educ 23(1):3

General Medical Council (2018) Outcomes for graduates. General Medical Council, London, p 28

Jiang H, Vimalesvaran S, Wang JK, Lim KB, Mogali SR, Car LT (2022) Virtual reality in medical students' education: scoping review. JMIR Med Educ 8(1):e34860

Katz D, Shah R, Kim E, Park C, Shah A, Levine A, Burnett G (2020) Utilization of a voice-based virtual reality advanced cardiac life support team leader refresher: prospective observational study. J Med Internet Res 22(3):e17425

Khan R, Plahouras J, Johnston BC, Scaffidi MA, Grover SC, Walsh CM (2019) Virtual reality simulation training in endoscopy: a Cochrane review and meta-analysis. Endoscopy 51(7):653–664

Kirkpatrick D, Kirkpatrick J (2006) Evaluating training programs: the four levels. Berrett-Koehler Publishers

Kolb DA (2014) Experiential learning: experience as the source of learning and development. FT Press

Krause KJ, Mullins DD, Kist MN, Goldman EM (2023) Developing 3D models using photogrammetry for virtual reality training in anatomy. Anat Sci Educ. https://doi.org/10.1002/ase.2301. PMID:37248365

Kyaw BM, Saxena N, Posadzki P et al (2019) Virtual reality for health professions education: systematic review and meta-analysis by the digital health education collaboration. J Med Internet Res 21(1):e12959. https://doi.org/10.2196/12959

Lam A (2022) Review of the future of surgery: technology enhanced surgical training report. Bull R Coll Surg Engl 104(6):308–309

Mahling M, Wunderlich R, Steiner D, Gorgati E, Festl-Wietek T, Herrmann-Werner A (2023) Virtual reality for emergency medicine training in medical school: prospective, large-cohort implementation study. J Med Internet Res 25:e43649

Mao RQ, Lan L, Kay J, Lohre R, Ayeni OR, Goel DP, Sa D (2021) Immersive virtual reality for surgical training: a systematic review. J Surg Res 268:40–58

Mathew RK, Mushtaq F, Collaboration, I. H (2021) Three principles for the progress of immersive technologies in healthcare training and education. BMJ Simul Technol Enhanc Learn 7(5):459–460

Mavrogiorgou P, Böhme P, Kramer M, Vanscheidt S, Schoppa T, Hooge V, Lüdike N, Pfeiffer T, Juckel G (2024) Virtual reality in teaching using mentally ill patient avatars. Nervenarzt 95(3):247–253. https://doi.org/10.1007/s00115-024-01610-y. PMID:38277046

McGaghie WC, Issenberg SB, Cohen ER et al (2011) Does simulation-based medical education with deliberate practice yield better results than traditional clinical education? A meta-analytic comparative review of the evidence. Acad Med 86(6):706–711. https://doi.org/10.1097/ACM.0b013e318217e119

McKinney B, Dbeis A, Lamb A, Frousiakis P, Sweet S (2022) Virtual reality training in unicompartmental knee arthroplasty: a randomized, blinded trial. J Surg Educ 79(6):1526–1535

Mills B, Dykstra P, Hansen S et al (2020) Virtual reality triage training can provide comparable simulation efficacy for Paramedicine students compared to live simulation-based scenarios. Prehosp Emerg Care 24(4):525–536. https://doi.org/10.1080/10903127.2019.1676345

Moro C, Štromberga Z, Raikos A, Stirling A (2017) The effectiveness of virtual and augmented reality in health sciences and medical anatomy. Anat Sci Educ 10(6):549–559. https://doi.org/10.1002/ase.1696

O'Sullivan DM, Foley R, Proctor K, Gallagher S, Deery A, Eidem BW, McMahon CJ (2021) The use of virtual reality echocardiography in medical education. Pediatr Cardiol 42(4):723–726

Padilha JM, Machado PP, Ribeiro A, Ramos J, Costa P (2019) Clinical virtual simulation in nursing education: a randomized controlled trial. Nurse Educ Today 75:75–83. https://doi.org/10.1016/j.nedt.2018.12.025

Pottle J (2019) Virtual reality and the transformation of medical education. Future Healthc J 6(3):181–185

Rothlind E, Fors U, Salminen H et al (2021) Virtual patients reflecting the clinical reality of primary care—a useful tool to improve cultural competence. BMC Med Educ 21(1):270. https://doi.org/10.1186/s12909-021-02701-z

Saalfeld P, Schmeier A, D'Hanis W, Rothkötter H-J, Preim B (2020) Student and teacher meet in a shared virtual reality: a one-on-one tutoring system for anatomy education. arXiv:2011.07926

Sakakibara J, Nasu K, Ikeda JI, Suzuki TH, Yokomizo J, Fujimoto H, Takada M, Nagashima T, Ohtsuka M (2025) Clinical application of vein visualization apparatus AccuVein® 500 in breast cancer surgery: a case report. J Med Case Rep 19(1):231

Sinha S, DeYoung V, Nehru A (2023) Determinants of learning anatomy in an immersive virtual reality environment—a scoping review. Med Sci Educ 33(1):287–297. https://doi.org/10.1007/s40670-022-01701-y. PMID:36573211

Stepan K, Zeiger J, Hanchuk S, Del Signore A, Shrivastava R, Govindaraj S, Iloreta A (2017) Immersive virtual reality as a teaching tool for neuroanatomy. Int Forum Allergy Rhinol 7(10):1006–1013. https://doi.org/10.1002/alr.21986. PMID:28719062

Vargas F, González A (2018) The use of virtual and augmented reality in anatomy teaching: a brief review. J Digit Imaging 31(6):667–674. https://doi.org/10.1007/s10278-018-0090-5. PMID:31937906

Vrillon A, Gonzales-Marabal L, Ceccaldi PF, Plaisance P, Desrentes E, Paquet C, Dumurgier J (2022) Using virtual reality in lumbar puncture training improves students learning experience. BMC Med Educ 22(1):244

Zahabi M, Abdul Razak AM (2020) Adaptive virtual reality-based training: a systematic literature review and framework. Virtual Reality 24(4):725–752

Zhang Y (2024) Virtual neurosurgery anatomy laboratory: a collaborative and remote cloud-based VR interface for surgical education. J Med Educ Innov 2(1):15–23. PMC10070459

4 Artificial Intelligence in Diagnosis

Emma Cox

Abstract

Artificial Intelligence (AI) is revolutionising diagnostics. It is already possible for Machine Learning models to accurately identify conditions from radiographic images; to answer medical questions effectively, and to combine different data sources to reach a diagnosis. This chapter explores the progress that has been made incorporating Artificial Intelligence into the diagnostic process, including its application to interpreting patient signs and symptoms, radiology and a combination of these and other inputs. This chapter also discusses some of the considerations and challenges facing the field and seeks to answer the question of whether AI is ready to replace clinicians.

Keywords

Artificial intelligence · AI-driven diagnostics · Multimodal AI · Large language models · Diagnostic imaging · Automated diagnosis

Diagnosis is the process of identifying that a patient's signs, symptoms and test results are caused by a particular condition. Diagnosis and treatment are the fundamental building blocks upon which modern healthcare and medical practice are founded. Until now, diagnosing patients has been an activity that is reserved solely for healthcare professionals, but artificial intelligence (AI) is starting to challenge this. Media outlets frequently report studies where Artificial Intelligence has outperformed clinicians, and there are even questions about whether AI will replace them. In this chapter, we will explore whether the claims are true and if AI is ready to start diagnosing patients. As part of this, we will explore what artificial intelligence is; how it works; what recent advances have been made; how different data modalities are used; and some of the main issues faced when implementing AI diagnostics.

4.1 Artificial Intelligence

The field of Artificial Intelligence consists of Machine Learning and Deep Learning (Google 2023). Both use algorithms that can make predictions and analyse data to find insights. Machine Learning refers to the ability to extract knowledge from data through simpler methods, such as decision trees and linear regression, whereas Deep Learning uses more advanced methods, such as artificial neural networks (Google 2023). The development of these algorithms involves

E. Cox (✉)
Medics.Academy, London, UK
e-mail: emma.cox@medics.academy

J. Malawana et al. (eds.), *Artificial Intelligence in Healthcare and Biomedical Visualization*, Biomedical Visualization 10, https://doi.org/10.1007/978-3-032-06520-9_4

training them on datasets, validating their outputs and adjusting the model as necessary (Campbell et al. 2020). One of the key differences between Machine Learning and Deep Learning is that in Deep Learning, the model can learn from its own mistakes, whereas in Machine Learning, a human is usually required to intervene and adjust the model (Google 2023). Once validated, the model can then be applied to other datasets, known as test datasets, to see how well it performs. How effective the model is, is largely determined by how well the training data represents the dataset or population that the model will ultimately be used on (Google 2023).

4.2 AI in Diagnostic Imaging

In this section, using glaucoma as an example, we will explore how Machine Learning can be applied to diagnose diseases from imaging. Glaucoma is a disease that causes gradual visual loss and changes to the optic disc. It is typically diagnosed through a combination of patient history, visual field testing, fundus imaging, intraocular pressure measurements and optical coherence tomography (OCT) (Bragança et al. 2024). Artificial Intelligence has been applied to many types of ophthalmic imaging—fundus images have featured prominently because of their availability, quality and low cost of acquisition. Machine Learning models have been created that can accurately categorise fundus images as either normal or having glaucomatous disease (accuracy 95% and above). Developing these models involves ophthalmologists and engineers using image processing, feature extraction techniques and applying a classifier to train the model to appreciate which images are normal and which show glaucoma. Initially, these Machine Learning models were trained to recognise disc cupping, but this proved problematic as there are other causes (e.g. Multiple Sclerosis and tumours) (Bragança et al. 2024). Another issue was that larger discs naturally have a bigger cup, which resulted in them being misclassified (Campbell et al. 2020). Disc cupping therefore, is suitable as an indicator of glaucoma but is not sufficient to diagnose it. As a result, feature extraction for these models was adapted to include the whole optic disc and multiple other features of glaucomatous disease (e.g. peripapillary atrophy and changes in the retinal nerve fibre layer) with great success (Bragança et al. 2024).

One difficulty with the glaucoma-classifier Machine Learning models is that they require feature vector extraction—this means that the relevant variables must be identified and extracted from the training data, which can be a laborious and time-consuming task (Bragança et al. 2024; Domino 2024). The resulting model output is also only as good as the input data and feature vector extraction (Bragança et al. 2024). Moreover, any model that relies upon specialists' labelling fundus images as glaucomatous or not is problematic, as there is often poor agreement between specialists about what constitutes glaucomatous disease. Indeed, in one study, six ophthalmologists were asked to diagnose glaucoma solely based on photographs: they only agreed 49% of the time. This causes difficulties for applying Machine Learning to detecting glaucomatous disease, as the classification that comes out of the model can only be as good as the classification that is provided in the training data set (Bragança et al. 2024).

As computing power has increased, Deep Learning models have been applied to detect glaucoma from fundal images with accuracies reaching over 99% (Bragança et al. 2024). Indeed, studies have consistently found that Deep Learning algorithms' performance is comparable to, if not superior to, ophthalmology experts (Campbell et al. 2020). The algorithms used in Deep Learning can extract their own features, saving ophthalmologists and engineers time (Lapka and Straňák 2024). Convolutional neural networks (CNNs) are frequently used in these models as they are the gold standard of Deep Learning image processing (Bragança et al. 2024). CNNs convert images into a form that is easier to process, without losing critical features that are needed for the algorithm to make accurate predictions. For Deep Learning algorithms to be able to accurately extract their own features and make accurate predictions, vast datasets are required. This has been problematic as fundus images datasets, whilst one of the more abundant, are often still insufficient (Lapka and Straňák 2024).

Unperturbed, researchers have come up with two different solutions to address the issue of insufficient datasets: Generative adversarial networks (GANs) and transfer learning (Bragança et al. 2024). GANS use Deep Learning to create images, and transfer learning involves training Deep Learning models on similar datasets and then transitioning them to the test data. GANs have started to be used to create and categorise retinal images (Bragança et al. 2024). GANs consist of two neural networks, one neural network is the generator and creates images, and the other is the discriminator, which evaluates how authentic the created images are (whether they are real or fake) (Brownlee 2019). If the generator fools the discriminator, the generator is rewarded and the discriminator model is updated. If the discriminator accurately identifies whether the image is real or fake, it is rewarded, and the generator model parameters are updated. Over time, the performance of both models improves (Brownlee 2019). GANs have started to be applied to differentiate glaucomatous retinae from normal ones and have achieved an area under the curve of 0.9017 (specificity 79.86%, sensitivity 82.9%) (Huang et al. 2023b). However, the uptake of GANs has been limited in glaucoma, perhaps because of the computing power required, and concern about the ethics of generating retinal images that aren't protected by data privacy laws but may contain elements of patient data (Huang et al. 2023b).

Transfer learning is also starting to be used in Deep Learning models, as it means that smaller datasets can be used to train the model (Bragança et al. 2024). Transfer learning involves pre-training the model with data that is similar, but slightly different from, the training data. In the case of glaucoma, pre-training has often involved using publicly available fundal images that may not be of the same quality as the selected dataset, which will be used to train the model (Bragança et al. 2024).

Increasingly, Machine and Deep Learning models are being applied together (Bragança et al. 2024). These models may use a combination of vector extraction and classification, and CNNs. They have achieved accuracies of 95–100% (Bragança et al. 2024).

4.3 Issues with AI in Diagnostic Imaging

Whilst the results of glaucoma Machine Learning and Deep Learning classification models are very promising, it is worth noting that there currently are not any software packages available for use in real clinical scenarios (Bragança et al. 2024). Moreover, many of the Machine Learning models have not been validated, so it is not possible to know their performance on 'unseen' data (Huang et al. 2023b). Models can perform very well on existing data but poorly on new data, a phenomenon known as 'overfitting' (Huang et al. 2023b). As a result, the accuracy rates achieved in many papers are unlikely to reflect real-world performance (Christopher et al. 2020; Zhu et al. 2024). Furthermore if a model is trained on images from one population, it is unlikely that the accuracy will be preserved when the model is applied to different racial, age or socio-demographic groups (Campbell et al. 2020). It is therefore vital to ensure training datasets fully represent the population, otherwise minorities are likely to be misdiagnosed and societal biases propagated (Christopher et al. 2020). When developing Machine Learning models for glaucoma, often only healthy or severe glaucomatous retinal images from glaucoma clinics are used (Campbell et al. 2020). As a result, the models are typically less able to identify mild glaucoma and may struggle to identify glaucoma in a patient who has other systemic diseases (Bragança et al. 2024). Given that glaucoma is a disease that usually presents in later years, this limitation significantly affects its applicability to clinical scenarios (Campbell et al. 2020).

It is not just patient factors that can affect model performance—the equipment used in training and test datasets also needs to be considered. Studies have shown that something as simple as changing the camera used for the test and training data can affect performance (Zhu et al. 2024). Moreover, many Machine Learning models are trained and tested on datasets that only contain high-quality images, rather than images that are more representative of a typical clinical scenario (Campbell et al. 2020; Bragança et al. 2024). A recent study has shown that including poor-quality images into the training data set can reduce the area under the curve by 0.1 (Campbell et al. 2020). To avoid overfitting and improve how models perform in real-world scenarios, it is vital to use varied training data. However, until the volume of available data sources increases, it is unlikely that this issue will be fully addressed. Whilst the use of GANs may help overcome the issue of insufficient data, they are unlikely to solve the homogeneity issue and may in fact contribute to it (Bragança et al. 2024).

Whilst factors that affect model performance are important, it is also necessary to consider how algorithms can be used in clinical settings. One consideration is that patients usually present to healthcare settings with symptoms, which means a wide variety of differential diagnoses will need to be considered. These diagnoses will then need to be interpreted in the context of any concurrent diseases. However, current Machine Learning models are not trained to recognise glaucoma if other disease processes are present. Indeed, they have been shown to give false negative results if there is concurrent high myopia or age-related macular degeneration (Campbell et al. 2020). Given the high prevalence of myopia and glaucoma in Asian populations, it is vital for models to be able to accurately process myopic eyes. Current models are also not trained to identify other diagnoses; as a result these diagnoses will be missed if they are applied to undifferentiated populations (Bragança et al. 2024).

One of the main challenges faced by implementing Deep Learning into clinical settings comes from the issue of explainability (Campbell et al. 2020). If a clinician diagnoses glaucomatous optic neuropathy during fundoscopy, they will use characteristic features such as RNFL thinning and excavation of the cup to reach that diagnosis. In contrast, it is not known what features a Deep Learning model has evaluated to reach its conclusion. As a result, Deep Learning models are often called 'black boxes' (Campbell et al. 2020). The opaqueness with which a conclusion is reached can affect the confidence patients and clinicians have in the conclusion (Zhu et al. 2024). To overcome this issue, models that allow humans to understand some of the workings of the algorithm are being developed, a phenomenon known as 'explainable AI'. An example of this is an AI model that reports which area of the retinal image the algorithm used to categorise the image (Zhu et al. 2024). Reassuringly, heatmap analysis has shown that the optic disc region is mainly used for glaucoma classification (Campbell et al. 2020). However, there are still concerns that other regions of images are used for classification. Indeed, one study looking at diabetic retinopathy found that changing only a few pixels in fundal images can cause the model to miscategorise images. The changes were undetectable to the human eye but were sufficient to cause the algorithm to miscategorise half of diabetic retinopathy images as normal (Campbell et al. 2020).

4.4 Other Diagnostic Imaging

Early Machine Learning models focussed upon determining whether a disease is present or not, as this is simpler than classifying multiple diseases. Arguably models that work in this way are best suited to screening. It is therefore unsurprising that a diabetic retinopathy screening device was the first fully automated medical AI system to be granted approval by the FDA (Parravano et al. 2024). In the trial that led to the device's approval, the model was compared to an independent standard that contained fundus and OCT images. It was found to meet the predefined superiority endpoint, with a sensitivity of 87.2% and a specificity of 90.7% for detecting referable diabetic retinopathy (Parravano et al. 2024).

Another notable use of Machine Learning in screening has been its application to mammograms. In a non-inferiority study, researchers demonstrated that having an AI model, rather than a radiologist, as the second reader of mammograms resulted in 20% more breast cancers being detected—notably without increasing the rate of false positives (Lång et al. 2023). Innovative approaches have been used to identify subtler breast cancers. One way this has been done has been to train the Machine Learning model to look for symmetry and differences between the left and right breast rather than just for the presence or absence of cancer (Xu et al. 2024).

When AI was first applied to chest radiographs, models were trained to simply determine whether a particular condition was present or not (Thakur et al. 2024). As Machine Learning models have evolved and more data have become available, models have been developed that can identify multiple conditions. Machine Learning models can now accurately diagnose many of the conditions visualised on chest radiographs, such as pulmonary nodules, pneumothoraces and pneumonia (Thakur et al. 2024). To accurately categorise images, models need to be trained on datasets that contain adequate representations of all the specified conditions (Yang et al. 2024). If a disease is not fully represented in the training data, the diagnostic accuracy for that disease will be significantly affected. Concerns have therefore been raised that rare diseases will be misdiagnosed, exacerbating existing issues with identifying patients suffering from rare diseases (Yang et al. 2024).

Machine Learning models are being applied to almost all image-based diagnostics. Whilst it is not possible to explore them all, some notable examples include using AI to: interpret prostate biopsies from suspected cancers; delineate brain tumour boundaries on MRIs for surgical planning; and detect and diagnose lung nodules on CT (Azadi Moghadam et al. 2024; Thakur et al. 2024). Novel inputs are also increasingly being incorporated into diagnostic models—examples include gait and facial expression analysis in Parkinson's Disease; and gaze-fixation, visual scanning and facial expression imitation in Autism Spectrum Disorders (Skaramagkas et al. 2023; Jia et al. 2024). The AI revolution is not just limited to healthcare settings: the FDA has approved a consumer Deep Learning algorithm that identifies atrial fibrillation from smartwatch data (Quer and Topol 2024). As models advance and more datasets become available, we will see more AI-driven diagnoses from healthcare and wearable data sources. Rather than replacing clinicians, it is likely that AI models will support clinicians to reach a diagnosis, a phenomenon known as computer-aided diagnosis (Zhou et al. 2021).

4.5 Large Language Models in Diagnostics

Whilst imaging may be an obvious target for implementing Artificial Intelligence in healthcare, the same principles are increasingly being applied to the written word. It is easy to see how classifying patients based on their reported symptoms or signs could help clinicians reach a diagnosis. Initially, the principles described above for images were applied to text: researchers would provide Natural Language Processing (NLP) and Machine Learning models with structured text about the signs and symptoms of medical conditions (training data), and the models would use it to effectively diagnose patients with these predefined conditions. Indeed, multiple studies have found that Machine Learning models can accurately differentiate different types of headaches (e.g. tension-type headache, migraine, medication overuse headaches) when provided with key demographics, headache characteristics and associated symptoms (Stubberud et al. 2024). The performance of these models varied, but the best model achieved an average accuracy of over 93.7% (Stubberud et al. 2024). Whilst structured patient data has been used in many studies, increasingly ML models are being applied to unstructured patient data. For instance, one ML model has been shown to successfully distinguish migraine and cluster headaches based on unstructured self-reported patient narratives (Stubberud et al. 2024). Being able to successfully apply ML classification models to unstructured data, means there can be far greater application of ML models to patient records and patient-reported symptoms.

As the training text datasets (corpora) have increased and ML models have improved, models known as Large Language Models (LLMs) have been developed. These models are trained on a particular Deep Learning architecture and are mainly used for interpreting and generating text (Yang et al. 2024). LLMs are specific NLP models that are capable of understanding, generating and manipulating a language (Biswas et al. 2024). LLMs are trained to predict the sequence of words in normal human language. One of the key things that sets them apart is their transformer architecture. This effectively is a 'self-attention' mechanism that the model uses to weigh up the importance of different words, or their positions within a sentence, whilst still processing each word itself. Prior to this, NLP had only focused upon processing the words that were adjacent to each other (Yang et al. 2024). For LLMs to be able to do this, they have to be trained on vast amounts of text data so that they can learn the patterns, context, semantics and grammar (Biswas et al. 2024). LLMs also possess the ability to learn and adapt. LLMs predict the next words in a sequence, evaluate their predictions against actual outcomes and adjust their parameters accordingly until they achieve a high level of proficiency (Pressman et al. 2024).

Whilst LLMs can be used to generate text, they have also been widely used to analyse clinical cases. Multiple studies have shown how LLMs can use transcripts from clinical interviews to predict the results of depression and PTSD assessments in terms of both diagnosis and severity scores (Malgaroli and McDuff 2024). Likewise, by analysing disorganised clinical notes, LLMs were able to effectively predict suicidal behaviour in mental health patients (Khan and Javed 2022). LLMs have also been found to have reasonable accuracy (but limited reliability) in diagnosing infectious diseases and some common cardiovascular and urinary conditions from patient notes (Pressman et al. 2024).

Whilst LLMs have shown great promise in classifying diseases, it is worth noting that their performance is better with common conditions and typical presentations—probably because these are better represented in the training data (Pressman et al. 2024). For instance, although the headache classifier mentioned above had an average accuracy of over 93.7%, it only had a sensitivity of 36.8% when classifying less common headaches such as secondary headaches, meaning that potentially serious conditions could be missed (Stubberud et al. 2024). The diagnosis of these conditions often relies upon nuance in the history, which may not be as effectively detected by an ML model. Indeed, even ML models that generate effective and accurate mental health assessments from patient narratives have been found to be inadequate for analysing more complex or challenging situations such as nuanced cases of postpartum depression (Omar et al. 2024). It is well documented that ML models often underperform when they are required to contextualise information and understand how different pieces of medical information fit together, and this affects their ability to diagnose complex conditions, rare disorders and common illnesses with atypical presentations (Pressman et al. 2024).

One of the more novel applications of LLMs has been to use its text classification capabilities to diagnose mental health disorders from social media data. When applying GPT-3 to Reddit data, researchers found that it was capable of diagnosing mental health disorders with an accuracy of around 87% (Omar et al. 2024). Likewise, researchers have found that other LLMs can diagnose schizophrenia from tweets with an average accuracy of 81%, and depression from YouTube vlogs with a precision of 65.57% (Iyortsuun et al. 2023). Whilst this may be an interesting application of LLMs, it has garnered a lot of criticism as there are fundamental differences between social media data and the traditional clinical data often used in healthcare research. For instance, social media data does not usually contain clinical history, existing diagnoses, treatment or social history and may not be a valid representation of mental state or experience (Merhbene et al. 2024).

Another area that has received a lot of interest is whether LLMs can pass medical exams

(Biswas et al. 2024). These studies are responsible for many of the sensationalist claims about Artificial Intelligence replacing clinicians. Indeed, LLMs have been shown to consistently pass the USMLE (86% accuracy), and to reach greater than an 80% accuracy when answering PubMed questions (Biswas et al. 2024). It is therefore easy to see where these claims come from, but it is important to note that human clinicians still outperform these LLMs (Biswas et al. 2024). Another consideration is that the examinations mentioned above are multiple choice—in real life, patients do not present as multiple-choice questions. Studies have found that Chat-GPT4 performance deteriorates when applied to open-ended questions or more difficult multiple-choice questions (Liu et al. 2024). Many of the studies looking at ChatGPT's performance in medical exams have used optimised prompts to improve the responses provided. Using optimised prompts involves including instructions such as, 'You are a medical student, and we will be using medical licensing examination questions to test you; please provide your best answers'. Indeed, studies have found that using prompts increased the accuracy of GPT-3.5 from 54% to 68%, and GPT-4 from 79% to 85%. This variation shows how the quality of the prompt or question significantly affects the model's performance, which is something that would need to be carefully considered before implementing LLMs into real-world scenarios (Liu et al. 2024).

Despite studies showing that LLMs perform worse with open-ended questions, much effort has been invested in applying LLMs to these scenarios. It is recognised that LLMs need to be able to do more than simply answer multiple-choice questions, if they are to be successfully integrated into clinical settings and workflows. Indeed, researchers have found that LLMs are able to diagnose common ocular diseases from clinical vignettes with an average accuracy of 71.1% (Biswas et al. 2024). ChatGPT-4, with an accuracy of 82%, was found to be superior to the other LLMs in this study. However, it is worth noting that its performance was still inferior to trained ophthalmologists (accuracy 86%, 63.6–95%) (Biswas et al. 2024). Sticking with ophthalmology, when ChatGPT-3.5 was given detailed clinical vignettes for subtypes of glaucoma, it was able to provide a provisional diagnosis with 72.7% accuracy (Yang et al. 2024). Likewise, ChatGPT-4 was shown to accurately diagnose corneal infections, dystrophies and degenerations with 85% accuracy when given clinical vignettes. However, it is worth noting that all these studies used publicly available online case reports for testing the LLMs. These case reports are very detailed and patient-specific. Given that we don't know exactly what training data is used for ChatGPT, it is possible that these exact cases were included in its training data, thus artificially inflating its performance (Yang et al. 2024).

When interpreting studies assessing how an LLM can diagnose a condition from a detailed clinical vignette, it is important to consider how closely these studies relate to real-world clinical scenarios. One study explored this issue by assessing ChatGPT-4's ability to correctly diagnose conditions based upon: the chief complaints alone; the chief complaints and history of present illness; and the chief complaints, history of present illness and descriptions of ophthalmic and other necessary examinations, including ocular imaging (Hu et al. 2023). When only the chief complaints were provided, the study found that ChatGPT-4 provided several possible diagnoses, none of which were correct. When the chief complaints and history of present illness were provided, 50% of responses were correct; when the chief complaints, history of present illness and descriptions of ophthalmic and other necessary examinations, including ocular imaging, were provided, 90% of responses were accurate (Hu et al. 2023). As in previous studies, this study used an online, publicly available clinical case to test the LLM, which may have overinflated its accuracy. The study does however, suggest that LLMs are reasonably well equipped to diagnose conditions if they are given all the information a specialist would have (including specialist investigations), but struggle when it isn't given as much clinical information. This obviously limits its real-world application. Arguably, patients and generalist medical practitioners stand to benefit most from ophthalmic diagnostic support devices, but as the model only has an accuracy of 50% when given the chief complaint and history of present illness, its real-world application to these clinical settings is currently limited (Hu et al. 2023).

Being a clinician requires far more than just interpreting sections of text that already contain all the necessary information. Clinicians are required to ascertain the relevant information from patients and to adjust and narrow their questioning accordingly (Yang et al. 2024). Over time, attempts have been made to simulate these typical medical consults. Before the development of LLMs, standard chatbots had been used for this purpose, but with limited success. These chatbots often couldn't deal effectively with the complexity of diseases and their presentations, resulting in key information being left out of the medical history. Moreover, limited language processing meant that the chatbots often generated questions that patients struggled to fully understand, and responses that were blunt. With the development of LLMs, some of these issues have been addressed—they are better able to deal with the complexity of disease and offer more human-like interactions. However, LLMs have still not been able to successfully simulate patient–clinician interactions. LLMs do not currently ask the precise follow-up enquiries that are required to gather all the information necessary for an accurate diagnosis to be made. This obviously limits their application to direct patient facing care, as patients may not be aware of all their symptoms and signs; may not know what is relevant and may not include all the necessary information. Nonetheless, it is technically possible for AI agents to be designed in this way, so there is promise that this issue will be addressed in the not-too-distant future (Yang et al. 2024).

4.6 Different LLMs

The release of ChatGPT, a publicly available LLM that has an intuitive interface, has meant that it is much easier to use and test LLMs (Liu et al. 2024). As a result, the application of ChatGPT has been vast. It has been applied to clinical activities that range from text classification to text generation and question answering (Yang et al. 2024). However, it is worth noting that ChatGPT may not be the best placed LLM for all these tasks (Nerella et al. 2024). ChatGPT, like most traditional LLMs, reads text sequentially (one word after the other) and then predicts the next word. This structure means that ChatGPT is optimised for text generation but may not perform as well on comprehension tasks (Yang et al. 2024). In contrast, the Bidirectional Encoder Representations from Transformers (BERT) LLM has been developed to read the entire sequence of words at the same time, enabling it to have a richer picture of the context and information conveyed in a passage of text (Nerella et al. 2024). BERT therefore excels in language understanding, and ChatGPT in text generation (Ding et al. 2023).

When considering which LLM to use for a study, it is important to consider the reference data the model uses. ChatGPT and BERT models, not originally designed for medical use, were trained on a wide range of materials, some of which may not be entirely accurate or reflective of current medical practice (Pressman et al. 2024). Steps have been taken to address this by developing the BioBERT, a BERT model that is pre-trained on PubMed Central articles and abstracts, and fine-tuned for popular biomedical NLP tasks (Nerella et al. 2024). Perhaps unsurprisingly, BioBERT has outperformed previous models when it comes to biomedical text mining tasks (Nerella et al. 2024). BERT models pre-trained on electronic health records have also been found to be effective at predicting the onset of conditions such as stroke, heart failure and diabetes (Nerella et al. 2024).

4.7 Issues with LLMs

Whilst LLMs can be optimised for different functions, there are some common difficulties they face when applied to healthcare. One issue is the problem of semantics in Medicine—words can have very different meanings depending upon the context. For instance, the word 'cold' can be used to describe a temperature or that the patient is suffering from coryzal symptoms. This nuance is often lost when LLMs are applied to the data, resulting in incorrect deductions and responses (Yang et al. 2024).

Whilst semantics might explain some of the inaccuracies in the answers provided by LLMs, it does not explain all of them. LLMs have been developed to predict the next word in a sentence. As a result, the response provided by the LLM is often very coherent and convincing, but it does not mean that it is correct (Nerella et al. 2024). When the answer to a query isn't provided in the training data, the LLM will invent what the response should be, creating fabrications which are known as 'hallucinations' (Biswas et al. 2024). Although some researchers now prefer the term 'confabulation' as 'hallucination' implies a sensory experience, whereas 'confabulation' refers to an erroneous memory (Yang et al. 2024). As the LLM is dependent upon its training data to generate an answer, it is less likely to hallucinate if the query requires only superficial knowledge or simple recall (Yang et al. 2024). Most clinical questions require deep understanding and synthesis of information. To try to overcome this issue, attempts have been made to make it easier for users to identify when an LLM is hallucinating. One such attempt asked ChatGPT to provide explanations for its answers. However, the study found that ChatGPT provided coherent explanations for both its incorrect and correct answers (Biswas et al. 2024). Not only that, ChatGPT-4 if prompted, would fabricate research and publications to support its answer (Kerr and McFarlane 2023). LLMs, unlike clinicians, do not recognise their knowledge limitations, which is concerning when applied to Medicine (Liu et al. 2024). One way to reduce hallucinations is to apply transfer learning to LLMs: pre-trained LLMs can be fine-tuned on specific data that is tailored to a particular task (Yang et al. 2024). For instance, Optha-LLaMA2 an LLM developed to diagnose ophthalmic conditions, was created by taking a pre-trained LLM and then fine-tuning it on reports of ophthalmic conditions. This fine-tuning reduced the frequency of hallucinations (Yang et al. 2024).

LLM training data can be another cause of inaccuracies. LLMs generate answers that are consensus-based rather than evidence-based (Biswas et al. 2024). As such, if there are inaccuracies within the training data, it is likely that they will be propagated. This is particularly likely where LLMs have been trained on open internet sources (Liu et al. 2024). Another difficulty associated with training data is that it can very quickly become out of date, thus affecting how applicable any LLM answers are to the current medical practice (Biswas et al. 2024). Indeed, ChatGPT training data is sourced before 2021 and many other models have capped their training data at 2023 (Yang et al. 2024). To prevent LLMs from becoming out of date, continuous updating of the training data would be required, but this is expensive and challenging.

Work has been undertaken to find alternative ways for LLMs to be kept up to date. One way that this could be done is by implementing an AI framework called Retrieval Augmented Generation (RAG) (Yang et al. 2024). RAG uses search algorithms to query external databases such as web pages or knowledge bases to find relevant information. This information is then processed through the pre-trained LLM to generate the overall answer (Google 2024). This method has been used by Aeyeconsult, an ophthalmology chatbot which has been shown to be more accurate than GPT4 at answering ophthalmology questions (Yang et al. 2024). Although there has been initial success in this field, one difficulty faced is the lack of large, high-quality databases that can be used for these medical models. Moreover, there is a risk that much of the context of the external data is lost during the retrieval and processing by the RAG and LLM. Another method that could be used to keep LLMs up to date would be to implement LLMs into everyday clinician workflows and to ask the clinicians to give feedback on the answers provided. The feedback provided could then be used to refine the LLM. This method is known as Reinforcement Learning from Human Feedback (RLHF). Difficulties with this method include potential inaccuracies or insufficiencies in the feedback provided by clinicians, and risks with LLMs potentially suggesting inaccurate answers to clinicians during their practice (Yang et al. 2024).

As mentioned above, the training data significantly affects the LLM's ultimate performance. One significant issue with this is that biases contained within the training data are propagated in the answers provided by LLMs (Pressman et al. 2024). The large datasets used for training are likely to be impacted by society's prejudices—unless action is taken, LLMs could perpetuate existing prejudices in areas such as ethnicity, gender and socioeconomic background. This could further widen inequalities in healthcare access, quality of care and clinical outcomes (Pressman et al. 2024). Indeed, in one study, ChatGPT-4 gave significantly different diagnoses and treatment recommendations when race or gender were the only factors changed in clinical vignettes (Yang et al. 2024). Another study found that an ML model that predicts postpartum depression gave less appropriate recommendations for black patients (Kerr and McFarlane 2023). Even if race was removed from the scenario, the model would use other evidence of poor social determinants of health as a proxy for race and would still make less appropriate recommendations (Kerr and McFarlane 2023). To prevent biases from being propagated, it is vital to train LLMs on diverse datasets (Yang et al. 2024). However, it is unlikely that diverse datasets will be enough, and so future LLMs are likely to include bias-detection mechanisms and clear ethical guidelines to prevent discrimination (Pressman et al. 2024). If these mechanisms are effectively implemented, it is possible that LLMs could be used to minimise healthcare disparities and counter individual preconceptions and prejudices (Pressman et al. 2024).

For LLMs to be effectively implemented in healthcare, they will need to be trained on vast quantities of patient data (Yang et al. 2024). The inherent workings of LLMs mean they remember their training data. As a result, LLMs are at risk of prompt attacks—attacks where specific templates are used to induce the LLM to provide confidential patient information. Indeed, it has been shown that even if anonymised sensitive patient information is used for training, some LLMs can reidentify the patients. It is therefore vital that adequate consideration is given to security when developing LLMs and that relevant guidance is followed (Yang et al. 2024).

Although LLMs can effectively mimic human responses, there are concerns about their ability to convey empathy and emotions (Pressman et al. 2024). Medicine is not just about facts and diagnoses; patients often need comfort, understanding and reassurance. There is concern that if this need isn't met, patient trust in technology and healthcare providers will be impacted. However, this has been effectively challenged by one study, which found that ChatGPT provided answers that participants deemed more empathetic than the responses given by clinicians (Pressman et al. 2024). Further investigation is therefore needed to reach a consensus on this issue.

Unsurprisingly, the challenges that are faced when implementing image interpretation ML models in the healthcare setting are also encountered when integrating LLMs into clinical care. One of these issues is the 'black box problem'. It is not clear how exactly an LLM reaches its answer, and there is no guarantee that the answer has been based upon clinical guidelines (Yang et al. 2024). In normal clinical practice, there can be disagreements between clinicians about the diagnosis and treatment plan. In such cases, a formal second opinion may be sought, and the reasoning behind the disagreement can be understood and challenged. With an LLM we do not know what a recommendation is based upon, so it is not possible to have this dialogue or shared understanding (Yang et al. 2024).

Other issues that affect both types of AI models include studies not using 'unseen' data to evaluate the model's performance, which may result in overly optimistic claims. There are very few studies evaluating the real-world clinical application of these models and so we cannot know how applicable the results are to the healthcare environment (Stubberud et al. 2024; Younis et al. 2024).

In the future, it is likely that LLMs will be embedded in patient journeys, but it is unlikely that it will be as a substitute for clinicians. Initially, they are likely to be used as tools to prompt clinicians or to triage patients, rather than as full patient-facing diagnostic (Rao et al. 2024). It is also unlikely that one LLM will do everything. Instead, it may be that different LLMs are used to generate patient summaries, flag important historical information to clinicians and make suggestions for particular treatment pathways (Yang et al. 2023).

4.8 Multimodal AI

We have already discussed how Artificial Intelligence can be used to interpret imaging and comprehend and generate text, but there is much more involved in diagnosing a patient than just these two aspects. During a patient consultation, a clinician will: take a history; examine the patient; and potentially interpret lab results and imaging, to reach a diagnosis. If AI is to accurately diagnose a patient, it will need to be able to evaluate and combine multiple data inputs.

Interest in Multimodal Machine Learning models is growing. Indeed, several institutions have developed innovative multimodal models that can accurately diagnose appendicitis in children (AUC >0.90) (Rey et al. 2024). These models combine demographic data, clinical data (such as physical exam findings), laboratory results and ultrasonography findings (Rey et al. 2024). Similarly, multimodal models have been applied to breast cancer detection. Combining pathology images and structured data from electronic medical records, these models have been shown to accurately classify malignant and benign breast cancer (Mohsen et al. 2022).

As may be expected, multimodal models often outperform unimodal models (Amal et al. 2022). Studies exploring ML model inputs have found that combining genetic and electronic medical record data gives a more accurate prediction of a patient's ischaemic heart disease risk than models only containing one of the modalities (Amal et al. 2022). Similarly, multiple studies have found Alzheimer's Dementia diagnostic models that combine imaging data with specific lab test results and demographic data, outperform single-source models (Mohsen et al. 2022).

Multimodal models have also been used to combine unique insights from different imaging modalities (Boehm et al. 2022). For instance, fusing digital mammography with diffusion contrast-enhanced MRI gave an AUROC (area under the receiver operating characteristic curve) of 0.87—higher than the respective unimodal AUROC values of 0.74 and 0.78. Similarly, multiple studies have found that combining imaging modalities such as MRI and PET scans improves the performance of ML models to differentiate patients with Alzheimer's Disease from healthy controls (Huang et al. 2023a). Likewise, the combination of histological imaging data and MRI outperformed unimodal models for classifying brain tumour subtypes (Boehm et al. 2022).

As one might expect, the specific modalities used in ML models are determined by the unique characteristics and features of each disease (Xu et al. 2024). For Alzheimer's Disease, PET and MRI imaging are the predominant modalities, supplemented by speech data—the imaging modalities give unique insights into early brain changes, and the speech changes convey any early functional impact. Contrastingly, breast cancer multimodal models contain genetic information, X-ray imaging, ultrasound and text information. The heterogeneity of breast cancer necessitates that different modalities are used to ensure that all the pathological aspects (such as family history and imaging findings) are fully assessed when making a diagnosis (Xu et al. 2024).

Novel data sources are increasingly being incorporated into multimodal models. Parkinson's Disease results in multiple physical signs that can be elicited during physical examination, such as a shuffling gait and voice changes. Efforts have been made to include these elements in multimodal models—indeed, gait, handwriting/drawing and speech data have been found to be the most effective combination with accuracies reported between 90% and 98% (Huang et al. 2023a). Increasingly, steps are being taken to ensure that we are making the most of the data that is currently available. At one institution, abdominopelvic CTs, which had been requested for any reason, were used to extract body composition biomarkers (e.g. hepatic steatosis and visceral-subcutaneous fat ratios) (Amal et al. 2022). These were then combined with electronic medical record data to accurately predict the risk of ischaemic heart disease at 1 and 5 years. Analysis found that the multimodal model outperformed models that only contained CT or electronic medical record data (Amal et al. 2022).

As with other Artificial Intelligence algorithms, there are several ways that multimodal models can be structured (Amal et al. 2022). One challenge researchers face during development is how to combine and concurrently analyse very different data modalities. The process of combining different modalities (data fusion) can occur at different points in the algorithm's process (Isavand et al. 2024). The time of fusion needs to be decided carefully, as it can significantly affect the model's performance:

1. Early fusion integrates the different data types (modalities) at the start of the model's learning process (Isavand et al. 2024). Each modality independently undergoes feature extraction. These features are then combined to form a representation of all the modalities, which is then passed into a single model. The multiple data sources are combined prior to analysis (Isavand et al. 2024).
2. In late fusion, each modality is fully processed by its own separate model to develop a prediction (Isavand et al. 2024). The predictions from the different models are then aggregated to generate a final prediction (Isavand et al. 2024).
3. Intermediate fusion, as the name suggests, involves combining different modalities somewhere between early and late fusion (Isavand et al. 2024). One way this is done is by following the initial steps of early fusion: independent feature extraction and combining the features together to form a representation of all the modalities; but rather than just passing that representation through a single model, the representation is propagated back to the feature extraction layers to further refine the representation. In this instance the features are further refined based upon the characteristics derived from the other modalities (Isavand et al. 2024).

The different fusion methods lend themselves to different tasks (Isavand et al. 2024). Early fusion is ideal for a holistic understanding of the data inputs, especially when interactions between different modalities are key to the diagnosis. Early integration can reduce the processing complexity and computational power required. However, it can be very challenging to integrate and align diverse data types, especially when there is variation in data scale or sample rates (Isavand et al. 2024). For instance, aligning tabular data (e.g. blood results) with 3D imaging data is not a straightforward process (Amal et al. 2022). One way this can be done is by normalising the data and assigning each datapoint a numerical value between 0 and 1. Another method is to extract multiple characteristics from each data input and then combine them in a way that aligns more with the other data's format. There is, however, a risk that some of the nuance of the data (e.g. CT scan images) is lost through these methods (Amal et al. 2022). If the data is not adequately aligned or is missing for a particular modality, it can affect model performance significantly and introduce significant bias (Isavand et al. 2024).

Conversely, late fusion is ideal for maximising the extraction from each modality as each one is analysed independently (Isavand et al. 2024). This can be particularly useful for diverse and complex datasets (Isavand et al. 2024). As the data sources are fused after analysis, less data is required and the model performance is impacted less if data is missing from one modality—this generally makes late fusion more robust than early fusion (Mohsen et al. 2022). However, late fusion means that subtle relationships between different modalities can be missed and that the overall understanding of complex interactions between modalities is less understood (Mohsen et al. 2022). Moreover, the complexity and computational power required are greater as a separate model has to be managed for each modality (Isavand et al. 2024).

In intermediate fusion, different modalities are combined during the learning process (Isavand et al. 2024). It is a compromise between early and late fusion—features are fully extracted and the interaction between the fused representation and the feature extraction layers means that relationships between modalities are more fully understood. Intermediate fusion leads to a much more comprehensive analysis and understanding of the data. However, it is often much harder to implement than early or late fusion as more advanced engineering techniques and even greater computational power are required (Isavand et al. 2024).

Ultimately, the choice of fusion method depends upon: the aim of the analysis; the nature and availability of the data sources; and the complexity of the required algorithms (Isavand et al. 2024). Roest et al. used Deep Learning methods to process prostate magnetic resonance images and combined this with clinical parameters such as PSA, patient age and prostate volume to accurately detect prostate cancer (Roest et al. 2024). They experimented with early and late fusion and found that early fusion resulted in superior performance. They also demonstrated that their multimodal model was superior to a model that included just one of the modalities. Indeed, on external validation, the early fusion multimodal model was found to significantly outperform radiologists in detecting prostate cancer (Roest et al. 2024). The process of diagnosing a patient with prostate cancer involves many dependent data points, so early fusion may mean that more nuanced relationships between the data modalities were detected (Roest et al. 2024). Early fusion was also effective in this instance because complete datasets (no 'missingness') were provided—the model wasn't required to exclude patients with incomplete datasets or to assume a median point for any missing data points, which would have affected its ability to discern relationships (Boehm et al. 2022).

Whilst not the focus of this chapter, it is worth noting that multimodal models are being increasingly used to predict patient outcomes and to guide treatment. For instance, Machine Learning models have been shown to predict prostate cancer outcomes more accurately than conventional markers (Azadi Moghadam et al. 2024). Improving our prostate cancer predictions has the potential to significantly impact patient experience and outcomes, as it can help them decide between active surveillance and definitive treatment. Indeed, a prognostic multimodal model has even been endorsed by the National Comprehensive Cancer Network for use in clinical guidelines for localised prostate cancer (Riaz et al. 2024). Similarly, colorectal cancer models have been developed that can accurately predict the response to specific therapies, overall survival and disease-free survival. The models can also identify clinically actionable genetic alterations. These models use patient age, sex, cancer stage and genomic, epigenetic, protein and metabolic profiles. They have been shown to outperform human pathologists in their predictions (Azadi Moghadam et al. 2024).

4.9 Issues with Multimodal Models

Multimodal models suffer from many of the same issues as unimodal Artificial Intelligence models, such as a lack of external validation, bias within training data sets, and the 'black box' problem. However, the biggest difficulty with developing effective and accurate multimodal models is the disparity between the amount of data needed to train and test the model on, and the actual availability of this data (Boehm et al. 2022). Often the data required for a medical AI model is not structured or stored in a way that makes it easy to access or include—radiological images are held on picture archiving and communication systems, and tissue specimens are often stored in laboratories as physical samples. Different data modalities often are not co-located and may have different patient identifiers, making them difficult to combine. As datasets are limited and multimodal models require more parameters, they are also more likely to suffer from overfitting (Boehm et al. 2022).

4.10 Ethical Issues with AI in Diagnostics

We have outlined several difficulties faced when developing diagnostic AI models. There are also fundamental issues that need to be addressed when implementing these models into real-world clinical settings. When a clinician makes a mistake, it is clear who is responsible, but when an ML model makes errors, it is less clear. It can be argued that it is difficult for clinicians to take responsibility if they do not understand how the algorithm has reached a diagnosis (Neri et al. 2020). Similarly, when a patient seeks a second opinion, it is possible for the two clinicians to discuss and understand how a conclusion was reached and to refine it as appropriate, but with AI, this level of discussion and refinement is very difficult if not impossible (Ploug and Holm 2023). Given these issues, it may be that AI models are used to augment rather than replace clinician diagnoses at least initially (Neri et al. 2020).

4.11 Conclusion

Artificial Intelligence is revolutionising diagnostics. It is already possible for Machine Learning models to identify pre-defined conditions from radiographic images with similar accuracy to radiologists; to answer medical questions effectively; and to combine different data sources to reach a diagnosis (Mohsen et al. 2022). With these capabilities, it may seem inevitable that Artificial Intelligence is going to replace clinicians, but there is a long way to go. Clinicians take histories from undifferentiated or poorly differentiated patients, often with multiple morbidities. They then elucidate important signs and symptoms, order and interpret investigations, and finally, they communicate and negotiate the management plan with the patient. AI models, on the other hand, are much more accustomed to dealing with differentiated patients and with only a small section of the patient journey. It is therefore much more likely that AI models will be used as a complementary tool for an aspect of the patient journey (Yang et al. 2023).

Unfortunately, many of the models mentioned in the literature have not undergone external validation and have only been appraised on limited test data (Huang et al. 2023b). Going forward, validation will need to be much more thorough, and there will need to be greater transparency around the training data used and measures taken to minimise biases. Ultimately, the burden of evidence for the effectiveness of AI models should be the same as for other diagnostic devices. Using randomised control trials to evaluate the impact of AI models in the real world is, therefore, a necessary next step (Yang et al. 2024).

In future, it is likely that we will see greater use of multimodal models in healthcare as models develop to more accurately represent the clinical picture and capture the nuances of conditions. For the potential advances in the field to be realised, there needs to be significant investments in data sharing and storage, computational power and security (Boehm et al. 2022). There also needs to be a clear delineation of how AI fits within existing ethical frameworks, including those concerning liability, patient choice and explainability.

References

Amal S, Safarnejad L, Omiye JA, Ghanzouri I, Cabot JH, Ross EG (2022) Use of multi-modal data and machine learning to improve cardiovascular disease care. Front Cardiovasc Med 9:840262

Azadi Moghadam P, Bashashati A, Goldenberg SL (2024) Artificial intelligence and pathomics: prostate cancer. Urol Clin North Am 51(1):15–26

Biswas S, Davies LN, Sheppard AL, Logan NS, Wolffsohn JS (2024) Utility of artificial intelligence-based large language models in ophthalmic care. Ophthalmic Physiol Opt 44(3):641–671

Boehm KM, Khosravi P, Vanguri R, Gao J, Shah SP (2022) Harnessing multimodal data integration to advance precision oncology. Nat Rev Cancer 22(2):114–126

Bragança CP, Torres JM, Macedo LO, Soares CPDA (2024) Advancements in glaucoma diagnosis: the role of AI in medical imaging. Diagnostics (Basel) 14(5):530

Brownlee J (2019) A gentle introduction to generative adversarial networks (GANs). Generative Adversarial Networks

Campbell CG, Ting DSW, Keane PA, Foster PJ (2020) The potential application of artificial intelligence for diagnosis and management of glaucoma in adults. Br Med Bull 134(1):21–33

Christopher M, Nakahara K, Bowd C, Proudfoot JA, Belghith A, Goldbaum MH, Rezapour J, Weinreb RN, Fazio MA, Girkin CA, Liebmann JM, De Moraes G, Murata H, Tokumo K, Shibata N, Fujino Y, Matsuura M, Kiuchi Y, Tanito M, Asaoka R, Zangwill LM (2020) Effects of study population, labeling and training on glaucoma detection using deep learning algorithms. Transl Vis Sci Technol 9(2):27

Ding X, Huang Y, Tian X, Zhao Y, Feng G, Gao Z (2023) Diagnosis, treatment, and management of otitis media with artificial intelligence. Diagnostics (Basel) 13(13):2309

Domino (2024) Feature extraction. Domino Data Lab Retrieved 2024, from https://domino.ai/data-science-dictionary/feature-extraction

Google (2023) What's the difference between deep learning, machine learning, and artificial intelligence? Google Cloud Topics 2024, from https://cloud.google.com/discover/deep-learning-vs-machine-learning#

Google (2024) What is Retrieval-Augmented Generation (RAG)? Google Cloud Topics, from https://cloud.google.com/use-cases/retrieval-augmented-generation

Hu X, Ran AR, Nguyen TX, Szeto S, Yam JC, Chan CKM, Cheung CY (2023) What can GPT-4 do for diagnosing rare eye diseases? A pilot study. Opthalmol Ther 12:3395–3402

Huang G, Li R, Bai Q, Alty J (2023a) Multimodal learning of clinically accessible tests to aid diagnosis of neurodegenerative disorders: a scoping review. Health Inf Sci Syst 11(1):32

Huang X, Islam MR, Akter S, Ahmed F, Kazami E, Serhan HA, Abd-Alrazaq A, Yousefi S (2023b) Artificial intelligence in glaucoma: opportunities, challenges, and future directions. Biomed Eng Online 22(1):126

Isavand P, Aghamiri SS, Amin R (2024) Applications of multimodal artificial intelligence in Non-Hodgkin Lymphoma B cells. Biomedicine 12(8):1753

Iyortsuun NK, Kim S-H, Jhon M, Yang H-J, Pant S (2023) A review of machine learning and deep learning approaches on mental health diagnosis. Healthcare 11(3):285

Jia SJ, Jing JQ, Yang CJ (2024) A review on autism spectrum disorder screening by artificial intelligence methods. J Autism Dev Disord 55(9):3011–3027

Kerr WT, McFarlane KN (2023) Machine learning and artificial intelligence applications to epilepsy: a review for the practicing Epileptologist. Curr Neurol Neurosci Rep 23(12):869–879

Khan NZJ, Javed MA (2022) Use of artificial intelligence-based strategies for assessing suicidal behavior and mental illness: a literature review. Cureus 14(7):e27225

Lång K, Josefsson V, Larsson A-M, Larsson S, Högberg C, Sartor H, Hofvind S, Andersson I, Rosso A (2023) Artificial intelligence-supported screen reading versus standard double reading in the Mammography Screening with Artificial Intelligence trial (MASAI): a clinical safety analysis of a randomised, controlled, non-inferiority, single-blinded, screening accuracy study. Lancet Oncol 24(8):936–944

Lapka M, Straňák Z (2024) The current state of artificial intelligence in neuro-ophthalmology. a review. Cesk Slov Oftalmol 3:1001–1012

Liu M, Okuhara T, Chang X, Shirabe R, Nishiie Y, Okada H, Kiuchi T (2024) Performance of ChatGPT across different versions in medical licensing examinations worldwide: systematic review and meta-analysis. J Med Internet Res 26:e60807

Malgaroli M, McDuff D (2024) An overview of diagnostics and therapeutics using large language models. J Trauma Stress 37:754

Merhbene G, Puttick A, Kurpicz-Briki M (2024) Investigating machine learning and natural language processing techniques applied for detecting eating disorders: a systematic literature review. Front Psych 15:1319522

Mohsen F, Ali H, El Hajj N, Shah Z (2022) Artificial intelligence-based methods for fusion of electronic health records and imaging data. Sci Rep 12(1):17981

Nerella S, Bandyopadhyay S, Zhang J, Contreras M, Siegel S, Bumin A, Silva B, Sena J, Shickel B, Bihorac A, Khezeli K, Rashidi P (2024) Transformers and large language models in healthcare: a review. Artif Intell Med 154:102900

Neri E, Coppola F, Miele V, Bibbolino C, Grassi R (2020) Artificial intelligence: who is responsible for the diagnosis? Radiol Med 125(6):517–521

Omar M, Soffer S, Charney AW, Landi I, Nadkarni GN, Klang E (2024) Applications of large language models in psychiatry: a systematic review. Front Psych 15:1422807

Parravano M, Cennamo G, Di Antonio L, Grassi MO, Lupidi M, Rispoli M, Savastano MC, Veritti D, Vujosevic S (2024) Multimodal imaging in diabetic retinopathy and macular edema: an update about biomarkers. Surv Ophthalmol 69:893

Ploug T, Holm S (2023) The right to a second opinion on artificial intelligence diagnosis-remedying the inadequacy of a risk-based regulation. Bioethics 37(3):303–311

Pressman SM, Borna S, Gomez-Cabello CA, Haider SA, Haider CR, Forte AJ (2024) Clinical and surgical applications of large language models: a systematic review. J Clin Med 13(11):3041

Quer G, Topol EJ (2024) The potential for large language models to transform cardiovascular medicine. Lancet Digit Health

Rao SJ, Isath A, Krishnan P, Tangsrivimol JA, Virk HUH, Wang Z, Glicksberg BS, Krittanawong C (2024) ChatGPT: a conceptual review of applications and utility in the field of medicine. J Med Syst 48(1):59

Rey R, Gualtieri R, La Scala G, Posfay Barbe K (2024) Artificial intelligence in the diagnosis and management of appendicitis in pediatric departments: a systematic review. Eur J Pediatr Surg 34(5):385–391

Riaz IB, Harmon S, Chen Z, Naqvi SAA, Cheng L (2024) Applications of artificial intelligence in prostate cancer care: a path to enhanced efficiency and outcomes. Am Soc Clin Oncol Educ Book 44(3):e438516

Roest C, Yakar D, Rener Sitar DI, Bosma JS, Rouw DB, Fransen SJ, Huisman H, Kwee TC (2024) Multimodal AI combining clinical and imaging inputs improves prostate cancer detection. Investig Radiol 59:854

Skaramagkas V, Pentari A, Kefalopoulou Z, Tsiknakis M (2023) Multi-modal deep learning diagnosis of Parkinson's disease-A systematic review. IEEE Trans Neural Syst Rehabil Eng 31:2399–2423

Stubberud A, Langseth H, Nachev P, Matharu MS, Tronvik E (2024) Artificial intelligence and headache. Cephalalgia 44(8):3331024241268290

Thakur GK, Thakur A, Kulkarni S, Khan N, Khan S (2024) Deep learning approaches for medical image analysis and diagnosis. Cureus 16(5):e59507

Xu X, Li J, Zhu Z, Zhao L, Wang H, Song C, Chen Y, Zhao Q, Yang J, Pei Y (2024) A comprehensive review on synergy of multi-modal data and AI technologies in medical diagnosis. Bioengineering (Basel) 11(3)

Yang R, Tan TF, Lu W, Thirunavukarasu AJ, Ting DSW, Liu N (2023) Large language models in health care: development, applications, and challenges. Health Care Sci 2(4):255–263

Yang Z, Wang D, Zhou F, Song D, Zhang Y, Jiang J, Kong K, Liu X, Qiao Y, Chang RT, Han Y, Li F, Tham CC, Zhang X (2024) Understanding natural language: potential application of large language models to ophthalmology. Asia Pac J Ophthalmol (Phila) 13:100085

Younis HA, Eisa TAE, Nasser M, Sahib TM, Noor AA, Alyasiri OM, Salisu S, Hayder IM (2024) A systematic review and meta-analysis of artificial intelligence tools in medicine and healthcare: applications, considerations, limitations, motivation and challenges. Diagnostics (Basel) 14(1)

Zhou Q, Zuley M, Guo Y, Yang L, Nair B, Vargo A, Ghannam S, Arefan D, Wu S (2021) A machine and human reader study on AI diagnosis model safety under attacks of adversarial images. Nat Commun 12(1):7281

Zhu Y, Salowe R, Chow C, Li S, Bastani O, O'Brien JM (2024) Advancing glaucoma care: integrating artificial intelligence in diagnosis, management, and progression detection. Bioengineering (Basel) 11(2)

Ethical Considerations in AI-Enabled Healthcare

5

Ezgi Aldemir, Carla Bloom, Susan Honeyman, and Robert Vardanyan

Abstract

The integration of artificial intelligence (AI) into healthcare systems presents significant opportunities to transform patient care, optimise resources, and advance education. However, the ethical implications of AI deployment demand equal scrutiny. This chapter provides a comprehensive examination of the ethical dimensions of AI-enabled healthcare, using both principled biomedical ethics and normative moral theories. The four foundational pillars (beneficence, non-maleficence, autonomy, and justice) are critically applied to areas such as data governance, algorithmic bias, patient consent, transparency, and accountability. Normative frameworks, including deontology, utilitarianism, and virtue ethics, further contextualise AI's moral challenges in clinical settings. Real-world applications are explored across diverse environments, including telemedicine, medical education, low-resource contexts, and space medicine, highlighting the nuanced ethical requirements of adaptability, inclusivity, and cultural sensitivity. The chapter also evaluates current regulatory frameworks and policy landscapes across global jurisdictions, identifying key gaps and offering recommendations for future-proof, ethically sound AI governance. Emphasising interdependency between ethical principles, the chapter argues for dynamic, collaborative, and patient-centred approaches to AI development. Ethical challenges are reframed not as barriers but as imperatives for innovation aligned with human dignity, societal equity, and professional integrity in an increasingly digital healthcare landscape.

Keywords

Artificial Intelligence · Ethics · Medical · Bioethical Issues · Autonomy · Beneficence · Nonmaleficence · Confidentiality · Informed Consent · Health Equity · Health Information Privacy · Decision Support Systems, Clinical · Health Services Accessibility · Healthcare Disparities · Regulatory Agencies · AI Regulation

E. Aldemir · C. Bloom
Department of Trauma and Orthopaedics, Jersey General Hospital, St Helier, Jersey

S. Honeyman · R. Vardanyan (✉)
Department of Neurosurgery, John Radcliffe Hospital, Oxford University Hospitals NHS Foundation Trust, Oxford, UK
e-mail: robert.vardanyan1@nhs.net

J. Malawana et al. (eds.), *Artificial Intelligence in Healthcare and Biomedical Visualization*, Biomedical Visualization 10, https://doi.org/10.1007/978-3-032-06520-9_5

Abbreviations

AI	Artificial Intelligence
CQC	Care Quality Commission
DRCF	Digital Regulation Cooperation Forum
FDA	Food and Drug Administration
GDPR	General Data Protection Regulation
HRA	Health Research Authority
IEC	International Electrotechnical Commission
IVDR	In Vitro Diagnostic Regulation
IOS	International Organisation for Standardisation
ITU	International Telecommunication Union
MDRF	Medical Device Regulators Forum
MHRA	Medicines and Healthcare products Regulatory Agency
NHS	National Health Service
NICE	National Institute for Health and Care Excellence
OECD	The Organisation for Economic Co-operation and Development
SaMD	Software as a Medical Device
UNESCO	United Nations Educational Scientific and Cultural Organisation
WEF	World Economic Forum
WHO	World Health Organisation
WIPO	World Intellectual Property Organisation

5.1 Introduction: Opportunities and Ethical Cautions

The transformative potential of AI in healthcare has been carefully detailed in previous chapters. From diagnostic support to surgical simulation, AI offers new frontiers for patient care and health education (Alam et al. 2023; Bhagat and Kanyal 2024; Hudda et al. 2024). In an era of growing demand for healthcare services, efficiency, automation, and fair resource allocation are paramount (Guindo et al. 2012). Though AI shows potential to address these needs (Eshwar 2023; Doupe et al. 2019), innovations must be both technologically sound and morally responsible.

This chapter examines the ethical dimensions of AI-enabled healthcare using established frameworks in biomedical ethics. Alongside promises of enhanced healthcare delivery, AI technologies pose challenges with biases, data breaches, opaque algorithms, and inconsistent legislation (World Health Organization 2023; Bekbolatova et al. 2024; Zhang et al. 2024a). By grounding technological endeavours in the ethical principles that underpin the healthcare profession, we ensure that they not only push the boundaries of medical possibility but also prioritise the best interests of patients and society.

Commitments to integrity and patient welfare have long shaped medical practice, from the Hippocratic Oath to today's robust standards and medical jurisprudence. The 'prima facie' principles (beneficence, non-maleficence, autonomy, and justice) (Page 2012) are identifiable in codes and covenants spanning centuries. In addition to these pillars, broader normative ethical theories are useful for evaluating ethical dilemmas in medicine (Jackson 2007).

The advancement of AI-enabled healthcare is not merely a technological or a medical endeavour, but a deeply ethical one. With the rapid evolution of AI technologies, the ethical issues faced today may entirely differ from those encountered tomorrow. As stewards of medical practice, stakeholders must engage in active ethical reflection and dynamic policymaking to uphold biomedical ethics in the digital age.

5.2 Overview of Ethical Frameworks

5.2.1 The Four Pillars of Ethics in AI-Enabled Healthcare

Brought to fame by Beauchamp and Childress in The Principles of Biomedical Ethics (Beauchamp and Childress 2013), the 'four pillars of ethics' are woven into medical education, clinical decision-making, and healthcare policies globally. The seminal Hippocratic Oath states: 'I will apply measures for the benefit of the sick…; I will keep them from harm and injustice'. (Stigall

2022). Though eclipsed by modern revisions, this covenant introduces the pillars of beneficence, non-maleficence, and justice. As the paternalism of earlier medical practice has waned, autonomy has joined these tenets to form the four pillars. Along with professional standards and policies, these pillars form the main ethical framework for healthcare dilemmas (Varkey 2021). Their implications for confidentiality, equity, and transparency are key in the era of AI.

Beneficence (acting in patients' best interests) and non-maleficence (avoiding harm to patients) have long been the cornerstone of medical ethics (Varkey 2021). AI technologies promise to optimise healthcare delivery and training for the benefit of patients and society (Yeasmin 2019). To be beneficent, AI tools must prioritise patient welfare, the benefits must be equitably distributed, and clinicians must be able to personalise care for individual best interests. AI can facilitate non-maleficence and patient safety through reducing errors and adverse events, predictive analytics, and decision support (Choudhury and Asan 2020). Nevertheless, AI algorithms could harm patients and other stakeholders through their propensity to perpetuate biases, produce erroneous results, or compromise data security (Abràmoff et al. 2023).

Tools facilitating shared decision-making, informed consent, and transparency are welcome additions to the changing healthcare landscape. However, we must address concerns around algorithmic paternalism or the loss of human agency in AI-generated decision-making to preserve patients' rights to informed consent and autonomy.

Justice in medical ethics consists of equity, adherence to law, and respect for the rights of individuals (Olejarczyk and Young 2024). AI can promote justice via improving access to healthcare through telemedicine, remote diagnosis, predictive healthcare, and advice services (Wahl et al. 2018). However, care must be taken to ensure equitable allocation and mitigate biases in algorithms that may disproportionately affect marginalised communities (Ferrara 2023). Furthermore, global collaboration and robust legislation are required to attenuate risks to wider society, such as cyberattacks.

By integrating these ethical pillars, the landscape of AI-enabled healthcare can be shaped to minimise negative impacts on patients and institutions whilst advancing human health.

5.2.2 Normative Ethical Principles in AI-Enabled Healthcare

Normative ethics, or moral philosophy, is concerned with formulating basic moral standards (Jackson 2007). Using normative ethical frameworks can highlight where advancements do, and do not, align with morality and societal values.

Deontology is a duty-based ethical theory that relies on adhering to inherent moral laws, distinct from their consequences (Misselbrook 2013). It is concerned with upholding absolute moral duties that can be applied universally, such as the four pillars of ethics. The four pillars and prioritising inherent morality are certainly important in the context of AI-enabled healthcare; however, its absolutist nature can hinder the ability of deontological ethics to address the complexity of modern healthcare. In novel situations (like AI-enabled healthcare), there is often conflict between duties, requiring a nuanced approach. Even in standard care provision, deontology may insufficiently address unique patient factors or broader contexts, such as cultural norms or institutional policies (Taylor 2013). Healthcare ethics are founded on intrinsic moral duties, but overlooking the consequences of adhering to moral rules may lead to unintended negative outcomes.

By contrast, consequentialist theories are concerned only with the value added by actions (Maggino 2023). One such theory is utilitarianism, which prioritises actions with the greatest total utility (the greatest good for the greatest number of people) and supports many healthcare practices aiming to maximise overall health outcomes in the context of resource limitations (Marseille and Kahn 2019). It is closely linked with concepts of distributive justice and legal justice, but provides a wider scope for analysing issues indirectly related to AI in healthcare. For example, it prompts consideration of the societal consequences of potentially enormous increases in energy usage by AI data centres (Vinuesa et al. 2020). Utilitarianism inherently prioritises population-level outcomes over individual needs, but this principle can be beneficial in optimising resource allocation and targeting public health interventions. However, the quantification of utility in healthcare is generally based on objective measures of quality of life (Bakker and van der Linden 1995), which may not capture the spectrum of benefits and harms of AI tools. Utilitarianism can offer valuable insights into ethical AI, but may require a combination with complementary frameworks (like deontology) to overcome its limitations (Emdad et al. 2023).

The applicability of virtue ethics to AI is less clear than that of deontology or utilitarianism, as virtue ethics emphasises the moral virtues and traits of the humans carrying out an action, rather than rules or consequences (Duffy et al. 2018). Virtue ethics can inform the use of AI in healthcare by highlighting the need for empathy, integrity, compassion, and honesty among stakeholders. The integration of virtue ethics into the design process could promote ethically sensitive and socially responsible AI (Giarmoleo et al. 2024). Furthermore, there is emerging discussion around virtue in 'human-AI intelligent caring', referring to the idea of compassion as a system of human and AI capabilities (Morrow et al. 2023). The role of moral responsibility cannot be overstated in ensuring AI-enabled healthcare tools are patient-centred and trustworthy.

5.2.3 Overlap and Conflict

Utilitarianism, deontology, and virtue ethics offer valuable frameworks with which to analyse the complexities of AI-enabled healthcare. These theories are interconnected and frequently conflict. For example, utilitarianism may align with justice by allocating resources where they can have the greatest impact on population health, or perpetuate existing disparities if algorithms prioritise serving the needs of majority groups over smaller marginalised populations (Hynninen et al. 2021; Silva et al. 2013). Therefore, a nuanced approach is necessary to ensure that technologies uphold ethical values while advancing the quality, accessibility, and equity of care.

5.3 Foundations of Ethical Considerations

5.3.1 Data Privacy

The functionality of AI-enabled healthcare applications relies on data-driven algorithms and machine learning models (Rajkomar et al. 2018; Sarker 2021a). AI systems, particularly deep learning models, extract intricate patterns from extensive datasets to 'learn' (Sarker 2021a, b). Healthcare is deeply complex, with infinitely variable presentations, genetics, environmental factors, and psychosocial contexts. The consequences of poorly performing AI in healthcare may be life-altering, so its reliability and accuracy are paramount (Festor et al. 2022). Ensuring accuracy and generalisability thus demands vast quantities of data—unparalleled in both volume and sensitivity (Rajkomar et al. 2019).

The digitalisation of health records has yielded extensive data, including entire medical histories, investigation results, and genomic profiling (Tresp et al. 2016). Data scope and granularity can be amplified by wearable devices providing real-time physiological data (Dinh-Le et al. 2019). With AI's power to discern new patterns, this data holds untold potential for advancements in healthcare delivery, population health, and research. If used appropriately, data collection on social determinants of health can aid us in mitigating inequities (Bompelli et al. 2021). Finally, global data sharing may aid in addressing global health risks, such as pandemics and climate events (Chattu et al. 2019; Adegoke et al. 2024).

Unfortunately, the same enormity and sensitivity of data that offers such a possibility also exposes AI-enabled healthcare to serious data security risks, such as misuse, breaches, and unauthorised access (Yadav et al. 2023). With reliance on AI, cyber-attacks targeting health organisations (or other causes of technological failure) may be catastrophic. Though data anonymisation may mitigate some risk to patient privacy, the aggregation of such vast datasets facilitates re-identification attacks, wherein data can be correlated with external information to reveal individuals' identities (Rahimzadeh 2021; El Emam et al. 2011). Finally, political issues (such as data sovereignty and international tensions) may complicate efforts to establish harmonised data protection standards and facilitate secure cross-border data sharing (Hadiyantina et al. 2022).

Given the nature of information gathered in confidential healthcare settings, the implications of these risks extend far beyond the immediate threat of data compromise. Breaches can disrupt healthcare operations, undermine public trust, and expose patients to exploitation and fraud (Johnson 2009). Loss of public trust could result in reluctance to seek medical care or share information, compromising patient outcomes and public health initiatives (Alanazi 2023; Kwon and Johnson 2015). Repercussions from breaches can financially burden healthcare organisations, impacting patients more broadly (Seh et al. 2020).

Robust data security safeguards are imperative if AI-enabled healthcare is to be integrated responsibly. By adhering to regulatory frameworks and best practices for ethical data stewardship, stakeholders can maintain the rights and trust of patients and wider communities.

5.3.2 Bias and Fairness

Bias in AI algorithms often originates from skewed training sets or flawed algorithmic design (Fazil et al. 2024). Though some forms of bias are useful (positive bias for differential optimal care) (Zechmeister-Koss et al. 2019), biases in AI models reinforcing suboptimal care for marginalised groups must be addressed. Creating demographic-unaware algorithms may achieve a utilitarian standard of meeting needs for the majority. However, achieving distributive justice and avoiding discrimination requires acknowledgement of differential presentations and responses across diverse groups (Andrus and Villeneuve 2022; Celi et al. 2022).

Training datasets are mainly derived from real-world data, so they reflect current and historic inequities (Celi et al. 2022; d'Elia et al. 2022). Barriers to healthcare access may result in underrepresentation or misrepresentation of marginalised groups in datasets, compounded by biased data collection (Celi et al. 2022; Cinnamon 2020). Biases are exacerbated by the inequitable global distribution of telemedicine, digital health records, and AI (Celi et al. 2022). Historic biases in research and public health also contribute to disparities (for instance, underrepresentation of women and people of colour in clinical trials) (Baylis 1996).

Design choices in AI applications can also introduce or exacerbate biases. Algorithms select variables from inputted data believed to be relevant for decision-making and predictions, so they can inadvertently perpetuate disparities if feature selection disproportionately weights biased variables (Abràmoff et al. 2023). For example, marginalised communities are disproportionately affected by socioeconomic disparities, so if these variables are more heavily weighted in predictive modelling, it may reinforce inequities (Oyeniran et al. 2022). Models also require reprocessing of raw data: if outliers or missing values are not handled carefully, or if data are normalised on arbitrary criteria, outputs will be skewed (Isgut et al. 2023). Training AI models also requires the adjustment of model parameters to maximise performance and minimise errors (Challen et al. 2019). Biased data or optimisation objectives may result in imbalanced outputs. For example, overrepresentation of one group in the data can result in the model learning to prioritise the outcomes of that group (Dhabliya et al. 2024). If biased outcomes are then reinforced via feedback loops and reinforcement algorithms, existing biases may be amplified and further entrenched in subsequent iterations (Dhabliya et al. 2024; Devillers et al. 2021). As the complexity of AI increases, its opacity and lack of interpretability may hinder efforts to detect and address inherent biases (Mensah 2023).

Clearly, biased outputs could impact the fairness of recommendations, predictions, and resource allocation. The intersectionality of biases further complicates this issue, as patients may experience multiple overlapping forms of discrimination that together result in disproportionate vulnerability, greater than their sum (Crenshaw 1989). In addition to these harms, biases can erode trust and confidence in AI tools, with potential implications for treatment adherence, healthcare outcomes, and public health (Olaoye and Frank 2024). Whilst humans have the agency to recognise and overcome these biases through reflection and training, AI algorithms are reliant on data, so careful design and regulation are imperative. Equitable design, deployment, and monitoring rely on interdisciplinary collaboration and proactive efforts to identify and mitigate biases (Chinta et al. 2024). Ultimately, addressing real-world inequities is vital to address current and future injustices.

5.3.3 Autonomy and Informed Consent

Truly informed consent and autonomy require transparency and understanding. Consent must extend beyond mere acknowledgement of AI tools, encompassing meaningful engagement about benefits and risks, including data privacy and bias. This is challenged by the complexity and algorithmic opacity of AI technologies. The 'black box' refers to the opacity of algorithms, largely due to their inherent mathematical and computational complexity (Burrell 2016). Coupled with technical terms and abstract machine learning concepts, this hinders their explainability, with implications for both patient autonomy and medicolegal accountability. If clinicians are unable to effectively explain AI tools, patients may be asked to consent to their use with only a superficial understanding of their function, risking scepticism and patient disempowerment (Durán and Jongsma 2021).

Given the pace of advancements, clinicians may also struggle to maintain up-to-date knowledge about AI tools and their changing performance characteristics (Schubert et al. 2025). AI algorithms continuously evolve, so informed consent requires continued education and communication.

By embracing principles of education, transparency, and open dialogue, the ethical imperative to involve patients as active partners in their care can be upheld (Amann et al. 2020).

5.3.4 Accountability and Transparency

As AI algorithms are integrated into workflows and clinical decision support, traditional accountability practices are challenged, as harm could occur due to several stakeholders and technological processes (Habli et al. 2020). The lack of transparency inherent to many AI systems also complicates finding the root cause of errors. Robust regulation and transparency measures to hold stakeholders accountable for errors and harm are imperative, as errors in an AI system may harm a much larger group than that of individual clinicians (Price 2019).

Determining the precise role of each stakeholder in AI-enabled healthcare errors is complicated. Multiple parties are involved in the production of accurate and reliable AI outputs. Though developers bear responsibility for algorithmic design and monitoring, clinicians provide critical input to train and develop AI models (Smith 2021). Healthcare institutions can also impact the comprehensiveness and accuracy of inputs via staffing levels and educational culture (Liu et al. 2021).

Once AI recommendations have been generated, clinicians are asked to bear the responsibility for integrating these insights, despite a lack of visibility and control over the algorithms used (Habli et al. 2020). This places clinicians in ethically murky waters, and such decisions may be affected by their risk aversion, technological literacy, institutional pressures, and psychological factors (such as confirmation bias, cognitive dissonance, overreliance, and decision-making adaptation) (Secinaro et al. 2021; Giordano et al.

2021). Though some argue that the 'black box problem' is less concerning than the proven accuracy of AI systems (Durán and Jongsma 2021), clinicians may feel apprehensive about hinging their trust on tools they do not understand (Shinners et al. 2020). Clinicians are challenged to accept their partial interpretation of AI technologies, recognising their capability to identify patterns not apparent to humans and trusting the accuracy of their outputs. Or, they can proceed with their usual decision-making strategies and attempt to integrate AI insights, arguably reducing the value added by such systems (Habli et al. 2020).

Accountability in AI-enabled healthcare is not a binary concept. Clinicians are responsible for the careful evaluation of AI recommendations in the context of their knowledge, experience, and understanding of algorithmic limitations (Giordano et al. 2021). Developers and regulatory bodies are responsible for developing and deploying ethically sound and reliable systems, working toward explainability, and ensuring appropriate oversight and auditing (Kiseleva et al. 2022). Attributing accountability extends beyond medicolegal liability, encompassing professional responsibilities and ethical standards. Ongoing ethical reflection, access to support and advice for clinicians, and guidance from regulatory bodies are vital (Mennella et al. 2024).

5.3.5 Ethical Interdependencies

In this section, data privacy, bias, autonomy, accountability, and transparency have been explored separately. However, these concepts are deeply interconnected, with interventions in one often influencing outcomes in others. These interdependencies can be leveraged to develop effective strategies for ethical AI-enabled healthcare (Sect. 5.5).

Enhancing data privacy safeguards patients' sensitive data and fosters trust and confidence in AI-enabled systems, empowering patients to share information confidently and engage actively in their care. This autonomy and trust can be enhanced by addressing biases and inequities, as accuracy and justice are upheld. Establishing accountability mechanisms promotes data privacy, equity, and fairness by ensuring AI systems are held to quality standards, and transparent reporting enables stakeholders to address errors and promote autonomy (Harishbhai Tilala et al. 2024). These examples demonstrate the necessity for a holistic approach to ethical AI, encompassing policies, practices, and technologies that prioritise integrity and patient welfare.

5.4 Exploring Specific AI Applications

5.4.1 Telemedicine and Patient Monitoring

AI-enabled telemedicine has grown rapidly since the COVID-19 pandemic (Page 2012; Mann et al. 2020), and a growing body of literature represents interest in AI's ability to meet changing healthcare needs (Zhang et al. 2024b). AI-enabled telemedicine has shown promise from cognitive behavioural therapy to dermatological examination and the management of inflammatory bowel disease (Pang et al. 2022; Fitzpatrick et al. 2017; Finnane et al. 2017). AI-powered assistants can use natural language processing capabilities for remote triage and assessment, and platforms can integrate deep learning algorithms and computer vision to remotely assess images (Bajwa et al. 2021). Patient monitoring can also be transformed as AI is integrated with real-time physiological data from wearable devices (Iqbal et al. 2023). Finally, predictive analytics and machine learning models offer opportunities for preventative medicine, identifying at-risk patients to facilitate timely targeted interventions (Xiao et al. 2018).

While telemedicine advancements are promising, they also pose challenges pertaining to data privacy and equity. Such tools also alter the therapeutic relationship, diminishing opportunities for face-to-face care, non-verbal communication, and human empathy (Sauerbrei et al. 2023).

5.4.1.1 Privacy and Data Management

Data security issues are particularly relevant to telemedicine. Remote communications (like video conferences or message platforms) are uniquely vulnerable if robust mechanisms are not in place to safeguard against interception, unauthorised access, data breaches, and data loss (Okereafor et al. 2020). The ethical implications of inadequate data privacy in telemedicine span the violation of autonomy, stigma, cybercrime, disrupted healthcare services, and erosion of trust (Akbar et al. 2024).

The complexity of anonymisation in AI data handling is mirrored here: differential privacy and anonymisation techniques (such as de-identification and pseudonymisation) compromise data utility and analysis (Williamson and Prybutok 2024). Protecting the confidentiality of telemedicine and remote monitoring involves encryption, secure authentication, and data protection compliance (Yadav et al. 2023). Encryption protocols may challenge interoperability between healthcare platforms, and the latency and computational overhead introduced may impact real-time monitoring and ease of use (Naveed et al. 2020; Odeh and Abu 2023). Telemedicine and remote monitoring tools should enhance the efficiency of healthcare delivery, so innovation in this field and efforts to integrate healthcare systems are paramount.

Commitment to patient-centred care and the foundational ethical principles requires cybersecurity measures, ethical data governance practices, and regulatory oversight.

5.4.1.2 The Digital Divide and Access Disparities

The 'digital divide' is a concept generally defined as the metaphorical division between those who do and do not have access to digital media, surmising a spectrum of digital inequity depending on their technological access, skills, and use (Hilbert 2011). It poses significant challenges to forming equitable AI systems and the fair distribution of services such as telemedicine. Causes of digital inequity include socioeconomic status, location and digital infrastructure, language and cultural barriers, technology literacy, and health literacy (van Dijk 2020). These factors are closely intertwined, and their intersectionality can result in disproportionate access limitations (Crenshaw 1989; Baah et al. 2019).

Those from lower socioeconomic backgrounds may experience significant barriers to accessing telemedicine, such as limited access to suitable devices and a reliable internet connection (due to cost or infrastructure). In paid healthcare systems, those with financial constraints or lacking health insurance coverage may prioritise basic needs over health costs (Haimi 2023).

Though remote care can aid accessibility, limited infrastructure in remote or rural communities may restrict access to reliable high-speed internet or network connectivity. Local healthcare facilities may also lack the resources to support electronic records or AI-enabled telemedicine, further limiting the reach of initiatives in traditionally underserved communities (Haimi 2023; Badr et al. 2024).

Older adults and those with limited formal education are disproportionately likely to have limited digital literacy, impeding access to telemedicine (Hilbert 2011; Haimi 2023). Disparities may be exacerbated by cultural beliefs, opinions, misconceptions, or poor health literacy (Badr et al. 2024). Poor health literacy means a reduced ability to understand and use health information to make informed decisions and engage with services, particularly in the context of increasingly complex healthcare technologies (Sørensen et al. 2012).

Marginalised or underserved communities are also more likely to be distrustful of healthcare providers and technology companies due to prior discrimination or cultural insensitivity, exacerbating inequities (Wesson et al. 2019). Moreover, access can be impeded by language and cultural barriers, particularly for linguistic minorities. It is essential that telemedicine platforms are culturally sensitive and available in multiple languages. Finally, inconsistent or restrictive regulations governing telemedicine use and licensure may restrict innovation and access (Haimi 2023; Raghu and Mehrotra 2023).

Evidently, the digital divide undermines justice and beneficence through inequitable distribution. Limited use of AI tools in populations already underserved in healthcare may exacerbate inequities, contributing to a poorer standard of care (Badr et al. 2024). Addressing this divide requires an integrated approach to tackle systemic inequalities. Leveraging the resources and expertise required to bridge the digital divide will likely require cross-sector collaboration representing healthcare, technology, government, philanthropy, and research.

5.4.2 Space Medicine and Low-Resource Settings

5.4.2.1 Unique Challenges

Deploying AI-enabled healthcare in challenging environments presents unique concerns, including the limitations of infrastructure, resources, and local medical knowledge. Developing ethical healthcare solutions requires careful consideration of technology appropriateness and prioritisation of scarce resources, such as infrastructure, equipment, funds, transport, medical personnel, infection control measures, and medications (Mahmoud et al. 2022). Leveraging AI tools could improve access, efficiency, and quality of care for patients in low-resource settings, including space (Dangi et al. 2024).

Though human specialist oversight is optimal, AI tools can certainly improve access to specialised care. AI algorithms can provide accurate clinical support to help standardise care and reduce errors, with roles ranging from radiological diagnosis of tuberculosis to improving adherence to evidence-based protocols for neonatal care (Shanmuga Priya et al. 2024; Amoakoh et al. 2020). AI could also be used to augment healthcare services despite resource constraints by automating routine tasks, providing educational resources, and streamlining healthcare workflows, so that trained staff can prioritise higher-order tasks (Siddiqui et al. 2023). If accessible, such tools could overcome geographic barriers to support timely care and epidemiological surveillance (Kerketta and Balasundaram 2024; Aljerian et al. 2022). AI predictive analytics and models could aid public health by forecasting disease outbreaks, identifying high-risk populations, and optimising resource allocation for disease prevention and control (Alowais et al. 2023).

Space medicine focuses on the health of astronauts and cosmonauts during spaceflight and the impact of space travel on human health (Hodkinson et al. 2017). Space is an extreme environment characterised by microgravity, radiation exposure, confinement, isolation, extreme temperatures, and resource limitation (White and Averner 2001). Advanced AI algorithms could aid in monitoring and optimal care for the challenges space presents to human physiology. For example, prolonged exposure to microgravity can induce muscle atrophy, bone density loss, and cardiovascular deconditioning (Hodkinson et al. 2017). AI technology could monitor changes in bone density and muscle mass, enabling timely intervention and personalised exercise regimes, and AI predictive modelling could guide countermeasures (Dimai 2023). AI radiation monitoring could continuously assess ionising radiation exposure and forecast health risks (Kuvvetli 2024). The psychological stressors of space travel may require mental health monitoring and support, which could be aided by AI-driven virtual chatbots, using natural language processing algorithms to engage in empathetic conversations or deliver confidential cognitive behavioural therapy (Greatbatch 2024). Furthermore, AI-driven sentiment analysis tools could be used to monitor communications for distress, facilitating early intervention and personalised support (Thakkar et al. 2024).

It appears that AI has the potential to address some of the challenges faced in low-resource settings and space. However, ensuring that technologies benefit the populations they serve requires careful consideration of local context, capacity, and ethical principles.

5.4.2.2 Adaptability and Appropriateness

The efficacy and feasibility of AI applications rely on their adaptability and appropriateness for the specific needs of their environment.

Low-resource settings may have significant infrastructure constraints, such as a lack of reliable electricity, basic healthcare infrastructure, or internet. Resource limitations are often accompanied by budget constraints and competing priorities, which can further challenge the feasibility, scalability, and sustainability of AI solutions (Pillai 2023; Abbas et al. 2017). Therefore, the cost-effectiveness of AI tools must be prioritised, considering the resources needed for deployment and long-term maintenance. Tools offering high impact with minimal resource requirements may be initially prioritised, but responsible innovation requires 'capacity-building' (Alami et al. 2020). This involves developing local infrastructure, resources, knowledge, and skills to ensure long-term sustainability (Alami et al. 2020; Khan et al. 2024; Ciecierski-Holmes et al. 2022).

Alongside limitations in health infrastructure and medical equipment, healthcare providers may have less access to specialised training and education. Co-developing AI solutions with local healthcare professionals can help to ensure that technologies are aligned with the needs of the workforce and complement existing workflows (Ciecierski-Holmes et al. 2022). Capacity-building training programs, educational resources, and knowledge-sharing platforms can then empower local healthcare professionals to use AI tools and adapt them to their evolving healthcare needs (Alami et al. 2020; Curioso 2019).

Space settings have limited access to healthcare supplies and personnel compared to terrestrial settings. Space missions operate within strict constraints of weight and power, exacerbated by long-duration spaceflight and planetary exploration (Simon et al. 2015). The finite resources and distance from Earth's infrastructure demand meticulous prioritisation and resource allocation (Asrar et al. 2022). AI tools must minimise power use, data storage requirements, and hardware footprint while maximising computational efficiency and diagnostic accuracy (Oche et al. 2024). Adaptations could include lightweight, energy-efficient algorithms and cloud computing for data processing and analysis (Waisberg et al. 2022). Extreme space environments may need radiation-hardened components, fail-safe mechanisms, robust hardware, and integration with onboard medical systems (Oche et al. 2024; Waisberg et al. 2022).

It is evident that space medicine and low-resource settings demand careful needs assessments to understand their unique challenges. Failure to adapt AI tools could exacerbate the risks inherent to such settings by wasting limited resources or compromising established practices. This violates beneficence, non-maleficence, and justice. To maintain reliability, safety, and public trust, AI-enabled healthcare interventions must be adapted to local needs (Okolo 2022; Okolo 2023). Finally, sociocultural ignorance may result in interventions that undermine patient dignity and autonomy, such as imposing Western models of care misaligned with local customs (Alami et al. 2020).

Sustainable AI-enabled healthcare requires the empowerment of communities, healthcare providers, and policymakers. It is vital that any initiatives are co-developed with relevant stakeholders. Responsible AI also requires mitigation of inequitable access and outcomes, particularly for vulnerable and marginalised populations (such as those in poverty or facing stigma for conditions such as HIV). Equity-focused AI in these settings involves prioritising accessibility, affordability, and cultural sensitivity when choosing AI tools and allocating resources (Berdahl et al. 2023). Developing practically appropriate, culturally sensitive, and impactful interventions requires adaptation to the specific circumstances of the communities involved.

5.4.2.3 Prioritising Interventions

Appropriate prioritisation enables a focus on interventions that maximise the impact of scarce resources in line with strategic priorities, health system capacities, and community needs. This is vital to ensure services can respond to emergencies (like infectious disease outbreaks and natural disasters) and address priority healthcare needs. Prioritisation can also support capacity-building investments and collaborations to leverage collective expertise and resources (Kaur et al. 2019).

Practical steps to ensure just prioritisation in low-resource settings include comprehensive needs assessments, strategic resource allocation, adaptation to technological constraints, capacity-building, risk assessment, and iterative adaptations (Berdahl et al. 2023; Kaur et al. 2019). Strategic resource allocation requires knowledge of the proposed interventions' cost-effectiveness, scalability, and feasibility, considered within the context of local technical infrastructure, workforce capacity, and regulations (Klaic et al. 2022). Ongoing evaluation of tools' usability, performance, and impact is required for refinement (Reddy et al. 2021).

Decisions must be guided by principles of distributive justice, ensuring that limited resources are distributed fairly and equitably to maximise health benefits for the population.

5.4.3 Surgical and Medical Training and Education

The role of AI in surgical and medical education and training is expanding, with capabilities including personalised learning, simulations and virtual reality, remote training, and even predictive modelling (Satapathy et al. 2023). Particularly in the context of competence-based surgical training, AI tools have shown initial promise in applications including laparoscopy, robotic surgery, and feedback (Bilgic et al. 2022). Furthermore, AI can optimise safe skills development and asynchronous learning (Kose and Koc 2015; Zarei et al. 2024). Against a background of increasing pressures on healthcare teaching services and increasing medical complexity, the development of evidence-based applications to enhance clinical readiness should be met with enthusiasm. However, the ethical issues raised by such innovation must be closely examined, as there are risks of unintended consequences on patient safety, learner competence, autonomy, and justice.

5.4.3.1 Assessment, Feedback, and Evaluation

AI technologies can support time-efficient training, reducing the burden on educators and healthcare services through automating objective performance assessments and personalised feedback, providing real-time insights on learners' clinical reasoning and procedural skills (Zarei et al. 2024). Real-time, objective feedback allows for errors to be identified early and can enhance skill acquisition (Nagaraj et al. 2023; Fazlollahi et al. 2022). Such feedback can be used to facilitate timely remediation that continuously adapts to evolving proficiency, curricular requirements, and evidence-based standards (Zhang et al. 2024a). Assessments and evaluations can be adapted to learners depending on their performance, identifying unique challenges and optimising learning outcomes (Chan and Zary 2019). The data collected from these personalised assessments could also be used for curriculum improvement and guiding teaching priorities. In addition to providing benefits for medical students and trainees, the life-long learning intrinsic to healthcare means that even the most senior clinicians may benefit from these adaptive learning technologies, pursuing mastery and up-to-date knowledge (Oh et al. 2023).

There are potential limitations to AI-generated feedback, such as the lack of emotional responsiveness and the possibility for intentional deception of algorithms (Zhang et al. 2024a). Furthermore, implementing AI into the curricula requires significant resources and investment, and educators may require training to effectively use AI tools in their teaching (Moldt et al. 2023; Kimmerle et al. 2023).

5.4.3.2 Learning Material Quality and Ethical Design

With ongoing concerns of inadequacy in medical education and training, AI tools may be able to offer learners improvements in efficiency, knowledge, and skills, and accessibility (Xu et al. 2024). Tools can promote the dissemination of up-to-date clinical knowledge, procedural protocols, and patient safety guidelines through simulations and knowledge-based platforms (Mir et al. 2023). AI technologies can facilitate learning for cases ranging from typical to vanishingly rare, providing valuable opportunities for learners to explore a greater breadth of clinical scenarios (Abdullahi et al. 2024). In addition to clinical knowledge, emerging AI-based communication training could also support learners in developing essential interpersonal and communication skills (Sallam et al. 2023; Stamer et al. 2023). If implemented successfully, AI-driven education tools could thus uphold the pillars of non-maleficence (through reductions in errors), beneficence (through evidence-based practice), and justice (through consistent care and redistribution of clinicians' time).

Conversely, inappropriate use or inadequate tools may result in inadequate preparation for the complexity of real clinical scenarios, over-reliance on AI technology, or a de-emphasis on humanistic care. To avoid errors, AI algorithms must be rigorously validated and regularly recalibrated to reflect evolving guidance. Furthermore, the appropriateness of AI technologies must be considered.

Simulations and virtual reality experiences aim to replicate real scenarios, facilitating readiness for practice via the development of procedural skills, teamwork, and clinical decision-making (Dhar et al. 2023). AI can be used to generate diverse simulations and improve the availability of simulations for self-directed learning (Hamilton 2024). To support inclusive care, simulations should reflect the diversity of patients, clinical conditions, and healthcare settings, and efforts must be made to address disparate learner access. Materials need to be accurate, relevant, and balance the need for immersive training with ethical design.

The use of generative AI for simulations can mitigate some of the ethical concerns associated with using real patient data in simulation (such as videos of surgery). Obtaining informed consent may be challenged by time constraints (such as in advance of emergency surgical intervention), retrospective data collection, and limited understanding of simulation. Furthermore, distribution of sensitive educational materials can introduce risks of unintentional exposure or misuse, misrepresentation, or sensationalisation, and unauthorised access. If AI-generated images, videos, or transcripts can be used to generate similar learning experiences without leveraging patient data, these risks may be avoided.

Ensuring the fidelity of AI-enabled simulations is appropriate to the stage of training is an important component of ethical design. High-fidelity simulations are hyper-realistic replications of complex scenarios (Carey and Rossler 2024). Alongside additional resource requirements, high-fidelity simulations pose several ethical concerns—particularly traumatic or sensitive scenarios. Prolonged exposure to simulated graphic or sensationalised content (without the gravitas of emotion underlying real patient care) may gradually desensitise learners to the emotional and ethical dimensions of healthcare (Bazmi et al. 2023). Less-experienced learners are generally aided by the reduced cognitive load of low-fidelity simulations (Carey and Rossler 2024; Norman et al. 2012). However, if high-fidelity simulations are suitable, trauma-informed design is recommended, including warnings, debriefs, well-being support, peer mentoring, ethical education, and reflection (Merkley et al. 2023). This is particularly relevant to AI-enabled simulations that are available for self-directed learning, as the usual support of an expert supervisor and peers is less accessible. Regardless of nature or fidelity, simulation design must be ethically sound, pedagogically relevant, and aligned with professional standards to provide meaningful learning without compromising safety or dignity.

Developing, deploying, and monitoring AI-enabled medical education tools ethically requires proactive identification of features undermining the deontological 'four pillars', such as biases, cultural insensitivity, and outdated or false information. It is imperative that safeguards are in place to balance learning needs with a culture of psychological safety, autonomy, resilience, and collaboration.

5.4.3.3 Appropriate Use and Critical Engagement

Without education on the limitations of AI tools, learners may struggle to discern truth from confidently-stated facts ('hallucinations') (Kitto et al. 2024) or feel over-certain in their accuracy (automation bias), risking clinical errors (Nguyen 2024). Learning tools must adhere to best practice guidelines, professional standards, and regulatory requirements to ensure clinical relevance and patient safety, with strict senior oversight and quality assurance mechanisms in place. Opportunities for learners, educators, and clinicians to provide iterative feedback on AI tools should be organised so that concerns can be proactively identified and resolved. Transparent reporting and education on AI algorithmic function, data sources, and development should be incorporated into medical curricula (Nguyen 2024; Paranjape et al. 2019; Grunhut et al. 2021).

Particularly for learners in the early stages of their career, a lack of critical engagement with AI may result in an over-confident approach to clinical practice and uncertainty, neglecting clinical reasoning, intellectual curiosity, and reflective practice (Kitto et al. 2024; Armitage 2023). Cautious innovation with consideration for real-world clinical scenarios and AI-critical literacy in learners can aid the integration of AI applications in medical education (Kitto et al. 2024). This requires an evidence-based, multidisciplinary approach to curriculum design, learner assessment, and continuous quality improvement. These tools must be used to complement traditional learning, as learners should be exposed to a variety of clinical settings to develop the situational awareness and clinical reasoning required for independent practice.

AI also has implications for medical and surgical career development. There is an ongoing dispute about the use of AI in assessments and research (Kung et al. 2023; Tan et al. 2024; GenAI et al. 2024). Healthcare professionals and learners are urged to act with integrity and transparency, adhering to guidance released by their institutions.

5.4.3.4 Collaboration and Responsibility

Collaborative efforts and transparency are required to navigate the ethics of AI-enabled health education. Subpar simulations may affect trainee competence or reinforce poor practice, risking harm and medico-legal action. Conversely, well-designed, evidence-based AI tools can enhance competence, confidence, and preparedness (Elendu et al. 2024). There are challenges allocating responsibility and accountability in AI-enabled healthcare, including medical education (World Health Organization 2021), but healthcare providers, educators, learners, and AI developers each hold moral responsibility for preventing patient safety, errors, and misconduct. Educational institutions are largely responsible for selecting appropriate AI educational tools, and educators play a critical role in designing and hosting relevant, accurate simulations. They are uniquely placed to identify and raise concerns. Developers must adhere to guidelines and industry standards, conducting validation studies, user testing, and iterative refinement. Working within the remits of standards set by regulatory and accreditation bodies is imperative. Ethical AI-enabled education is a shared responsibility, and stakeholders must uphold professionalism, integrity, and accountability.

5.4.4 Integration Across Applications

AI technologies certainly offer opportunities in addressing specific challenges across multiple settings, and enhancing societal well-being and equitable health outcomes. However, careless or hasty integration may pose risks to patients and society, such as data breaches, perpetuating inequities, and patient disenfranchisement. Integrating ethical reflection into every stage of the AI lifecycle is paramount for advancements to serve the collective good (Li et al. 2022).

Ethical AI extends beyond addressing immediate challenges in isolation: it requires broader consideration of societal and systemic implications. By fostering collaboration, ethical advocacy, and transparency, stakeholders can strive toward the betterment of patient care and medical knowledge. Evident in the challenges and promises across contexts ranging from medical schools to Mars, ethical AI is not just a moral imperative, but a practical necessity for ensuring the sustainable, responsible integration of AI into healthcare systems globally.

5.5 Navigating Ethical Challenges

5.5.1 Regulatory and Policy Frameworks

Though several international and multilateral organisations provide guidance and recommendations to support the regulation of AI-enabled healthcare, national or regional jurisdictions are responsible for their own legislative and regulatory frameworks (Palaniappan et al. 2024).

Internationally, the World Health Organisation provides global leadership on public health issues and has published guidance on the ethical use of AI technologies for governments, AI developers, companies, regulatory bodies, and international organisations (World Health Organization 2021). The Organisation for Economic Co-operation and Development (OECD) promotes policies for the global economic and social good, including the use of AI (Organisation for Economic Co-operation and Development (OECD) 2019). The OECD AI Principles provide a framework for developing robust, safe, fair, trustworthy AI (OECD 2023). With 47 current adherents, the OECD AI Principles aim to guide policymakers and developers by value-based principles (OECD 2023). A further OECD contribution is their AI Policy Observatory, which tracks AI policies to provide insights and best practices for policymakers (OECD 2022). Furthermore, the International Organisation for Standardisation and International Electrotechnical Commission have developed standards for AI, addressing risk management, system architecture, and standardisation (Genovesi et al. 2024). The International Medical Device Regulators Forum aims to harmonise regulation for medical devices, which can include AI technologies (Hubner et al. 2021). The Global Partnership on AI promotes collaboration on AI policy and regulation (Jelinek et al. 2021). Specialised United Nations agencies, UNESCO (the UN Educational, Scientific, and Cultural Organisation) and ITU (International Telecommunication Union) have promoted standards and recommendations for sustainable, safe, just AI (Liao et al. 2023; Hanushchak-Yefimenko and Hrytsun 2024). The ITU develops global standards for AI's interoperability, safety, and security, and its AI for Good initiative promotes the use of AI to achieve sustainable development goals (De Lange 2020). Furthermore, the World Economic Forum addresses public–private cooperation and agendas, and the World Intellectual Property Organisation addresses patents and intellectual property (Maggioncalda 2024).

The European Commission is responsible for proposing legislation and implementing decisions in the European Union (EU) (Christoforaki and Beyan 2022). The European Commission has proposed a trailblazing 'AI Act': comprehensive legislation that categorises AI by risk and imposes strict security, transparency, and quality standards for high-risk applications (including those in healthcare) (Bhatnagar and Gajjar 2024; Wang 2024). Though awaiting formal EU Council endorsement, this 2024 proposition has been endorsed by all 27 EU states in the European Parliament (Kalpakos 2023). This act applies extraterritorially, meaning non-EU providers seeking to provide their services within the EU will also need to comply (Siegmann and Anderljung 2022).

The European Commission's High-Level Expert Group on AI has also published guidance advocating for technical robustness, privacy, accountability, and human agency in AI (European Commission 2024). Medical Device Regulation (MDR) and In Vitro Diagnostic Regulation (IVDR) are EU regulations requiring conformity assessments, marking, and post-market surveillance for medical devices, which can include AI-enabled healthcare tools (Melvin and Torre 2019). Further requirements may arise for technologies falling within regulations such as the EU Digital Services Act (World Health Organization 2024), which mandates transparency reporting for online platforms. GDPR is a critical regulation on data protection and privacy, upholding stringent data protection and privacy standards to safeguard patient data both within the EU and extraterritorially (Hoofnagle et al. 2019). GDPR mandates explicit patient consent, data minimisation, and personal data autonomy (Kirwan et al. 2021).

In the United Kingdom (UK), there is no current body of law regulating AI-enabled healthcare (Bhatnagar and Gajjar 2024). The AI and Digital Regulations Service compiles the mandatory regulations and best-practice recommendations for AI-enabled healthcare. It was launched by a multi-agency partnership aiming to guide AI use in the National Health Service (NHS), comprised of the National Institute for Health and Care Excellence (NICE), Care Quality Commission (CQC), Medicines and Healthcare products Regulatory Agency (MHRA), and Health Research Authority (HRA) (AI and Digital Regulations Service for health and social care [Internet] 2024a). Separately, NICE evaluates the efficacy and cost-effectiveness of interventions to guide NHS use, CQC regulates the quality and safety of England's health services, HRA provides standards for health research, and MHRA provides standards for the safety, quality, and efficacy of medicines and health products, including Software as a Medical Device (SaMD) technologies (NHS Transformation Directorate [Internet] 2024). AI health tools are often classified as SaMD, though the WHO has outlined challenges discerning clinical from 'wellness' applications (World Health Organization 2021). The Digital Regulation Cooperation Forum (DRCF) is a multi-agency partnership aiming to facilitate a coordinated approach to responsive online regulation, comprising four digital regulators in the UK (Bhatnagar and Gajjar 2024). In April 2024, DRCF launched a pilot AI and Digital Hub to support developers with the complexity of UK regulations (DRCF 2024). The DRCF advocates a 'pro-innovation' approach to AI regulation, emphasising safety, security, robustness, transparency and explainability, fairness, accountability and governance, contestability, and redress (Bhatnagar and Gajjar 2024).

AI integration is guided by several other frameworks in the UK. Compliance with the UK Data Protection Act and General Data Protection Regulation (GDPR) is monitored by the Information Commissioner's Office (Bhatnagar and Gajjar 2024). Adherence to the Human Rights Act 1998 and Equality Act 2010 is enshrined in UK law to preserve human rights and equity (Bhatnagar and Gajjar 2024). Goods also require UK Conformity Assessed marking to prove adherence to safety and performance standards (AI and Digital Regulations Service for health and social care [Internet] 2024b). The Digital Technology Assessment Criteria evaluates the safety, data protection, and NHS interoperability of digital health tools (AI and Digital Regulations Service for health and social care [Internet] 2024b).

In the United States of America (USA), regulation is largely governed by the Food and Drug Administration (FDA). The FDA released an action plan in 2021 for AI and machine learning software, which focused on the need for regulation accounting for the iterative nature of software updates and developments, emphasising transparency, safety, equity, and efficacy (U.S. Food and Drug Administration 2021). The FDA's Digital Health Program suggests a risk-based approach for AI SaMDs, with variable requirements for pre-market submissions (Lal et al. 2022). Additionally, the FDA encourages developers to adhere to Good Machine Learning Practices, with a lifecycle approach to performance, safety, and transparency (Lal et al. 2022). The Federal Trade Commission is also involved in regulating AI tools, prioritising the fairness and equity of algorithms and enforcing consumer protection laws to prevent deceptive practice (Wagner 2020). Consumer protection laws have been used by other agencies in the USA to tackle bias in AI (World Health Organization 2024). Recent propositions include the October 2023 Executive Order for safe and trustworthy AI, which mandates standards to address bias, privacy, education, and job displacement (Bhatnagar and Gajjar 2024). The White House Office of Science and Technology Policy has also released a 'Blueprint for an AI Bill of Rights' framework, which outlines five principles: data privacy, algorithmic discrimination protections, notice and explanation, safe and effective systems, and human alternatives, consideration, and fallback (The White House 2022). The use of personal health data is further regulated by the Health Insurance Portability and Accountability Act (Bergren 2001).

Alongside the USA, UK, and Europe, innovative AI-enabled healthcare regulations are noted in Australia, China, Brazil, and Singapore (Palaniappan et al. 2024). The Government of China's regulations for generative AI were implemented in August 2023, with the Cyberspace Administration of China mandating measures to avoid bias, ensure high-quality data collection and processing, and protect data privacy (Gong and Qu 2023). In December 2023, Singapore updated its 2019 National AI Strategy for responsible AI, including a commitment to regularly update its frameworks to reflect emerging concerns and advancements (Lawrence Wong 2023). Brazil has also proposed new AI regulations to establish new laws and a national strategy integrating rights- and risk-based frameworks (Belli et al. 2023). Australia's approach involves risk-based regulation of SaMDs by the Therapeutic Goods Administration, with additional guidance on ethical AI-enabled healthcare from the Royal Australian and New Zealand College of Radiologists (Palaniappan et al. 2024).

5.5.2 Regulatory Challenges and Recommendations for Ethical AI

5.5.2.1 Standardisation and Compliance

Despite common themes, the lack of regulation standardisation and interoperability across jurisdictions and healthcare systems can impede ethical governance, cross-border initiatives, and the development of compliant AI technologies(World Health Organization 2024). International standards should thus form the basis of jurisdictional legislation and regulation to ensure the consistent protection of human rights and ethics (Mennella et al. 2024; Bouderhem 2024). WHO has released detailed guidance on the ethics and governance of AI, consisting of a 2021 consensus statement (World Health Organization 2021) and a 2024 revision for large multi-modal models (World Health Organization 2024). This is the suggested framework for consistent international regulation (World Health Organization 2021).

Their guidance highlights six principles for ethical AI: protect autonomy; promote human well-being, safety, and the public interest; ensure transparency, explainability, and intelligibility; foster responsibility and accountability; ensure inclusiveness and equity; and promote responsive, sustainable AI (World Health Organization 2024). Developers are reminded of their responsibility to address bias, misinformation, data privacy, cybersecurity, labour concerns, the environmental footprint, exclusivity, and oversight (World Health Organization 2024). They are advised to engage trained scientific/programming personnel in design, align with medical profession standards and data protection laws, complete data protection impact assessments, and use high-quality data (World Health Organization 2024). Advice for governments and regulatory bodies includes obligating developers to find and mitigate ethical risks, requiring strict auditing, and encouraging open-source data for public oversight (World Health Organization 2024). The need for ethical design and stakeholder involvement is stressed throughout (World Health Organization 2024).

Ethical stewardship of AI requires international collaboration to deliver these standards (Dods and Erskine 2024). However, WHO has raised concerns that many AI technologies (particularly large-language models) will be inherently unable to uphold autonomy, equity, transparency, and data privacy due to their structure and functional requirements (World Health Organization 2024). Consequently, the guidance explains that AI-enabled healthcare may depend on 'the willingness of a country to forego certain human rights': a stark warning on the risks of inconsistent global regulation (World Health Organization 2024). Similarly, legislative lag and the optional nature of many recommendations mean responsible development relies on the ethical commitment of developers. Companies can choose to collaborate with governments or the Frontier Model Forum to support ethical innovation, but WHO experts outline examples of corporations ousting their ethics teams in favour of profit and pace of development (World Health Organization 2024). Despite these concerns, the appeal of optional guidance is that it can be flexibly applied and quickly adapted to evolving technologies, avoiding the protracted process of establishing enforceable legislation and standards. If international collaboration for ethical AI continues, one method of streamlining the regulatory process is mutual recognition agreements, allowing AI tools approved in one jurisdiction to be recognised in others (Regulatory Horizons Council 2021).

5.5.2.2 Transparency, Understanding, and Responsibility

Issues of explainability and interpretability are ongoing, with implications for autonomy, informed consent, and accountability (Amann et al. 2020). GDPR includes the right to an explanation, so limited explainability and interpretability of complex AI technologies may inherently violate this law (Kirwan et al. 2021). AI developers must prioritise these values for trustworthiness and informed consent (Solanki et al. 2023). Strategies may include model interpretability techniques, visualisation tools, and blockchain and federated learning technologies (Lopez-Ramos et al. 2024). Clear standards for explainable AI and transparent design should be created (Balasubramaniam et al. 2023).

As with any healthcare intervention, AI tools have benefits and risks, so patients must be empowered to make informed decisions about its use (Iserson 2024). Clinicians should counsel patients on AI tools in a clear, accessible, and culturally sensitive manner. Education materials and decision aids may be useful to demystify AI and promote health literacy (Shick et al. 2024). There is concern that AI-enabled healthcare may result in the erosion of autonomy if healthcare systems become dependent on AI, either due to resource constraints or changing clinician competencies (Akinrinmade et al. 2023). Therefore, long-term sustainability must be considered during the development and deployment of AI technologies.

Transparency is necessary for accountability. Emerging research suggests that even the most comprehensive current regulations are far too vague to ensure transparent AI, and there is a need for regulatory revision (Bommasani et al. 2024). Proactive efforts to enhance transparency, accuracy, regulations, and education may aid in alleviating clinicians' concerns around accountability and safety (Marseille and Kahn 2019). There is debate on whether corporations should make AI code 'open access': ensuring AI codes are publicly accessible and modifiable would enhance transparency and external scrutiny, but may leave code vulnerable to malice (Bhatnagar and Gajjar 2024). Other strategies include consistent information sharing, standardised testing, digestible counselling, regulatory oversight, and audits (Ferrara 2023). Human factors research should also be considered (Sujan et al. 2019). Broader ethical oversight and monitoring are imperative.

An accountability culture requires standardised protocols for reporting and addressing harms, risk assessments, and stakeholder feedback mechanisms (Grote et al. 2024). Post-market surveillance is required to continuously monitor performance and safety, and regular impact assessments should be conducted on the implications of AI systems (World Health Organization 2023). Current legislation seeks to hold healthcare professionals to set standards of practice, but attributing accountability for errors or harm in the age of AI requires a novel approach, considering stakeholder liabilities, the foreseeability of AI risks, and the evolving nature of AI technology and regulations (World Health Organization 2023). The delineation of responsibility necessitates transparency around the use of AI algorithms and their accuracy and reliability, clear contractual agreements, and focused legal frameworks (World Health Organization 2023).

5.5.2.3 Data Privacy and Protection

Regulations to protect data privacy and security are extensive, but complications arise due to inconsistencies, vast dataset aggregation, real-time processing, dubious data quality, augmentation practices, and transnational data flow (World Health Organization 2021; World Health Organization 2024). Many regulations were implemented before advanced AI tools, so policymakers are advised to revise frameworks for relevance and enforceability (World Health Organization 2021). AI tools such as large-language models also challenge data collection laws, such as the need for informed consent, as they often rely on 'web-scraped' or proprietary data and may lack facilities for timely data destruction or minimisation (World Health Organization 2024; Competition and Markets Authority 2024).

Mitigating risks to data privacy and integrity requires robust data protection measures and a deontological commitment to ethical data stewardship (World Health Organization 2021). Prevention of breaches demands encryption techniques, access controls, risk monitoring, and data anonymisation or pseudonymisation where possible (World Health Organization 2023). Encryption protocols and end-to-end encryption can safeguard data (at rest and in transit), preventing unauthorised access or interception (Atri 2024). Auditing and monitoring to ensure regulatory compliance are vital. Furthermore, role-based access control mechanisms, multi-factor authentication protocols, and monitoring aids prevent unauthorised access to patient data and support accountability (Fareed and Yassin 2022). Other privacy-preserving techniques include blockchain technologies, federated learning (algorithmic training on decentralised datasets), and differential privacy techniques (Torkzadehmahani et al. 2022).

AI-enabled healthcare can increase the vulnerability to and impact of cyberattacks (Sanmorino 2023; Damar et al. 2024), with some tools posing unique risks such as data manipulation and 'kidnapping' or alterations to system behaviour (World Health Organization 2023). International collaboration and regulatory compliance are necessary to address the global health and political risks from breaches and cyberattacks (Radanliev 2024).

5.5.2.4 Bias, Access, and Inclusion

The equity and fairness of AI models rely on the equity and fairness of underlying datasets (Choudhury and Asan 2020). Mitigating biases in algorithms demands the collection of diverse, representative data, so efforts to address systemic inequalities in real-world healthcare remain core in tackling injustice and harm (Celi et al. 2022; Sreerama and Krishnamoorthy 2022). Fairness-aware algorithmic design incorporates fairness metrics into its optimisation objectives to prevent harmful bias (Cruz et al. 2021). The use of fairness-aware design must also consider the differing needs of underserved populations (Abràmoff et al. 2023), which may be aided by techniques such as adoption, re-sampling, and adversarial learning (Olejarczyk and Young 2024). The explainability of AI algorithms is crucial to allow biases to be identified and mitigated (Xivuri and Twinomurinzi 2023). Alongside transparency from AI developers, proposed methods include causal inference analysis, sensitivity analysis, and model-agnostic interpretability techniques (Molnar et al. 2020). Prior to use, AI models should be validated with bias audits and sensitivity analyses (Mohsin et al. 2023). After deployment, continuous evaluation should include human oversight and equity testing (Gichoya et al. 2023). Algorithmic performance may be aided by regular retraining with feedback and diverse datasets (Gichoya et al. 2023). Equality, diversity, and inclusion training in AI development teams could promote ethical design.

In addition to addressing discrimination and bias in the AI algorithms themselves, the inequities in accessing AI technologies must be addressed (Okolo 2023). Understanding the needs of underserved communities requires multidisciplinary involvement (Alami et al. 2020). Insights from stakeholders (such as community leaders, faith organisations, advocacy groups, and local healthcare professionals) can be reinforced with the engagement of epidemiologists and data scientists (Alami et al. 2020). Additionally, collaboration with international organisations (such as the UN) and industry partners (such as pharmaceutical or technology companies) can support technical assistance, capacity-building, and scalable innovations (Khan et al. 2024). Co-development of appropriate, ethical, and impactful healthcare solutions in underserved communities promotes autonomy and equity, and partnerships should continue for iterative feedback to ensure interventions meet the needs of targeted communities (Khan et al. 2024; Božić 2023).

Addressing inequities requires broader ethical activism for policy change and targeted interventions. Expanding access could include advocacy for investment in digital infrastructure, providing subsidised or free devices through collaboration with non-profits or technology manufacturers (such as distributing donated or refurbished devices), technology transfer, and telehealth expansion (Storeng et al. 2021; Durocher et al. 2021).

Adaptations to the design of AI solutions may include offline capabilities, minimal bandwidth requirements, or low-power consumption (Wahl et al. 2018; Williams et al. 2021). Leveraging mobile technology and cloud-based solutions may also help overcome infrastructure challenges by providing scalable and accessible platforms for AI use (Wahl et al. 2018; Karavatselou et al. 2019). Long-term, capacity-building investments in technology, data management systems, internet, and telecommunications could narrow the digital divide (Celi et al. 2022; Alami et al. 2020). Accessible initiatives to enhance digital literacy and health literacy among underserved populations are recommended (Celi et al. 2022). Furthermore, AI platforms should prioritise accessibility, usability, and inclusivity via tools such as text-to-speech. Finally, research and program evaluations should be conducted to evaluate the impact of interventions on disparities and inform future strategies for equitable care.

Tackling inequity and promoting distributive justice requires the strategic use of AI tools based on the specific needs of various healthcare settings. Ethical prioritisation involves navigating competing needs for the available resources with the greatest respect for justice, beneficence, non-maleficence, and autonomy. In healthcare, there are often disparities in resource allocation and access to advanced technologies, which can exacerbate existing inequities in outcomes (Celi et al. 2022; Reddy et al. 2022). Utilitarian principles suggest that AI tools should be prioritised per their ability to address pressing health needs and maximise positive outcomes to the greatest extent for the greatest number of individuals. Balancing this with the need for social justice and minimising the harm from inaction can be complicated, particularly if resources are scarce. Recommendations include developing transparent prioritisation criteria and monitoring patient outcomes and equality metrics (Kim et al. 2023; Hamam 2024; Nazer et al. 2023).

5.5.2.5 Future-Proofing and Responsive Regulation

The regulatory frameworks for AI-enabled healthcare are still evolving, but the dynamic nature of machine learning will continue to place a significant burden on regulators and demand cross-sector ethical engagement (Bhatnagar and Gajjar 2024). AI systems often undergo rapid iterations, which can introduce new risks not captured by existing frameworks (Kim et al. 2023). As technologies develop, new ethical challenges are likely to emerge. For example, sophisticated AI systems may be able to make autonomous decisions on diagnosis and management (Abràmoff et al. 2018). GDPR mandates that individuals have the right not to be subject to solely automated decision-making, and the need for human oversight is reflected across guidance for ethical AI, but detailed standards are necessary (Van Kolfschooten 2024). A further example is the potential role of AI in precision medicine and gene editing technologies such as CRISPR, raising concerns around genetic privacy, ensuring informed consent for interventions and the long-term impact on patients and their children, and maintaining social equity (Omeye 2024). Stringent policies and frameworks will be required for genetic data governance, alongside long-term research projects and ethical development.

It is vital that regulations and policies are adaptive and responsive, such as the evolving life-cycle approaches demonstrated by the FDA's framework for AI and machine-learning SaMDs (Lal et al. 2022). Fostering innovation whilst minimising the regulatory lag may be further aided by regulatory sandboxes, where developers can test their tools in a controlled environment under regulatory supervision so that guidelines are responsive to new advancements (Yordanova and Bertels 2024).

To anticipate and respond to future ethical concerns, collaboration among healthcare professionals, ethicists, policymakers, developers, and patient groups is crucial (World Health Organization 2021). For example, dedicated interdisciplinary ethics committees or boards comprised of representatives from these diverse fields may be established to provide guidance and oversight, or perhaps undertake collaborative research on the sociocultural and ethical implications of AI technologies (World Health Organization 2021).

Fostering ethical innovation could also involve the incentivisation of ethical research, such as funding or competitions for innovations in ethical AI (Gurzawska 2021). Public awareness campaigns may aid in informing public discourse. For AI technologies to align with the values of medical ethics, stakeholders must accept the need for continued oversight, robust regulation, auditing, education, and interdisciplinary collaboration.

5.6 Conclusion

This chapter has explored the complex ethical terrain of AI-enabled healthcare, introducing challenges with data governance, bias and fairness, autonomy, transparency, and accountability. These are identifiable across healthcare sectors, ranging from telemedicine and education to space and low-resource settings. Each of these issues is interconnected, and the ethical dynamics of each can be significantly impacted by advancements or setbacks in others.

As the field evolves, new challenges will emerge, requiring ongoing dialogue, research, and policy adaptation. Sustained collaboration among healthcare professionals, AI developers, ethicists, policymakers, laypeople, and patients is essential. Regulatory and policy frameworks must keep pace with innovation to ensure technologies align with ethical standards and societal values. International collaboration is vital for globally consistent standards.

Ethical issues should not be seen as mere obstacles, but as opportunities to build a future where AI technologies enhance patient care and sustain the highest ethical standards.

References

Abbas JJ, Smith B, Poluta M, Velazquez-Berumen A (2017) Improving health-care delivery in low-resource settings with nanotechnology: challenges in multiple dimensions. Nanobiomed 4:1849543517701158. https://doi.org/10.1177/1849543517701158

Abdullahi T, Singh R, Eickhoff C (2024) Learning to make rare and complex diagnoses with generative AI assistance: qualitative study of popular large language models. JMIR Med Educ 10:e51391

Abràmoff MD, Lavin PT, Birch M, Shah N, Folk JC (2018) Pivotal trial of an autonomous AI-based diagnostic system for detection of diabetic retinopathy in primary care offices. Npj Digit Med. 1(1):39

Abràmoff MD, Tarver ME, Loyo-Berrios N, Trujillo S, Char D, Obermeyer Z et al (2023) Considerations for addressing bias in artificial intelligence for health equity. Npj Digit Med 6(1):170

Adegoke B, Odugbose T, Adeyemi C (2024) Data analytics for predicting disease outbreaks: a review of models and tools. Int J Life Sci Res Updat 2(2):001–009

AI and Digital Regulations Service for health and social care [Internet] (2024a) Home. Available from: https://digitalregulations.innovation.nhs.uk/

AI and Digital Regulations Service for health and social care [Internet] (2024b) Using the Digital Technology Assessment Criteria (DTAC). cited 2024 Aug 24. Available from: https://digitalregulations.innovation.nhs.uk/regulations-and-guidance-for-developers/all-developers-guidance/using-the-digital-technology-assessment-criteria-dtac/

Akbar MF, Tianwin J, Devano E, Kartawiguna D (2024) Assessing the impact of medical ethics violations on the effectiveness of artificial intelligence in telemedicine. In: 2024 12th International Conference on Cyber and IT Service Management (CITSM) [Internet], IEEE, Batam, pp 1–6. 2024 [cited 2024 Dec 23]. https://doi.org/10.1109/CITSM64103.2024.10775891

Akinrinmade AO, Adebile TM, Ezuma-Ebong C, Bolaji K, Ajufo A, Adigun AO et al (2023) Artificial intelligence in healthcare: perception and reality. Cureus. https://doi.org/10.7759/cureus.45594

Alam F, Lim MA, Zulkipli IN (2023) Integrating AI in medical education: embracing ethical usage and critical understanding. Front Med 10:1279707. https://doi.org/10.3389/fmed.2023.1279707

Alami H, Rivard L, Lehoux P, Hoffman SJ, Cadeddu SBM, Savoldelli M et al (2020) Artificial intelligence in health care: laying the foundation for responsible, sustainable, and inclusive innovation in low- and middle-income countries. Glob Health 16(1):52

Alanazi AT (2023) Clinicians' perspectives on healthcare cybersecurity and cyber threats. Cureus 15(10):e47026. 2023 Oct 14 [cited 2024 Sep 12]. https://doi.org/10.7759/cureus.47026

Aljerian N, Arafat M, Aldhubib A, Almohaimeed I, Alsultan A, Alhosaini A et al (2022) Artificial intelligence in health care and its application in Saudi Arabia. Int J Innov Res Med Sci 7(11):666–670

Alowais SA, Alghamdi SS, Alsuhebany N, Alqahtani T, Alshaya AI, Almohareb SN et al (2023) Revolutionizing healthcare: the role of artificial intelligence in clinical practice. BMC Med Educ 23(1):689

Amann J, Blasimme A, Vayena E, Frey D, Madai VI (2020) Explainability for artificial intelligence in healthcare: a multidisciplinary perspective. BMC Med Inform Decis Mak 20(1):310

Amoakoh HB, Klipstein-Grobusch K, Agyepong IA, Amoakoh-Coleman M, Kayode GA, Reitsma JB et al (2020) Can an mhealth clinical decision-making support system improve adherence to neonatal healthcare protocols in a low-resource setting? BMC Pediatr 20(1):534

Andrus M, Villeneuve S (2022) Demographic-reliant algorithmic fairness: characterizing the risks of demographic data collection in the pursuit of fairness. In: 2022 ACM Conference on Fairness, Accountability, and Transparency [Internet], ACM, Seoul Republic of Korea, pp 1709–21. 2022 [cited 2024 Sep 20]. https://doi.org/10.1145/3531146.3533226

Armitage RC (2023) ChatGPT: the threats to medical education. Postgrad Med J 99(1176):1130–1131

Asrar FM, Saint-Jacques D, Williams D (2022) Outer space assets offer benefits to health care: family doctors play a key role in supporting innovative work. Can Fam Physician 68(11):797–798, 800

Atri P (2024) Enhancing big data security through comprehensive data protection measures: a focus on securing data at rest and in-transit. Int J Comput Eng 5(4):44–55

Baah FO, Teitelman AM, Riegel B (2019) Marginalization: conceptualizing patient vulnerabilities in the framework of social determinants of health—an integrative review. Nurs Inq 26(1):e12268

Badr J, Motulsky A, Denis JL (2024) Digital health technologies and inequalities: a scoping review of potential impacts and policy recommendations. Health Policy 146:105122

Bajwa J, Munir U, Nori A, Williams B (2021) Artificial intelligence in healthcare: transforming the practice of medicine. Future Healthc J 8(2):e188–e194

Bakker C, van der Linden S (1995) Health related utility measurement: an introduction. J Rheumatol 22(6):1197–1199

Balasubramaniam N, Kauppinen M, Rannisto A, Hiekkanen K, Kujala S (2023) Transparency and explainability of AI systems: from ethical guidelines to requirements. Inf Softw Technol 159:107197

Baylis F (1996) Women and Health Research: working for change. J Clin Ethics 7(3):229–242

Bazmi S, Samadi F, Department of Medical Ethics, Iran University of Medical Sciences, Tehran, Iran, Forouzandeh M, Department of Medical Ethics, Iran University of Medical Sciences, Tehran, Iran (2023) Investigating the moral sensitivity of medical students in the preclinical and late clinical courses Shabnam Bazmi. Med J Islam Repub Iran. https://doi.org/10.47176/mjiri.37.39

Beauchamp TL, Childress JF (2013) Principles of biomedical ethics, 7th edn. Oxford University Press, New York, p 459

Bekbolatova M, Mayer J, Ong CW, Toma M (2024) Transformative potential of AI in healthcare: definitions, applications, and navigating the ethical landscape and public perspectives. Healthcare 12(2):125

Belli L, Curzi Y, Gaspar WB (2023) AI regulation in Brazil: advancements, flows, and need to learn from the data protection experience. Comput Law Secur Rev 48:105767

Berdahl CT, Baker L, Mann S, Osoba O, Girosi F (2023) Strategies to improve the impact of artificial intelligence on health equity: scoping review. JMIR AI 2:e42936

Bergren MD (2001) HIPAA hoopla: privacy and security of identifiable health information. J Sch Nurs 17(6):336–341

Bhagat SV, Kanyal D (2024) Navigating the future: the transformative impact of artificial intelligence on hospital management- A comprehensive review. Cureus. https://doi.org/10.7759/cureus.54518

Bhatnagar A, Gajjar D (2024) Policy implications of artificial intelligence (AI) [Internet]. Parliamentary Office of Science and Technology. 2024 Jan [cited 2024 May 5]. Available from: https://post.parliament.uk/research-briefings/post-pn-0708

Bilgic E, Gorgy A, Yang A, Cwintal M, Ranjbar H, Kahla K et al (2022) Exploring the roles of artificial intelligence in surgical education: a scoping review. Am J Surg 224(1):205–216

Rishi Bommasani, Kevin Klyman, Shayne Longpre, Betty Xiong, Sayash Kapoor, Nestor Maslej, et al. (2024) Foundation model transparency reports. arXiv. https://doi.org/10.48550/arXiv.2402.16268

Bompelli A, Wang Y, Wan R, Singh E, Zhou Y, Xu L et al (2021) Social and behavioral determinants of health in the era of artificial intelligence with electronic health records: a scoping review. Health Data Sci 2021:9759016

Bouderhem R (2024) Shaping the future of AI in healthcare through ethics and governance. Humanit Soc Sci Commun. 11(1):416

Božić V (2023) Risks of digital divide in using Artificial Intelligence (AI). https://doi.org/10.13140/RG.2.2.18156.13443

Burrell J (2016) How the machine 'thinks': understanding opacity in machine learning algorithms. Big Data Soc 3(1):205395171562251

Carey JM, Rossler K (2024) The how when why of high fidelity simulation. In: StatPearls [Internet]. StatPearls Publishing, Treasure Island. 2024 [cited 2024 May 4].

Available from: http://www.ncbi.nlm.nih.gov/books/NBK559313/
Celi LA, Cellini J, Charpignon ML, Dee EC, Dernoncourt F, Eber R, et al. (2022) Sources of bias in artificial intelligence that perpetuate healthcare disparities—a global review. Fraser HS (ed) PLOS Digit Health 1(3):e0000022
Challen R, Denny J, Pitt M, Gompels L, Edwards T, Tsaneva-Atanasova K (2019) Artificial intelligence, bias and clinical safety. BMJ Qual Saf 28(3):231–237
Chan KS, Zary N (2019) Applications and challenges of implementing artificial intelligence in medical education: integrative review. JMIR Med Educ 5(1):e13930
Chattu VK, Nanda A, Chattu SK, Kadri SM, Knight AW (2019) The emerging role of blockchain technology applications in routine disease surveillance systems to strengthen global health security. Big Data Cogn Comput 3(2):25
Chinta SV, Wang Z, Zhang X, Viet TD, Kashif A, Smith MA, et al. (2024) AI-driven healthcare: a survey on ensuring fairness and mitigating bias [Pre-Print]. arXiv. https://doi.org/10.48550/arXiv.2407.19655
Choudhury A, Asan O (2020) Role of artificial intelligence in patient safety outcomes: systematic literature review. JMIR Med Inform 8(7):e18599
Christoforaki M, Beyan O (2022) AI ethics—a bird's eye view. Appl Sci 12(9):4130
Ciecierski-Holmes T, Singh R, Axt M, Brenner S, Barteit S (2022) Artificial intelligence for strengthening healthcare systems in low- and middle-income countries: a systematic scoping review. Npj Digit Med 5(1):162
Cinnamon J (2020) Data inequalities and why they matter for development. Inf Technol Dev 26(2):214–233
Competition & Markets Authority (2024) AI foundation models: technical update report, pp 40–44
Crenshaw K (1989) Demarginalizing the intersection of race and sex: a black feminist critique of antidiscrimination doctrine, feminist theory and antiracist politics. U Chi Leg F 1989:139
Cruz AF, Saleiro P, Belem C, Soares C, Bizarro P (2021) Promoting fairness through hyperparameter optimization. In: 2021 IEEE International Conference on Data Mining (ICDM). IEEE, Auckland, pp 1036–1041. https://doi.org/10.1109/ICDM51629.2021.00119
Curioso WH (2019) Building capacity and training for digital health: challenges and opportunities in Latin America. J Med Internet Res 21(12):e16513
d'Elia A, Gabbay M, Rodgers S, Kierans C, Jones E, Durrani I et al (2022) Artificial intelligence and health inequities in primary care: a systematic scoping review and framework. Fam Med Community Health 10(Suppl 1):e001670
Damar M, Özen A, Yılmaz A (2024) Cybersecurity in the health sector in the reality of artificial intelligence, and information security conceptually. J AI 8(1):61–82
Dangi RR, Sharma A, Vageriya V (2024) Transforming healthcare in low-resource settings with artificial intelligence: recent developments and outcomes. Public Health Nurs. https://doi.org/10.1111/phn.13500
De Lange DE (2020) Responsible artificial intelligence and partnerships for the goals. In: Leal Filho W, Azul AM, Brandli L, Lange Salvia A, Wall T (eds) Partnerships for the goals, Encyclopedia of the UN Sustainable Development Goals. Springer International Publishing, Cham, pp 1–13
Devillers L, Fogelman-Soulié F, Baeza-Yates R (2021) AI & Human values: inequalities, biases, fairness, nudge, and feedback loops, Lecture Notes in Computer Science, vol 12600. Springer International Publishing, Cham, pp 76–89. https://doi.org/10.1007/978-3-030-69128-8_6
Dhabliya D, Dari SS, Dhablia A, Akhila N, Kachhoria R, Khetani V (2024) Addressing bias in machine learning algorithms: promoting fairness and ethical design. Li G, Subramaniam U, Sekar M (ed) E3S Web Conf 491:02040. https://doi.org/10.1051/e3sconf/202449102040
Dhar E, Upadhyay U, Huang Y, Uddin M, Manias G, Kyriazis D et al (2023) A scoping review to assess the effects of virtual reality in medical education and clinical care. Digit Health 9:20552076231158O
van Dijk J (2020) The digital divide. Polity, Cambridge Medford, p 184
Dimai HP (2023) New horizons: artificial intelligence tools for managing osteoporosis. J Clin Endocrinol Metab 108(4):775–783
Dinh-Le C, Chuang R, Chokshi S, Mann D (2019) Wearable health technology and electronic health record integration: scoping review and future directions. JMIR Mhealth Uhealth 7(9):e12861
Dods S, Erskine M (2024) The role of standards and stewardship in the co-evolution of AI and humans. GHD. Available from: https://www.ghd.com/en-gb/insights/the-role-of-standards-and-stewardship-in-the-co-evolution-of-ai-and-humans
Doupe P, Faghmous J, Basu S (2019) Machine learning for health services researchers. Value Health 22(7):808–815
DRCF (2024) The DRCF launches informal advice service to support innovation and enable economic growth [Internet]. Available from: https://www.drcf.org.uk/publications/press-releases/the-drcf-launches-informal-advice-service-to-support-innovation-and-enable-economic-growth/
Duffy J, Gallagher J, Holmes S (2018) Virtue ethics. Rhetor Rev 37(4):321–392
Durán JM, Jongsma KR (2021) Who is afraid of black box algorithms? On the epistemological and ethical basis of trust in medical AI. J Med Ethics. https://doi.org/10.1136/medethics-2020-106820
Durocher K, Boparai N, Jankowicz D, Strudwick G (2021) Identifying technology industry-led initiatives to address digital health equity. Digit Health 7:20552076211056156
El Emam K, Jonker E, Arbuckle L, Malin B (2011) A systematic review of re-identification attacks on health data. Scherer RW (ed) PLoS ONE 6(12):e28071
Elendu C, Amaechi DC, Okatta AU, Amaechi EC, Elendu TC, Ezeh CP et al (2024) The impact of

simulation-based training in medical education: a review. Medicine (Baltimore) 103(27):e38813

Emdad FB, Ho SM, Ravuri B, Hussain S (2023) Towards a unified utilitarian ethics framework for healthcare artificial intelligence. College of Communication & Information, Florida State University, Tallahassee. https://doi.org/10.48550/arXiv.2309.14617

Eshwar MS (2023) Exploring the potential of artificial intelligence in healthcare: possibilities and challenges. Int Sci J Eng Manag 2(4). https://doi.org/10.55041/ISJEM00408

European Commission (2024) Ethics guidelines for trustworthy AI [Internet]. European Union. 2024 [cited 2024 Aug 22]. Available from: https://digital-strategy.ec.europa.eu/library/ethics-guidelines-trustworthy-ai

Fareed MA, Yassin A (2022) Privacy-preserving multi-factor authentication and role-based access control scheme for the E-healthcare system. Bull Electr Eng Inform 11(4):2131–2141

Fazil A, Hakimi M, Shahidzay A (2024) A comprehensive review of bias in AI algorithms. Nusant Hasana J 3(8):1–11

Fazlollahi AM, Bakhaidar M, Alsayegh A, Yilmaz R, Winkler-Schwartz A, Mirchi N et al (2022) Effect of artificial intelligence tutoring vs expert instruction on learning simulated surgical skills among medical students: a randomized clinical trial. JAMA Netw Open 5(2):e2149008

Ferrara E (2023) Fairness and bias in artificial intelligence: a brief survey of sources, impacts, and mitigation strategies. Sci 6(1):3

Festor P, Jia Y, Gordon AC, Faisal AA, Habli I, Komorowski M (2022) Assuring the safety of AI-based clinical decision support systems: a case study of the AI Clinician for sepsis treatment. BMJ Health Care Inform. 29(1):e100549

Finnane A, Dallest K, Janda M, Soyer HP (2017) Teledermatology for the diagnosis and management of skin cancer: a systematic review. JAMA Dermatol 153(3):319

Fitzpatrick KK, Darcy A, Vierhile M (2017) Delivering cognitive behavior therapy to young adults with symptoms of depression and anxiety using a fully automated conversational agent (Woebot): a randomized controlled trial. JMIR Ment Health 4(2):e19

GenAI BA et al (2024) Cocreation, authorship, ownership, academic ethics and integrity in a time of generative AI. Open Prax 16(1):1–10

Genovesi S, Mönig JM, Schmitz A, Poretschkin M, Akila M, Kahdan M et al (2024) Standardizing fairness-evaluation procedures: interdisciplinary insights on machine learning algorithms in creditworthiness assessments for small personal loans. AI Ethics 4(2):537–553

Giarmoleo FV, Rocchi M, Ferrero I (2024) Ethics of artificial intelligence a virtue ethics approach. In: Disruptive digitalisation and platforms: risks and opportunities of the great transformation of politics, socio-economic models, work and education [Internet], 1st edn. Routledge, pp 57–74. 2024 [cited 2024 Nov 22]. https://doi.org/10.4324/9781032617190-6

Gichoya JW, Thomas K, Celi LA, Safdar N, Banerjee I, Banja JD et al (2023) AI pitfalls and what not to do: mitigating bias in AI. Br J Radiol 96(1150):20230023

Giordano C, Brennan M, Mohamed B, Rashidi P, Modave F, Tighe P (2021) Accessing artificial intelligence for clinical decision-making. Front Digit Health 3:645232

Gong J, Qu H (2023) What you need to know about China's new generative AI measures. Bird & Bird. Published August 3. Available from: https://www.twobirds.com/en/insights/2023/china/what-you-need-to-know-about-china's-new-generative-ai-measures

Greatbatch C (2024) The role of artificial intelligence in space medicine. J Australas Soc Aerosp Med 3(1):1–5

Grote G, Parker SK, Crowston K (2024) Taming artificial intelligence: a theory of control-acountability alignment among AI developers and users. Acad Manag Rev. https://doi.org/10.5465/amr.2023.0117

Grunhut J, Wyatt AT, Marques O (2021) Educating future physicians in artificial intelligence (AI): an integrative review and proposed changes. J Med Educat Curri Develop 8:238212052110368

Guindo LA, Wagner M, Baltussen R, Rindress D, Van Til J, Kind P et al (2012) From efficacy to equity: literature review of decision criteria for resource allocation and healthcare decisionmaking. Cost Eff Resour Alloc 10(1):9

Gurzawska A (2021) Responsible innovation in business: perceptions, evaluation practices and lessons learnt. Sustainability 13(4):1826

Habli I, Lawton T, Porter Z (2020) Artificial intelligence in health care: accountability and safety. Bull World Health Organ 98(4):251–256

Hadiyantina S, Ayub ZA, Mohamed Yusoff Z (2022) Transborder data flows. J Int Stud [Internet] 18. 2022 [cited 2024 Dec 24]. https://doi.org/10.32890/jis

Haimi M (2023) The tragic paradoxical effect of telemedicine on healthcare disparities- a time for redemption: a narrative review. BMC Med Inform Decis Mak 23(1):95

Hamam H (2024) Guest editorial achieving health equity through AI for diagnosis and treatment and patient monitoring. IEEE J Biomed Health Inform 28(2):702–706

Hamilton A (2024) Artificial intelligence and healthcare simulation: the shifting landscape of medical education. Cureus. https://doi.org/10.7759/cureus.59747

Hanushchak-Yefimenko L, Hrytsun V (2024) Foreign experience of managing the development of entrepeneurship using artificial intelligence. Management 38(2):157–167

Harishbhai Tilala M, Kumar Chenchala P, Choppadandi A, Kaur J, Naguri S, Saoji R et al (2024) Ethical considerations in the use of artificial intelligence and machine learning in health care: a comprehensive review. Cureus. 16(6):e62443

Hilbert M (2011) The end justifies the definition: the manifold outlooks on the digital divide and their practical usefulness for policy-making. Telecommun Policy 35(8):715–736

Hodkinson PD, Anderton RA, Posselt BN, Fong KJ (2017) An overview of space medicine. Br J Anaesth 119:i143–i153

Hoofnagle CJ, Van Der Sloot B, Borgesius FZ (2019) The European Union general data protection regulation: what it is and what it means. Inf Commun Technol Law 28(1):65–98

Hubner S, Maloney C, Phillips SD, Doshi P, Mugaga J, Ssekitoleko RT et al (2021) The evolving landscape of medical device regulation in east, central, and Southern Africa. Glob Health Sci Pract 9(1):136–148

Hudda S, DrR K, DrN N (2024) The changing landscape of healthcare with state of the art AI technology. Int J Res Appl Sci Eng Technol 12(5):1700–1705

Hynninen Y, Vilkkumaa E, Salo A (2021) Operationalization of utilitarian and egalitarian objectives for optimal allocation of health care resources. Decis Sci 52(5):1169–1208

Iqbal J, Cortés Jaimes DC, Makineni P, Subramani S, Hemaida S, Thugu TR et al (2023) Reimagining healthcare: unleashing the power of artificial intelligence in medicine. Cureus 15(9):e44658. https://doi.org/10.7759/cureus.44658

Iserson KV (2024) Informed consent for artificial intelligence in emergency medicine: a practical guide. Am J Emerg Med 76:225–230

Isgut M, Gloster L, Choi K, Venugopalan J, Wang MD (2023) Systematic review of advanced AI methods for improving healthcare data quality in post COVID-19 era. IEEE Rev Biomed Eng 16:53–69

Jackson F (2007) The Oxford handbook of contemporary philosophy. Oxford University Press, Oxford, pp 31–62

Jelinek T, Wallach W, Kerimi D (2021) Policy brief: the creation of a G20 coordinating committee for the governance of artificial intelligence. AI Ethics 1(2):141–150

Johnson ME (2009) Data hemorrhages in the health-care sector. In: Dingledine R, Golle P (ed) Financial cryptography and data security, Lecture Notes in Computer Science, vol 5628. Springer Berlin Heidelberg, Berlin, Heidelberg, pp 71–89. 2009 [cited 2024 Sep 12]. https://doi.org/10.1007/978-3-642-03549-4_5

Kalpakos ME (2023) Defining the future: the AI act's potential in equitably safeguarding fundamental rights and promoting AI innovation. UFITA 87(1):128–172

Karavatselou E, Fengou MA, Mantas G, Lymberopoulos D (2019) Profile management system in ubiquitous healthcare cloud computing environment. In: Sucasas V, Mantas G, Althunibat S (eds) Broadband communications, networks, and systems, Lecture Notes of the Institute for Computer Sciences, Social Informatics and Telecommunications Engineering, vol 263. Springer International Publishing, Cham, pp 105–114. https://doi.org/10.1007/978-3-030-05195-2_11

Kaur G, Prinja S, Lakshmi PVM, Downey L, Sharma D, Teerawattananon Y (2019) Criteria used for priority-setting for public health resource allocation in low- and middle-income countries: a systematic review. Int J Technol Assess Health Care 35(6):474–483

Kerketta A, Balasundaram S (2024) Leveraging AI tools to bridge the healthcare gap in rural areas in India [Pre-Print]. 2024 Aug [cited 2024 Dec 24]. https://doi.org/10.1101/2024.07.30.24311228

Khan MS, Umer H, Faruqe F (2024) Artificial intelligence for low income countries. Humanit Soc Sci Commun 11(1):1422

Kim JY, Hasan A, Kellogg K, Ratliff W, Murray S, Suresh H et al (2023) Development and preliminary testing of Health Equity Across the AI Lifecycle (HEAAL): a framework for healthcare delivery organizations to mitigate the risk of AI solutions worsening health inequities. Health Policy. https://doi.org/10.1371/journal.pdig.0000390

Kimmerle J, Timm J, Festl-Wietek T, Cress U, Herrmann-Werner A (2023) Medical students' attitudes toward AI in medicine and their expectations for medical education. J Med Educat Curri Develop 10:23821205231219346

Kirwan M, Mee B, Clarke N, Tanaka A, Manaloto L, Halpin E et al (2021) What GDPR and the Health Research Regulations (HRRs) mean for Ireland: "explicit consent"—a legal analysis. Ir J Med Sci 1971 190(2):515–521

Kiseleva A, Kotzinos D, De Hert P (2022) Transparency of AI in healthcare as a multilayered system of accountabilities: between legal requirements and technical limitations. Front Artif Intell 5:879603

Kitto S, Ng YY, Cleland J (2024) 'Slowing down when you should': optimising the translation of artificial intelligence into medical school curricula. Singapore Med J 65(3):186–189

Klaic M, Kapp S, Hudson P, Chapman W, Denehy L, Story D et al (2022) Implementability of healthcare interventions: an overview of reviews and development of a conceptual framework. Implement Sci 17(1):10

Kose U, Koc D (2015) In: Ordóñez De Pablos P (ed) Artificial intelligence applications in distance education, Advances in Mobile and Distance Learning. IGI Global, pp 1–11. https://doi.org/10.4018/978-1-4666-6276-6

Kung TH, Cheatham M, Medenilla A, Sillos C, De Leon L, Elepaño C, et al. (2023) Performance of ChatGPT on USMLE: potential for AI-assisted medical education using large language models. Dagan A (ed) PLOS Digit Health 2(2):e0000198

Kuvvetli I (2024) New space-based technology has huge potential for applications on earth. DTU Space. 2024 Jun 18 [cited 2024 Oct 31]. Available from: https://www.space.dtu.dk/english/newsarchive/2024/06/new-space-based-technology-has-huge-potential-for-applications-on-earth

Kwon J, Johnson ME (2015) "The market effect of healthcare security: do patients care about data breaches?" Workshop on the Economics of Information Security

Lal A, Dang J, Nabzdyk C, Gajic O, Herasevich V (2022) Regulatory oversight and ethical concerns surrounding software as medical device (SaMD) and digital twin technology in healthcare. Ann Transl Med 10(18):950

Lawrence Wong (2023) AI for the public good for Singapore and the world [Internet]. Government of the Republic of Singapore. Available from: https://file.go.gov.sg/nais2023.pdf

Li F, Ruijs N, Lu Y (2022) Ethics & AI: a systematic review on ethical concerns and related strategies for designing with AI in healthcare. AI 4(1):28–53

Liao HT, Pan CL, Zhang Y (2023) Smart digital platforms for carbon neutral management and services: business models based on ITU standards for green digital transformation. Front Ecol Evol 11:1134381

Liu CF, Huang CC, Wang JJ, Kuo KM, Chen CJ (2021) The critical factors affecting the deployment and scaling of healthcare AI: viewpoint from an experienced medical center. Healthcare 9(6):685

Lopez-Ramos LM, Leiser F, Rastogi A, Hicks S, Strümke I, Madai VI, et al. (2024) Interplay between federated learning and explainable artificial intelligence: a scoping review [Pre-Print]. arXiv. https://doi.org/10.48550/arXiv.2411.05874

Maggino F (ed) (2023) Encyclopedia of quality of life and Well-being research, 2nd edn. Springer International Publishing, Cham. https://doi.org/10.1007/978-3-031-17299-1

Maggioncalda J (2024) 4 ways public-private partnerships can bridge the AI opportunity gap [Internet]. World economic forum - emerging technologies. 2024 [cited 2024 Aug 22]. Available from: https://www.weforum.org/stories/2024/01/public-private-partnerships-ai-reskilling/

Mahmoud K, Jaramillo C, Barteit S (2022) Telemedicine in low- and middle-income countries during the COVID-19 pandemic: a scoping review. Front Public Health 10:914423

Mann DM, Chen J, Chunara R, Testa PA, Nov O (2020) COVID-19 transforms health care through telemedicine: evidence from the field. J Am Med Inform Assoc 27(7):1132–1135

Marseille E, Kahn JG (2019) Utilitarianism and the ethical foundations of cost-effectiveness analysis in resource allocation for global health. Philos Ethics Humanit Med 14(5):5

Melvin T, Torre M (2019) New medical device regulations: the regulator's view. EFORT Open Rev 4(6):351–356

Mennella C, Maniscalco U, De Pietro G, Esposito M (2024) Ethical and regulatory challenges of AI technologies in healthcare: a narrative review. Heliyon 10(4):e26297

Mensah GB (2023) Artificial Intelligence and ethics: a comprehensive review of bias mitigation, transparency, and accountability in AI systems. https://doi.org/10.13140/RG.2.2.23381.19685/1

Merkley C, Bright K, Mack AD (2023) Trauma informed simulation-based education: scoping review protocol. https://doi.org/10.17605/OSF.IO/N9H2F

Mir MM, Mir GM, Raina NT, Mir SM, Mir SM, Miskeen E et al (2023) Application of artificial intelligence in medical education: current scenario and future perspectives. J Adv Med Educ Prof 11(3):133–140

Misselbrook D (2013) Duty, Kant, and deontology. Br J Gen Pract J R Coll Gen Pract 63(609):211

Mohsin SN, Gapizov A, Ekhator C, Ain NU, Ahmad S, Khan M et al (2023) The role of artificial intelligence in prediction, risk stratification, and personalized treatment planning for congenital heart diseases. Cureus. https://doi.org/10.7759/cureus.44374

Moldt JA, Festl-Wietek T, Madany Mamlouk A, Nieselt K, Fuhl W, Herrmann-Werner A (2023) Chatbots for future docs: exploring medical students' attitudes and knowledge towards artificial intelligence and medical chatbots. Med Educ Online 28(1):2182659

Molnar C, Casalicchio G, Bischl B (2020) Interpretable machine learning -- a brief history, State-of-the-Art and Challenges. https://doi.org/10.1007/978-3-030-65965-3_28

Morrow E, Zidaru T, Ross F, Mason C, Patel KD, Ream M et al (2023) Artificial intelligence technologies and compassion in healthcare: a systematic scoping review. Front Psychol 13:971044

Nagaraj MB, Namazi B, Sankaranarayanan G, Scott DJ (2023) Developing artificial intelligence models for medical student suturing and knot-tying video-based assessment and coaching. Surg Endosc 37(1):402–411

Naveed A, Sigwele T, Yim Fun H, Kamala M, Misfa SA (2020) Addressing semantic interoperability, privacy and security concerns in electronic health records. J Eng Sci Res 2(1)

Nazer LH, Zatarah R, Waldrip S, Ke JXC, Moukheiber M, Khanna AK, et al. (2023) Bias in artificial intelligence algorithms and recommendations for mitigation. Kalla M (ed) PLOS Digit Health 2(6):e0000278

Nguyen T (2024) ChatGPT in medical education: a precursor for automation bias? JMIR Med Educ 10:e50174

NHS Transformation Directorate [Internet] (2024) The AI and digital regulations service. Available from: https://transform.england.nhs.uk/ai-lab/ai-lab-programmes/regulating-the-ai-ecosystem/the-ai-and-digital-regulations-service/

Norman G, Dore K, Grierson L (2012) The minimal relationship between simulation fidelity and transfer of learning. Med Educ 46(7):636–647

Oche PA, Ewa GA, Ibekwe N (2024) Applications and challenges of artificial intelligence in space missions. IEEE Access 12:44481–44509

Odeh A, Abu Al-Haija Q (2023) Medical image encryption techniques: a technical survey and potential challenges. Int J Electr Comput Eng IJECE 13(3):3170

OECD (2022) Harnessing the power of AI and emerging technologies: background paper for the CDEP Ministerial meeting. (OECD Digital Economy Papers; vol 340). Report No.: 340. https://doi.org/10.1787/f94df8ec-en

OECD (2023) The state of implementation of the OECD AI Principles four years on. (OECD Artificial Intelligence Papers; vol 3). Report No.: 3. https://doi.org/10.1787/835641c9-en

Oh N, Choi GS, Lee WY (2023) ChatGPT goes to the operating room: evaluating GPT-4 performance and its potential in surgical education and training in the era of large language models. Ann Surg Treat Res 104(5):269

Okereafor K, Manny P, Sabri MS (2020) Understanding cybersecurity challenges of telecommuting and video conferencing applications in the COVID-19 pandemic. SSRN Electron J 8(6):13–23

Okolo CT (2022) Optimizing human-centered AI for healthcare in the global south. Patterns 3(2):100421. https://doi.org/10.1016/j.patter.2021.100421

Okolo CT (2023) Addressing global inequity in AI development. In: Lindgren S (ed) Handbook of critical studies of artificial intelligence. Edward Elgar Publishing, pp 378–389. https://doi.org/10.4337/9781803928562.00040

Olaoye G, Frank E (2024) The impact of bias and fairness issues on the robustness and security of AI systems [Pre-Print]. EasyChair Prepr 13461 [Internet]. 2024 [cited 2024 Aug 22]. Available at: https://easychair.org/publications/preprint/98Sb/open

Olejarczyk JP, Young M (2024) Patient rights and ethics. In: StatPearls. StatPearls Publishing, Treasure Island. 2024 [cited 2024 May 5]. Available from: http://www.ncbi.nlm.nih.gov/books/NBK538279/

Omeye FI (2024) Ethical considerations in AI-driven genome editing. Res output. J Public Health Med 3(1):14–18

Organisation for Economic Co-operation and Development (OECD) (2019) Recommendation of the council on artificial intelligence. OECD Legal Instruments. 2019 May 22 [cited 2024 Dec 10]. Available from: https://legalinstruments.oecd.org/en/instruments/oecd-legal-0449

Oyeniran OC, Adewusi AO, Adeleke AG, Akwawa LA, Azubuko CF (2022) Ethical AI: addressing bias in machine learning models and software applications. Comput Sci IT Res J 3(3):115–126

Page K (2012) The four principles: can they be measured and do they predict ethical decision making? BMC Med Ethics 13(1):10

Palaniappan K, Lin EYT, Vogel S (2024) Global regulatory frameworks for the use of Artificial Intelligence (AI) in the healthcare services sector. Healthcare 12(5):562

Pang L, Liu H, Liu Z, Tan J, Yuan ZL, Qiu Y et al (2022) Role of telemedicine in inflammatory bowel disease: systematic review and meta-analysis of randomized controlled trials. J Med Internet Res 24(3):e28978

Paranjape K, Schinkel M, Nannan Panday R, Car J, Nanayakkara P (2019) Introducing artificial intelligence training in medical education. JMIR Med Educ 5(2):e16048

Pillai AS (2023) Artificial intelligence in healthcare systems of low- and middle-income countries: requirements, gaps, challenges, and potential strategies. IJAHA [Internet] 8(3):19–33. 2023 Mar 6 [cited 2024 Aug 29]. Available from: http://norislab.com/index.php/IJAHA/article/view/72

Price WN (2019) Risks and remedies for artificial intelligence in health care | Brookings [Internet]. 2019 [cited 2024 May 3]. Available from: https://www.brookings.edu/articles/risks-and-remedies-for-artificial-intelligence-in-health-care/

Radanliev P (2024) Cyber diplomacy: defining the opportunities for cybersecurity and risks from Artificial Intelligence, IoT, blockchains, and quantum computing. J Cyber Secur Technol:1–51

Raghu G, Mehrotra A (2023) Licensure laws and other barriers to telemedicine and telehealth: an urgent need for reform. Lancet Respir Med 11(1):11–13

Rahimzadeh V (2021) A policy and practice review of consumer protections and their application to hospital-sourced data aggregation and analytics by third-party companies. Front Big Data 3:603044

Rajkomar A, Oren E, Chen K, Dai AM, Hajaj N, Hardt M et al (2018) Scalable and accurate deep learning with electronic health records. Npj Digit Med 1(1):18

Rajkomar A, Dean J, Kohane I (2019) Machine learning in medicine. N Engl J Med 380(14):1347–1358

Reddy S, Rogers W, Makinen VP, Coiera E, Brown P, Wenzel M et al (2021) Evaluation framework to guide implementation of AI systems into healthcare settings. BMJ Health Care Inform 28(1):e100444

Reddy H, Shiv Joshi, Joshi A, Wagh V (2022) A critical review of global digital divide and the role of technology in healthcare. Cureus [Internet]. 2022 Sep 29 [cited 2024 May 4]. https://doi.org/10.7759/cureus.29739

Regulatory Horizons Council (2021) Report on medical devices. Regulatory Horizons Council, London. Viewed 14th December 2024. https://assets.publishing.service.gov.uk/media/611d11f1d3bf7f63aeb66cb3/rhc-medical-report.pdf

Sallam M, Salim N, Barakat M, Al-Tammemi A (2023) ChatGPT applications in medical, dental, pharmacy, and public health education: a descriptive study highlighting the advantages and limitations. Narra J 3(1):e103

Sanmorino A (2023) Emerging trends in cybersecurity for health technologies. J Ilm Inform Glob 14(3):76–81

Sarker IH (2021a) Machine learning: algorithms, real-world applications and research directions. SN Comput Sci 2(3):160

Sarker IH (2021b) Deep learning: a comprehensive overview on techniques, taxonomy, applications and research directions. SN Comput Sci 2(6):420

Satapathy P, Hermis AH, Rustagi S, Pradhan KB, Padhi BK, Sah R (2023) Artificial intelligence in surgical education and training: opportunities, challenges, and ethical considerations—correspondence. Int J Surg 109(5):1543–1544

Sauerbrei A, Kerasidou A, Lucivero F, Hallowell N (2023) The impact of artificial intelligence on the person-centred, doctor-patient relationship: some problems and solutions. BMC Med Inform Decis Mak 23(1):73

Schubert T, Oosterlinck T, Stevens RD, Maxwell PH, Van Der Schaar M (2025) AI education for clinicians eClin-

icalMedicine 79:102968. https://doi.org/10.1016/j.eclinm.2024.102968
Secinaro S, Calandra D, Secinaro A, Muthurangu V, Biancone P (2021) The role of artificial intelligence in healthcare: a structured literature review. BMC Med Inform Decis Mak 21(1):125
Seh AH, Zarour M, Alenezi M, Sarkar AK, Agrawal A, Kumar R et al (2020) Healthcare data breaches: insights and implications. Healthc Basel Switz 8(2):133
Shanmuga Priya K, Mani AP, Geethalakshmi S, Yadav S (2024) Advancements in artificial intelligence for the diagnosis of multidrug resistance and extensively drug-resistant tuberculosis: a comprehensive review. Cureus 16(5):e60280. https://doi.org/10.7759/cureus.60280
Shick AA, Webber CM, Kiarashi N, Weinberg JP, Deoras A, Petrick N et al (2024) Transparency of artificial intelligence/machine learning-enabled medical devices. Npj Digit Med 7(1):21
Shinners L, Aggar C, Grace S, Smith S (2020) Exploring healthcare professionals' understanding and experiences of artificial intelligence technology use in the delivery of healthcare: an integrative review. Health Informatics J 26(2):1225–1236
Siddiqui R, Zafar A, Qazi SA (2023) Artificial intelligence and the future of healthcare in Pakistan: opportunities and challenges. J Pak Med Assoc 73(10):1944–1946
Siegmann C, Anderljung M (2022) The Brussels effect and artificial intelligence. Politics and International Relations. https://doi.org/10.33774/apsa-2022-vxtsl
Silva DS, Smith MJ, Upshur REG (2013) Disadvantaging the disadvantaged: when public health policies and practices negatively affect marginalized populations. Can J Public Health 104(5):e410–e412
Simon MA, Wald SI, Howe AS, Toups L (2015) Evolvable mars campaign long duration habitation strategies: architectural approaches to enable human exploration missions. In: AIAA SPACE 2015 conference and exposition. American Institute of Aeronautics and Astronautics, Pasadena. https://doi.org/10.2514/6.2015-4514
Smith H (2021) Clinical AI: opacity, accountability, responsibility and liability. AI Soc 36(2):535–545
Solanki P, Grundy J, Hussain W (2023) Operationalising ethics in artificial intelligence for healthcare: a framework for AI developers. AI Ethics. 3(1):223–240
Sørensen K, Van Den Broucke S, Fullam J, Doyle G, Pelikan J, Slonska Z et al (2012) Health literacy and public health: a systematic review and integration of definitions and models. BMC Public Health 12(1):80
Sreerama J, Krishnamoorthy G (2022) Ethical considerations in AI addressing bias and fairness in machine learning models. J Knowl Learn Sci Technol ISSN 2959-6386 Online 1(1):130–138
Stamer T, Steinhäuser J, Flägel K (2023) Artificial intelligence supporting the training of communication skills in the education of health care professions: scoping review. J Med Internet Res 25:e43311
Stigall W (2022) The Hippocratic Oath. Linacre Q 89(3):275–286
Storeng KT, Fukuda-Parr S, Mahajan M, Venkatapuram S (2021) Digital technology and the political determinants of health inequities: special issue introduction. Glob Policy 12(S6):5–11
Sujan M, Furniss D, Grundy K, Grundy H, Nelson D, Elliott M et al (2019) Human factors challenges for the safe use of artificial intelligence in patient care. BMJ Health Care Inform 26(1):e100081
Tan LF, Heng JJY, Teo DB (2024) Response to: 'The next paradigm shift? ChatGPT, artificial intelligence, and medical education'. Med Teach 46(1):151–152
Taylor RM (2013) Ethical principles and concepts in medicine. In: Handbook of clinical neurology. Elsevier, pp 1–9. https://doi.org/10.1016/B978-0-444-53501-6.00001-9
Thakkar A, Gupta A, De Sousa A (2024) Artificial intelligence in positive mental health: a narrative review. Front Digit Health 6:1280235
The White House (2022). Blueprint for an AI Bill of Rights [Internet]. White House Office of Science and Technology Policy. 2022 [cited 2024 Aug 22]. Available from: https://www.whitehouse.gov/wp--content/uploads/2022/10/Blueprint-for-an-AI-Bill-of-Rights.pdf
Torkzadehmahani R, Nasirigerdeh R, Blumenthal DB, Kacprowski T, List M, Matschinske J et al (2022) Privacy-preserving artificial intelligence techniques in biomedicine. Methods Inf Med 61(S 01):e12–e27
Tresp V, Marc Overhage J, Bundschus M, Rabizadeh S, Fasching PA, Yu S (2016) Going digital: A survey on digitalization and large-scale data analytics in healthcare. Proc IEEE 104(11):2180–2206
U.S. Food and Drug Administration (2021) FDA releases Artificial Intelligence/Machine Learning Action Plan. FDA Newsroom, Press Announcements, 12 January. Accessed 2nd February 2025
Van Kolfschooten HB (2024) A health-conformant reading of the GDPR's right not to be subject to automated decision-making. Med Law Rev 32(3):373–391
Varkey B (2021) Principles of clinical ethics and their application to practice. Med Princ Pract 30(1):17–28
Vinuesa R, Azizpour H, Leite I, Balaam M, Dignum V, Domisch S et al (2020) The role of artificial intelligence in achieving the sustainable development goals. Nat Commun 11:233. https://doi.org/10.1038/s41467-019-14108-y
Wagner JK (2020) The Federal Trade Commission and consumer protections for mobile health apps. J Law Med Ethics 48(S1):103–114
Wahl B, Cossy-Gantner A, Germann S, Schwalbe NR (2018) Artificial intelligence (AI) and global health: how can AI contribute to health in resource-poor settings? BMJ Glob Health 3(4):e000798
Waisberg E, Ong J, Paladugu P, Kamran SA, Zaman N, Lee AG et al (2022) Challenges of artificial intelligence in space medicine. Space Sci Technol 2022:9852872

Wang Y (2024) The impact of the artificial intelligence act on ChatGPT. Lect Notes Educ Psychol Public Media 44(1):185–192

Wesson DE, Lucey CR, Cooper LA (2019) Building trust in health systems to eliminate health disparities. JAMA 322(2):111

White RJ, Averner M (2001) Humans in space. Nature 409(6823):1115–1118

Williams D, Hornung H, Nadimpalli A, Peery A (2021) Deep learning and its application for healthcare delivery in low and middle income countries. Front Artif Intell 4:553987

Williamson SM, Prybutok V (2024) Balancing privacy and progress: a review of privacy challenges, systemic oversight, and patient perceptions in AI-driven healthcare. Appl Sci 14(2):675

World Health Organization (2021) Ethics and governance of artificial intelligence for health: WHO guidance. World Health Organization, Geneva. Licence: CC BY-NC-SA 3.0 IGO

World Health Organization (2023) Regulatory considerations on artificial intelligence for health. World Health Organization, Geneva

World Health Organization (2024) Ethics and governance of artificial intelligence for health: large multi-modal models. WHO Guidance, 1st edn. World Health Organization, Geneva, p 1

Xiao C, Choi E, Sun J (2018) Opportunities and challenges in developing deep learning models using electronic health records data: a systematic review. J Am Med Inform Assoc 25(10):1419–1428

Xivuri K, Twinomurinzi H (2023) How AI developers can assure algorithmic fairness. Discov Artif Intell 3. https://doi.org/10.21203/rs.3.rs-2820618/v1

Xu Y, Jiang Z, Ting DSW, Kow AWC, Bello F, Car J et al (2024) Medical education and physician training in the era of artificial intelligence. Singapore Med J 65(3):159–166

Yadav N, Pandey S, Gupta A, Dudani P, Gupta S, Rangarajan K (2023) Data privacy in healthcare: in the era of artificial intelligence. Indian Dermatol Online J 14(6):788–792

Yeasmin S (2019) Benefits of artificial intelligence in medicine. In: 2019 2nd International Conference on Computer Applications & Information Security (ICCAIS). IEEE, Riyadh, pp 1–6. https://doi.org/10.1109/CAIS.2019.8769557

Yordanova K, Bertels N (2024) Regulating AI: challenges and the way forward through regulatory sandboxes. In: Sousa Antunes H, Freitas PM, Oliveira AL, Martins Pereira C, Vaz De Sequeira E, Barreto Xavier L (eds) Multidisciplinary perspectives on artificial intelligence and the law, Law, Governance and Technology Series, vol 58. Springer International Publishing, Cham, pp 441–456. https://doi.org/10.1007/978-3-031-41264-6

Zarei M, Eftekhari Mamaghani H, Abbasi A, Hosseini MS (2024) Application of artificial intelligence in medical education: a review of benefits, challenges, and solutions. Med Clínica Práctica 7(2):100422

Zechmeister-Koss I, Stanak M, Wolf S (2019) The status of health economic evaluation within decision making in Austria. Wien Med Wochenschr 169(11–12):271–283

Zhang W, Cai M, Lee HJ, Evans R, Zhu C, Ming C (2024a) AI in medical education: global situation, effects and challenges. Educ Inf Technol 29(4):4611–4633

Zhang X, Ma L, Sun D, Yi M, Wang Z (2024b) Artificial intelligence in telemedicine: a global perspective visualization analysis. Telemed E-Health. https://doi.org/10.1089/tmj.2023.0704

6 The Role of Artificial Intelligence in Medical Education

Aida Kafai Golahmadi, Arian Arjomandi Rad, and Thanos Athanasiou

Abstract

The chapter explores the groundbreaking role of Artificial Intelligence (AI) in medical education, highlighting its potential to enhance learning outcomes, streamline processes, and prepare future healthcare professionals for the complexities of modern medicine. The integration of AI-driven technologies, such as adaptive learning platforms, virtual simulations, and predictive analytics, offers personalized educational experiences tailored to the unique needs of individual students. By analyzing vast datasets, AI can identify knowledge gaps, recommend targeted resources, and facilitate mastery of clinical skills through immersive simulations.

We delve into how AI fosters collaborative learning environments, enabling students and educators to engage in meaningful interactions and peer-to-peer exchanges. Case studies illustrate successful implementations of AI tools in various medical schools, demonstrating significant improvements in student performance and retention rates. Ethical considerations surrounding the use of AI in education, including data privacy and the need for human oversight, are also addressed, ensuring a balanced perspective on technology's impact.

Ultimately, this chapter advocates for the continued integration of AI in medical education, emphasizing its capacity to cultivate a more effective, efficient, and equitable learning landscape that equips future healthcare professionals with the skills necessary to thrive in an increasingly complex medical environment.

Keywords

Artificial Intelligence · Medical Education · Learning Enhancement · Simulation · Data-Driven · Personalized Training

6.1 Introduction

6.1.1 Overview of the Current State of Medical Education

Contemporary medical education is moving away from the traditional didactic approach and standardized curricula towards individualized

A. Kafai Golahmadi (✉)
The Whittington Hospital, London, UK
e-mail: a.kafaigolahmadi@nhs.net

A. Arjomandi Rad
Department of Cardiothoracic Surgery, Maastricht University Medical Center, Maastricht, The Netherlands

Department of Cardiothoracic Surgery, John Radcliffe Hospital, Oxford University Hospitals NHS Foundation Trust, Oxford, UK

T. Athanasiou
Department of Surgery and Cancer, Imperial College London, London, UK

J. Malawana et al. (eds.), *Artificial Intelligence in Healthcare and Biomedical Visualization*, Biomedical Visualization 10, https://doi.org/10.1007/978-3-032-06520-9_6

learning trajectories that accommodate diverse learning styles and cognitive frameworks (Piumatti et al. 2021). This paradigm shift is driven by the rapidly evolving and multifaceted nature of modern healthcare, coupled with an increasingly nuanced understanding of social determinants of health, which demands the integration of technological innovations, such as virtual reality, simulation, and online learning platforms, to facilitate a comprehensive and holistic approach to medical education (Elendu et al. 2024; Sato et al. 2024). Key challenges of this transition include the implementation of competency-based education (CBE), the promotion of interprofessional education, and the effective integration of technology (Frank et al. 2010; Kosiol et al. 2024).

Despite the persistent underfunding of research into medical education, which delays quality assurance and accreditation processes (Majumder et al. 2023), the advent of the Covid-19 pandemic has accelerated these implementations and has forced educators across the globe to adopt an open mind towards technological advances (Chen and Mullen 2020). On the other hand, these recent reforms, whilst enhancing the delivery of a personalized and flexible learning experience, risk inadvertently diminishing the depth of foundational biomedical science knowledge, which is fundamental to the formation of the future physician–scientist working in a multidisciplinary team (Challa et al. 2021). This, combined with transitioning from traditional grading systems to pass/fail evaluations, generates unintended negative consequences, including a potential decline in physicians who practice bench to bedside (Buja 2019).

6.1.2 Introduction to AI and Its Relevance in Medical Education

AI-powered platforms leverage machine learning and big data analytics to deliver educational content tailored to the individual's needs and learning style, and AI-driven assessment tools facilitate comprehensive competency-based evaluations and generate real-time, customized constructive feedback (Chan and Zary 2019). The three main emerging applications of AI in medical education include AI-driven learning support systems, assessment methodologies, and curriculum review tools; however, several reservations persist among academic institutions regarding their efficacy and proficiency and the ethical implications (Chan and Zary 2019).

Virtual inquiry systems, distance learning platforms, and AI-generated teaching videos are improving access to diversified educational resources, and we are witnessing AI's potential to enhance both the analytical and humanistic dimensions of medical education, particularly for the growing population of digitally native learners (Mir et al. 2023). Nonetheless, we have encountered several challenges, including the ethical implications of AI use, the need to overcome technical hurdles, and the necessity to provide comprehensive training to both educators and students on AI's applications, benefits, and limitations, to effectively integrate it into their practice (Mir et al. 2023; Ali et al. 2024a, b). These steps require strong organizational support and a commitment from all stakeholders to embrace this transformative technology (Narayanan et al. 2023).

AI is also automating the scoring of objective tests, analyzing complex written responses, and offering detailed feedback on procedural skills using virtual reality simulations and sophisticated analysis of recorded procedures (Narayanan et al. 2023). On the academic front, AI is streamlining research, supporting literature reviews and complex data analysis, and improving administrative efficiency by automating tasks such as admissions, record-keeping, and budgeting (Narayanan et al. 2023; Mizumoto and Eguchi 2023). While recognizing challenges such as the need for substantial datasets and the imperative to mitigate biases, the responsible integration of AI offers a substantial potential for improving efficiency and efficacy in medical education (Narayanan et al. 2023; Mennella et al. 2024).

A staged curriculum approach should integrate foundational mathematical and data science concepts in preclinical years and then progress to clinical applications and ethical considerations, to prepare future physicians for the complexities of AI-driven healthcare (Paranjape et al. 2019).

6.1.3 Purpose of the Chapter and an Overview of Emerging Trends

This chapter delves into the burgeoning field of artificial intelligence (AI) applications within medical education, aiming to provide a comprehensive and nuanced understanding of its transformative potential. Its primary purpose is to showcase the diverse ways AI is being integrated into various aspects of medical training, moving beyond simple technological descriptions to explore the pedagogical implications and challenges inherent in its implementation. The chapter will not only catalogue the existing applications of AI but will critically analyze their effectiveness, limitations, and ethical considerations. It will also examine AI's role in personalizing learning experiences, moving beyond the "one-size-fits-all" approach of traditional didactic methods towards AI-powered tutoring systems that adapt to individual learning styles and provide tailored feedback, intelligent assessment tools that offer richer insights into student understanding, and AI-driven simulations that create immersive and realistic clinical scenarios for practice.

Furthermore, the chapter will address how AI is employed to curate and update medical knowledge bases, ensuring curricula remain current and relevant to the ever-evolving field of medicine. The integration of AI into assessment is another key focus, examining the use of automated scoring systems, AI-powered essay grading, and the development of AI-driven tools to evaluate clinical reasoning and procedural skills. This analysis will extend beyond purely technical applications, considering the impact of AI on the assessment of soft skills, communication, and teamwork, essential qualities for effective medical practice.

Beyond these applications, the chapter will critically address the ethical and practical considerations surrounding the use of AI in medical education, carefully examining issues related to data privacy and security, algorithmic bias and fairness, and the need for transparency and accountability in the use of AI-driven tools. We will also discuss the necessary infrastructure and resources required to effectively integrate AI into medical education programs, including the need for faculty development, robust technical support, and equitable access for all learners. Ultimately, this chapter aims to provide medical educators, administrators, and policymakers with a clear and insightful understanding of the transformative potential, limitations, and ethical implications of AI in medical education, fostering informed decision-making and responsible implementation of this powerful technology.

6.2 The Evolution of Medical Education

6.2.1 Historical Perspective on Medical Education

The history of medical education reflects the broader evolution of society, with its roots extending back to ancient civilizations where knowledge was passed orally from practitioners to apprentices (Buja 2019). One of the earliest formal medical schools emerged in ancient Greece around 400 BC, with Hippocrates pioneering the practice of observation and documentation: his empirical methodology laid the groundwork for systematic diagnoses and the pillars of medical ethics, which remain integral to the profession (Kleisiaris et al. 2014).

The formalization of medical education gained momentum during the Middle Ages with the establishment of the University of Salerno in Italy in the nineteenth century, widely regarded as Europe's first medical school, which introduced a structured curriculum integrating theoretical learning with practical applications (Della Monica et al. 2013). This foundation was further strengthened during the Renaissance by Andreas Vesalius's seminal work, *De humani corporis fabrica*, which underscored the importance of dissection and hands-on learning, advancing evidence-based approaches to medical sciences (Vasalius 1543; Zampieri et al. 2015).

In the nineteenth century, institutions such as Johns Hopkins University introduced more rigorous medical training and, with the transformative Abraham Flexner's 1910 report, standardized medical education across North America by establishing stringent admissions and training requirements and emphasizing the integration of biomedical research into medical practice (Flexner 1910; Duffy 2011).

The introduction of problem-based learning (PBL) in the 1960s represented a paradigm shift, fostering critical thinking and the application of knowledge to clinical scenarios, promoting active learning and patient–centered care (Gwee 2009). Meanwhile, the advances in pedagogy led to the incorporation of organ-system-based curricula, promoting integration across disciplines and a multidisciplinary approach to the cases (Obi et al. 2021).

Medical education's development during the twentieth century can be categorized into three distinct eras: the master-apprentice model before 1910, the Flexnerian period (1910–1970) focused on science-based learning, and the contemporary emphasis on society-centered education (Balcioglu et al. 2015). Current undergraduate medical programs aim to equip students with critical thinking skills, professionalism, and an awareness of the social determinants of health, whilst encouraging lifelong self-development and reflective practices in a holistic, evidence-based framework (Lim et al. 2023).

The twenty-first century global healthcare systems are increasingly under pressure to optimize clinical training provision due to the growing number of healthcare professionals and tighter regulations for using patients and human specimens in clinical training, such as The Human Tissue Act 2004 (Taylor and Wilson 2007). These, coupled with the changes brought into education worldwide by the COVID-19 pandemic, have led to innovative solutions such as simulated case-based learning, where clinical scenarios are replicated at lower costs and without the need of real patients, online lectures, which exponentially grow the audience without added costs, and virtual reality sets which can replicate any reality in a 3D version giving an immersive and tangible experience of the event (Papapanou et al. 2022).

While not replacing real-world experience, simulations allow for deliberate, sequenced learning that promotes skill acquisition and diagnostic reasoning, leveraging situated learning and communities of practice (Norman 2012). These frameworks view learning as an inherently social and context-driven activity. Where students begin as peripheral participants in professional communities, gradually assuming greater responsibilities and developing expertise (Mann 2011).

Other technological advances, namely mobile applications and social media platforms, have enabled interactive and personalized learning experiences, which align with the broader shift toward distance learning and student-centered education, fostering engagement and adaptability (Kerimbayev et al. 2023).

6.2.2 From Traditional to Technology-Enhanced Medical Education: The Role of AI

The early twenty-first century marked the beginning of the medical education technology (MedTech) era, driven by the adoption of computer-based tools and online resources, which facilitated the dissemination and accessibility of knowledge at a greater scale and faster rate; despite disparities in digital access and faculty resistance to adopting new technologies (Chowdhury et al. 2024; O'Doherty et al. 2018). Early innovations, such as photographic slides, film strips, and overhead projectors, were promptly followed by the integration of multimedia tools, online platforms, virtual reality (VR), and augmented reality (AR) simulations from the early 2010s, which fundamentally revolutionized the field, enabling interactive and personalized learning experiences (Chowdhury et al. 2024; Kuehn 2018).

Future trends point toward AI-driven platforms, adaptive learning, and immersive simulations to further personalize learning and overcome geographical barriers, however, we must also ensure traditional bedside teaching to support the development of *soft skills* as well as solid basic science knowledge (Chowdhury et al. 2024) and maintain the human dimension in doctor-patient relationships (Tokuç and Varol 2023).

A successful example of this is the A.T. Still University's (ATSU) technology-enhanced active learning for medical education (TEAL-MEd), which integrated games and virtual patient simulations into its curriculum to adapt to evolving student learning styles; employing four platforms (McCoy et al. 2015):

1. TurningPoint for interactive pauses.
2. Bravo for quiz games.
3. Prognosis-ATSU for mobile clinical simulations.
4. DecisionSim for virtual patient scenarios.

The program received overwhelmingly positive feedback from the students, which led to its successful integration into various courses, and the team is currently aiming to expand TEAL-MEd to encompass community health center care delivery (McCoy et al. 2015).

On the other hand, a review of journal articles from 1998 to 2016 on mobile technology-enhanced medical education reveals that while mobile learning applications are increasing, they remain less prevalent than other methods, as they predominantly focus on knowledge comprehension and skills acquisition, with less emphasis on higher-order thinking skills and hands-on skills (Chang and Hwang 2018).

As technology continues its rapid advancement, AI emerges as a transformative force poised to further revolutionize medical education (Dignum 2021; Knopp et al. 2023; Sapci 2020), owing to its potential to personalize learning, enhance assessment methods, and support immersive training environments. However, addressing the ethical implications of AI while maintaining the centrality of human teaching elements will be critical in creating a balanced and effective learning environment for future healthcare providers (Dignum 2021; Knopp et al. 2023; Sapci 2020).

Similarly, challenges such as ensuring equitable access to technology and concerns about misinformation must be proactively addressed; thus, a hybrid model of medical education, combining traditional methods with innovative technologies, is currently believed to be the ideal way of effectively preparing future doctors for the complexities of modern healthcare (Tokuç and Varol 2023).

6.3 Personalized Learning Experiences

6.3.1 Definition and Importance of Personalized Learning

Personalized learning (PL) has emerged as a transformative educational approach, grounded in metacognitive principles, that adapts to the unique needs, preferences, and learning styles of individuals. Personalized learning encompasses diverse methods such as mentoring, tutoring, and coaching, which foster development across emotional, intellectual, and physical dimensions (Skrzypek et al. 2016). It is a dynamic process, continuously adapting instruction to align with learners' progress and characteristics, ensuring relevance and effectiveness (Tetzlaff et al. 2020).

A review by Walkington et al., exploring PL across various subjects and educational levels, revealed that while PL is widely adopted, it often lacks clear conceptualization and robust theoretical underpinnings due to the challenges in promoting learner agency (Walkington and Bernacki 2020).

In a critical interpretive synthesis of 71 empirical studies (2006–2019) to examine PL implementation in K-12 settings, two major themes emerged: the pivotal role of technology and the influence of contextual factors (Zhang et al. 2020).

Several studies then demonstrated that personalized learning enhanced academic success in medical education by tailoring educational strategies to students' metacognitive profiles—such as "Active," "Pragmatic," "Theoretical," and "Reflective"—which significantly improved engagement, satisfaction, and performance, especially in challenging subjects such as anatomy (Stambuk-Castellano et al. 2024).

Large language models, like ChatGPT, are also being used to personalize learning in medical education as they can offer tutoring, patient simulation, and examination question generation, enhancing tailored learning through evidence-based strategies like active recall and memory cues (Arango-Ibañez et al. 2023).

Personalized learning has become a cornerstone of competency-based medical education (CBME), which seeks to balance individual learner needs with standardized outcomes (Gifford et al. 2020) and technology plays an integral role in advancing this field. Adaptive educational technologies create responsive learning environments that cater to individual needs, optimizing clinical performance and delivering timely feedback (Stambuk-Castellano et al. 2024; Sandars and Patel 2018). Emerging tools, including artificial intelligence, enhance accessibility and engagement, offering unprecedented opportunities to transform educational experiences (Castro et al. 2024).

6.3.2 Adaptive Learning Systems, Learning Analytics, and Data-Driven Insights

Adaptive learning systems personalize the learning experience by leveraging data-driven insights to tailor educational content, whilst learning analytics involves the measurement, collection, analysis, and reporting of data about learners and their contexts. The AI-driven integration of adaptive learning with learning analytics (LA) allows for a more nuanced understanding of student interactions and performance, enabling educators to provide targeted interventions and support, enhancing learning efficiency and effectiveness (Bojic et al. 2023; Mavroudi et al. 2018; Menon et al. 2017).

The implementation of competency-based medical education (CBME) has led to the accumulation of vast amounts of data, which can be analyzed to assess trainee performance and identify areas for improvement (Chan et al. 2018; Saqr 2015; Sundaram et al. 2024). LA also helps in understanding how students interact with digital platforms and the relationship between these interactions and their academic performance, hence allowing us to have a deeper understanding of whether these technological advances are having the desired outcome(Bojic et al. 2023; Chan et al. 2018).

Notably, the School of Medicine and Health Sciences at Tecnologico de Monterrey in Mexico developed a personalized learning model to address differences in students' entry-level knowledge. This model includes diagnostic tests to tailor learning paths in cell biology and chemistry, allowing students to learn at their own pace and improve their academic performance (Cardenas et al. 2022).

The use of big data from adaptive learning platforms provides valuable insights into student behavior and learning patterns and allows educators to identify factors that contribute to better learning outcomes. For instance, studies have shown that factors such as mobile device usage and group membership can influence student engagement with adaptive learning platforms (Menon et al. 2017; Liu et al. 2017; Sparrow et al. 2024; Sense et al. 2021).

In particular, we know that adaptive and intelligent systems support collaborative learning by facilitating peer interactions and domain-specific activities, hence improving both knowledge acquisition and collaboration skills (Magnisalis et al. 2011).

Despite the several advantages of these analytic systems, their integration into practice remains laborious due to concerns regarding data privacy, system complexity, and the need for a clear adaptation strategy (Renz and Hilbig 2020).

6.4 AI Tutors: Enhancing the Learning Experience

AI tutors and chatbots leverage advanced technologies such as natural language processing and machine learning to create interactive and engaging learning experiences that simulate real-life clinical scenarios, allowing students to apply theoretical knowledge in a practical context, whilst fostering independent learning and analytical skills.

Interestingly, in a study by Fazlollahi et al. (2022), AI tutoring systems outperformed remote expert instruction in teaching simulated surgical skills, providing effective metric-based assessments and feedback.

Chatbots, like ChatGPT, are being utilized by students as virtual teaching assistants, helping them with complex concepts, creating mnemonics, and summarizing research articles (Ghorashi et al. 2023; Guo and Li 2023), but they also assist educators in preparing the teaching materials and evaluating student performance (Mondal et al. 2023), in an almost symbiotic relationship.

Medical educators must adapt to these technologies while ensuring that AI tools are used as assistive rather than primary educational resources, due to their novelty and the difficulty in assessing the effectiveness of AI in education (Ghorashi et al. 2023; Chan and Zary 2019).

6.4.1 AI Tutors in Medical Schools: Case Studies

In recent years, the integration of artificial intelligence (AI) into educational settings has seen significant advancements, particularly within medical schools for practical and clinical skills training, and the following case studies highlight the varied implementations and outcomes of AI tutors that are revolutionizing the way healthcare students learn, practice, and prepare for their professional careers.

1. AI Medical School Tutor (MST): MST is designed to tutor medical students through interactions with Digital Virtual Patients, a natural language interface with realistic clinical cases authored by experts, which enables students to explore complex medical concepts dynamically, focusing on clinical reasoning, foundational knowledge application, and adaptive learning experiences. Field trials with third and fourth-year medical students showed positive outcomes, indicating MST's effectiveness in enhancing clinical reasoning skills (Afzal et al. 2020).
2. LearnGuide: a specialized ChatGPT tool that supports self-directed learning among medical students by providing problem-based training, and in a 14-week randomized trial, it showed significant improvements in self-directed learning and critical thinking, when compared to traditional methods, directly improving educational outcomes (Wang et al. 2024).
3. AI-Tutoring in Ophthalmology Clerkship: AI-tutoring module used in an ophthalmology clerkship to teach congenital cataracts. Students interacted with an AI diagnosis platform, which enhanced their understanding of disease signs and diagnosis, and they reported higher satisfaction and improved performance, particularly in understanding disease signs, compared to traditional lecture methods (Wu et al. 2020).
4. BotMD: an AI-powered chatbot designed specifically for healthcare professionals, which functions as a virtual assistant that streamlines the process of finding drug information, clinical guidelines, and answers to frequently asked medical questions. It can be customized to provide tailored responses based on an institution's internal protocols, hence it saves time for doctors and nurses, allowing them to focus more on patient care. Additionally, BotMD can assist with administrative tasks, such as scheduling and documentation, further alleviating the burden on healthcare providers.
5. PubMed Health: an AI-driven tool that enhances the capabilities of traditional PubMed searches by offering more refined and contextually relevant search results. It also provides summaries of the studies, making it easier to find pertinent information quickly, and it aids in understanding complex medical topics by presenting data and outcomes in user-friendly formats, thus supporting informed decision-making by helping users keep abreast of the latest medical evidence-based options.

6.4.2 Benefits of AI Tutors

The integration of AI tutors into medical education has garnered widespread appreciation across various specialties for several compelling reasons and as AI technology continues to evolve, its integration into medical curricula will likely expand.

Below, we explore the most widely appreciated benefits of AI tutors, which have led to their implementation in medical education.

1. Personalized Learning Experience
   Unlike traditional teaching methods that often follow a one-size-fits-all approach, AI tutors analyze students' performance and learning styles to deliver customized content and resources, which facilitates mastery of complex concepts at each student's own pace, leading to improved retention and understanding (Arango-Ibañez et al. 2023).
2. Immediate Feedback and Assessment
   AI tutors offer real-time personalized feedback, allowing students to identify areas of strength and weakness instantly, which allows learners to adjust their study strategies accordingly, fostering a more adaptive learning environment. The ability to receive timely responses to questions and quizzes enhances the learning process, enabling students to correct mistakes and solidify their understanding as they go along (Chan and Zary 2019; Nagi et al. 2023; Stamer et al. 2022).
3. Access to Vast Resources
   AI tutors have access to extensive databases of medical literature and clinical guidelines, allowing students to explore topics beyond their coursework and engage with current medical issues, hence supporting their evidence-based training (Lozano et al. 2023). This offers a unique opportunity to apply their curiosity and challenge existing concepts which may no longer be valid, as medicine and science are evolving fields where recommendations often change based on the latest available evidence.
4. Simulation of Real-World Scenarios
   Many AI tutors are designed to simulate real-world medical scenarios, providing students with the opportunity to practice clinical skills in a safe, controlled environment where they can build their confidence and competence before entering clinical practice. For example, virtual patient interactions allow learners to hone their diagnostic and communication skills without the risk of impacting patient safety (Kononowicz et al. 2019). In one study, where ChatGPT was used to generate patient information and simulate clinical scenarios, students reported high levels of satisfaction and learning progress, indicating the potential of AI to improve educational outcomes (Thomae et al. 2024).
5. Enhanced Collaboration and Communication Skills
   AI tutors are utilized to foster collaborative learning environments, where small groups of students interact with an AI-powered chatbot and each other, to enhance teamwork and communication skills. The learners discuss cases and challenge each other's thinking, and the AI-powered tutor mediates resolution and offers innovative solutions to challenging scenarios, like a real clinical tutor, preparing students for the interdisciplinary nature of modern healthcare, where teamwork and leadership are integral to the functioning of the system (Wu et al. 2020; Patiño and Peñafiel 2023).
6. Time Efficiency for Educators
   The implementation of AI tutors also benefits educators by automating and streamlining administrative tasks such as grading and providing feedback, so that instructors can devote more time to mentoring and coaching, ultimately enhancing the educational experience (Ahmad et al. 2022; Zawacki-Richter et al. 2019).

The myriad benefits of AI tutors—ranging from personalized learning experiences to efficiently accessing educational resources—not only enhance the knowledge and skills of medical students but also prepare them for a future where they can deliver high-quality patient care. As AI technology continues to evolve, its integration into medical training will likely expand, opening new avenues for educational excellence and improved healthcare outcomes.

Nevertheless, it is important to acknowledge the several challenges this implies, mostly related to the technical difficulties in developing AI applications, assessing their effectiveness, as well as addressing ethical concerns, such as algorithmic bias and data privacy, to ensure equitable access to AI-driven educational tools (Chan and Zary 2019; Abd-Alrazaq et al. 2023; McLean 2024).

6.4.3 Integration of AI in Curriculum Design

The integration of artificial intelligence (AI) into medical education is transforming the way medical students learn and interact with complex medical concepts, and it has now become necessary to include AI-specific competencies in the medical curricula to teach students the correct way of using these tools. A recent scoping review identified several educational programs and frameworks that focus on teaching AI principles to medical students, residents, and practicing physicians, providing them with a comprehensive understanding of AI applications in medicine and the theoretical design of these algorithms (Tolentino et al. 2024).

Stakeholders highlight the importance of standardized AI learning objectives in medical curricula, and currently, the emphasis is on developing AI competencies, which include understanding AI technologies, programming skills, and clinical applications through innovative teaching methods (Moldt et al. 2024).

Up to this date, specific curricula have been developed to address AI's role in a particular medical speciality, namely ophthalmology (Tolentino et al. 2024); however, these will need to be expanded to other specialties and preclinical sciences as well, to ensure a comprehensive understanding of AI applications.

The need for standardized frameworks and competencies to guide AI curriculum development is complicated by the current lack of consensus on content and delivery methods, which also impedes the development of standardized assessments of AI theories (Lee et al. 2021).

An increasing number of medical schools are now integrating AI as a longitudinal theme across their curricula, including an exploration of a diverse array of AI tools, alongside a comprehensive framework for the engineering and design of AI solutions, whilst emphasizing the critical role that data plays in driving innovations within the domain of AI (Grunhut et al. 2021).

Simultaneously, various programs are emphasizing the teaching of AI ethics, incorporating principles such as autonomy, beneficence, nonmaleficence, and justice, alongside public health ethics principles like efficiency and common good orientation to ensure ethical dilemmas are addressed comprehensively (Weidener and Fischer 2023; Weidener and Fischer 2024a, b).

The University of Illinois College of Medicine (UICOM) implemented a modular 4-week AI elective for fourth-year medical students in 2019, integrating AI with evidence-based medicine and employing a competency-based, constructivist approach. They developed online modules simulating real-world healthcare tasks to teach AI applications without requiring prior technical skills, with a focus on both clinical and preclinical subjects. This initiative was evaluated across two cohorts (40 students total), and the program yielded significant improvements in both knowledge and practical application skills, as evidenced by high quiz and assignment scores, and student feedback highlighted the course's effectiveness in bridging theory and practice (Krive et al. 2023). The authors ultimately propose integrating AI education longitudinally, spanning preclinical and clinical years to maximize impact, and they suggest a phased approach, starting with foundational knowledge and progressing to real-world application, addressing the need for dedicated curricular time and faculty involvement (Krive et al. 2023).

The University of Toronto has taken a proactive approach to incorporating artificial intelligence (AI) education within its medical degrees by integrating substantial data science components into foundational health research curricula and a variety of extracurricular programs, utilizing advanced technological tools that students can practice using (McCoy et al. 2020).

The Massachusetts Institute of Technology (MIT) has also introduced the Critical Data initiative, which features a unique series of events known as "datathons," tailored to enhance the educational experience of medical students by immersing them in practical, data-driven challenges that underscore the significance of data science in medical education. Through these hands-on events, students gain valuable insights into the application of AI in healthcare settings, fostering a harmonious blend of theoretical knowledge and practical skills essential for the evolving landscape of medicine (McCoy et al. 2020).

Although the positive results are encouraging, limitations in the course delivery format and resource requirements pose challenges to widespread implementation. Future research should focus on integrating AI education into required curricula and assessing its long-term impact on students' clinical practice.

6.4.4 The Use of AI in Assessment and Evaluation

AI technologies, in addition to enriching the learning experience, are progressively being employed to transform conventional assessment practices: by automating evaluations and delivering real-time feedback, these tools enable the adoption of more dynamic and continuous assessment models, thereby streamlining and enhancing the efficiency of the evaluation process (Varma et al. 2023; Narayanan et al. 2023).

This shift is particularly evident in competency-based medical education (CBME), where AI aids in creating continuous feedback loops that promote assessment for learning rather than merely an assessment of learning, allowing the students to act on the feedback in real-time and apply the acquired knowledge and skills as they go along (Lentz et al. 2021).

AI technologies, such as Artificial Neural Networks (ANN) and Convolutional Neural Networks (CNN), are being used to develop innovative assessment methods in anatomy, where traditional teaching, heavily reliant on cadaveric dissection, faces challenges like resource limitations, time constraints, and potentially hazardous working conditions (Abdellatif et al. 2022). While various technological advancements, such as 3D models, virtual and augmented reality, and even body painting, have been incorporated to improve learning, these methods often lack robust evaluation and comprehensive integration into existing curricula, and the COVID-19 pandemic further underscored the need for adaptable and flexible teaching strategies (Abdellatif et al. 2022). Abdellatif et al. suggest several novel applications of AI in anatomy education, including virtual reality simulations, deep learning tools for complex anatomical structures, and AI-powered assessment systems (Abdellatif et al. 2022).

AI can automate the assessment of written responses and provide feedback on medical image interpretations with high reliability, thus improving the efficiency and accuracy of evaluations and reducing the time and workforce required to mark the assessments (Tolsgaard et al. 2023). Moreover, AI facilitates authentic assessments by enabling immersive, project-based learning experiences that are more aligned with real-world applications, to not only accommodate diverse learning styles but also foster critical thinking and creativity among medical students (Fatima et al. 2024).

In a study conducted in multiple institutions in Pakistan, AI was integrated into the anatomy curriculum to provide students with personalized feedback on their dissection techniques by using machine learning algorithms to analyze video recordings of dissections and provide students with detailed feedback on their performance. This approach not only improved students' practical skills but also enhanced their understanding of anatomical structures, owing to the ability to analyze every fine movement that may have escaped the human eye due to human factors, such as distraction (Fatima et al. 2024).

The Humanitas University Medical School in Milan, Italy, implemented an AI-driven natural language processing to evaluate students' interactions with patients in clinical settings and, provided real-time feedback on communication skills and clinical decision-making, essential competencies which are traditionally honed through repeated practice and feedback with a clinical tutor (Gordon et al. 2024). One could argue that this system allows us to minimize bias when providing feedback, as a human tutor may have certain communication style preferences or may even have an unconscious bias towards a specific scenario, whilst the automated system will be more objective, facilitating authentic assessments.

Current barriers to fully implementing these models include difficulties in developing AI applications, ensuring data integrity, the need for faculty training, resource requirements, and addressing ethical concerns such as algorithmic transparency and data privacy (Chan and Zary 2019; Abdellatif et al. 2022; Turner et al. 2023). Additionally, there is a need for continuous co-production and evaluation of AI technologies with diverse stakeholders to ensure that AI systems are objective and value-free (Lentz et al. 2021).

6.5 Ethical Considerations and Challenges in the Integration of AI in Medical Education

The integration of Artificial Intelligence (AI) into medical education presents a transformative opportunity, yet it also introduces a myriad of ethical considerations and challenges that must be addressed to ensure responsible and effective implementation.

AI systems in medicine can perpetuate or even exacerbate existing biases, leading to potential discrimination against certain patient groups, especially when these tools are increasingly used in diagnostics and treatment planning, where biased algorithms could result in unequal healthcare outcomes (Weidener and Fischer 2023; D'Souza et al. 2024).

Moreover, the opacity of AI algorithms, often referred to as "black box" systems, poses challenges in understanding how decisions are made and the resulting lack of transparency can hinder accountability, making it difficult to trace errors or biases back to their source (Zhui et al. 2024; D'Souza et al. 2024).

Another important consideration of the use of AI in patient care is the question of informed consent, as patients may not fully understand how AI is used in their treatment and, it is crucial to ensure patient autonomy in this process, as it involves navigating complex ethical landscapes where traditional consent processes may not suffice (Weidener and Fischer 2023; Katznelson and Gerke 2021; Lu et al. 2024).

Additionally, AI systems require vast amounts of data, raising concerns about patient privacy and data security, and the potential for data breaches or misuse of sensitive health information necessitates robust data protection measures (Zhui et al. 2024; D'Souza et al. 2024).

Equally, understanding and managing the interaction between humans and AI systems is crucial to prevent overreliance and ensure effective use, and in a recent scoping review, valid concerns have been identified, such as concerns about academic integrity (cheating), data accuracy, the propagation of misinformation ("hallucinations"), and the potential for over-reliance on AI, hindering critical thinking and problem-solving skills (Preiksaitis and Rose 2023). Based on these findings, the authors propose three crucial areas for future research: developing learners' critical evaluation skills for AI-generated content, rethinking assessment methodologies in light of AI capabilities, and investigating the dynamics of human-AI interaction in educational settings (Preiksaitis and Rose 2023).

The deployment of AI in medical education must be managed carefully to avoid widening educational disparities, and while AI can provide broader access to medical knowledge, it must be implemented in a way that ensures equitable access for all students (McLean 2024; Zhui et al. 2024).

Abd-Alrazaq et al., also critically examine the challenges associated with large language models (LLM), such as those in GPT series, further reflecting on ethical issues such as academic dishonesty (plagiarism) and copyright concerns, and they advocate for a responsible and effective use of LLMs while mitigating potential risks, with a robust ethical guidelines as a backbone of their development, to augment rather than replace human expertise (Abd-Alrazaq et al. 2023).

When it comes to replacing human clinical tutors with AI tutors, we must be wary of exacerbating existing social inequalities due to AI's potential to displace jobs, particularly in low-income countries, in addition to its unequal access based on socio-economic factors (Farhud and Zokaei 2021).

In conclusion, Artificial Intelligence, while potentially beneficial for certain tasks, cannot replicate the human element of human empathy and compassion in medical training, particularly in situations requiring emotional support and nuanced understanding. It is therefore of paramount importance to balance technological progress with ethical considerations, ensuring equitable access, upholding patient autonomy, and preserving the fundamental human element of healthcare (Farhud and Zokaei 2021).

6.5.1 Teaching AI Ethics

To address the ethical complexities discussed above, there is an emerging consensus on the importance of adopting a principled framework for AI ethics and embedding it into medical education in line with the pillars of medical ethics—autonomy, beneficence, nonmaleficence, and justice—and with the public health ethics tenets of efficiency, the common good and proportionality (Weidener and Fischer 2024a, b).

Incorporating real-world examples and case-based learning would facilitate a deeper understanding of the practical implications of AI ethics in medicine; thus, it would be beneficial to teach AI ethics using case-based discussion and simulated scenarios, in addition to theoretical and practical knowledge, to encourage critical thinking and problem-solving skills (Weidener and Fischer 2023; Weidener and Fischer 2024a, b; Katznelson and Gerke 2021).

Given the inherently interdisciplinary nature of AI's ethical challenges, multidisciplinary collaboration with fields such as computer science, law, and social sciences is essential to ensure a comprehensive understanding of the ethical landscape and equip students to navigate complex issues (Lu et al. 2024).

As AI technologies continue to advance, so must educational strategies and content; thus, ongoing research is required to develop competency-based learning objectives and adapt medical curricula to the rapidly evolving role of AI in healthcare (Weidener and Fischer 2024a, b; Lee 2023).

A recent scoping review identified a scarcity of publications focused on teaching AI ethics in medical education, with very recent and primarily theoretical studies, which unanimously agree on the need for incorporating AI ethics into medical curricula; however, their recommendations regarding the teaching content and methods are very different. Some advocate for a complete curriculum overhaul, emphasizing empathy and knowledge management, while others propose integrating AI ethics within existing ethical frameworks. (Weidener and Fischer 2023).

Due to a lack of empirical studies, further research on the development of standardized teaching content and methodologies, and on a clearer understanding of the ethical dimensions of AI in medicine is mandatory to bridge these gaps (Weidener and Fischer 2023).

By equipping future medical professionals with the necessary knowledge and skills to address these challenges, we can ensure that the integration of AI into medicine is both ethical and beneficial.

6.5.2 Future Directions and Innovations in Medical Education

The growing need to incorporate AI into medical curricula has prompted medical schools to embed AI as a longitudinal thread across their existing modules, to provide students with a comprehensive experience of AI tools, understanding of the engineering of AI solutions, and an appreciation of the ethical implications of AI in clinical practice (Grunhut et al. 2021; Bohler et al. 2024), fostering a patient-centered digital future in medicine (Ejaz et al. 2022).

To address the qualitative differences AI introduces, such as concerns about explainability, health equity, and data security, educators must focus on developing robust data science competencies, practically integrating data science-focused content into existing medical curricula and offering extracurricular programs to cultivate leadership in AI (McCoy et al. 2020). The University of Toronto Faculty of Medicine and MIT Critical Data's "datathons" serve as exemplary models for such initiatives, emphasizing the importance of a dual-focused approach in AI education (McCoy et al. 2020).

Generative AI technologies, such as Chat GPT and Bard, present new opportunities for self-directed learning, simulation scenarios, and writing assistance; however, they also pose challenges related to academic integrity and data accuracy. Future research should focus on developing learners' skills to critically evaluate AI, rethinking assessment methodologies, and studying human–AI interactions to maximize the benefits of generative AI while mitigating its risks (Preiksaitis and Rose 2023).

As AI becomes a mainstay in healthcare settings, it is crucial for medical educators to address the ethical implications of AI-driven clinical decision-making, and physicians must practice incorporating AI predictions ethically and effectively into their professional capabilities. This requires a curriculum that includes study cases with AI recommendations, fostering critical decision-making skills and an understanding of the ethical landscape of AI in medicine (Grunhut et al. 2021).

The global perspective on AI in medical education highlights the need for interregional collaboration to enhance research quality: the United States, along with institutions like Harvard Medical School and the University of Toronto, is leading the way in AI research in medical education (Wang et al. 2023). Furthermore, there is an urgent need to bolster collaboration across regions to ensure that advancements in AI are accessible and beneficial to medical students worldwide, by providing foundational technology and robust AI teaching in low- and middle-income countries to drive innovation in their healthcare settings (Ejaz et al. 2022).

The future of medical education lies in the seamless integration of AI into healthcare curricula, fostering a new generation of healthcare providers who are proficient in AI technologies and competencies. By addressing ethical considerations and promoting global collaboration, medical education can harness the full potential of AI to enhance learning and ultimately improve patient care; hence, ongoing research and innovation will be essential to navigate the challenges and opportunities this new technology presents.

6.6 Conclusion

6.6.1 Summary of the Transformative Impact of AI in Medical Education

The transformative impact of Artificial Intelligence (AI) in medical education is profoundly reshaping traditional teaching and learning paradigms with innovative methods that enhance the didactic experience for students and educators alike. AI applications range from personalized learning support to advanced assessment tools, offering tailored educational experiences that cater to individual student needs and learning styles, as the complexity and volume of information require efficient and effective learning strategies (Gordon et al. 2024; Chan and Zary 2019; Nagi et al. 2023). AI also plays a significant part in curriculum development and review, although this area has seen less emphasis due to challenges in digitalization and the sensitive nature of examinations (Chan and Zary 2019). The ability of AI to provide real-time feedback and guided learning pathways is particularly beneficial in medical training, where knowledge retention is paramount and constructive feedback must be continuously provided to enhance practical skills (Nagi et al. 2023; Arango-Ibañez et al. 2023). These capabilities not only improve educational outcomes but also prepare students for the dynamic nature of medical practice.

To address the need for continuous adaptation to new medical knowledge and practices, AI tools, such as large language models, have been designed to facilitate the generation of examination questions and patient simulations, which are essential for developing critical thinking and decision-making skills (Arango-Ibañez et al. 2023). These technologies help bridge the gap between theoretical knowledge and practical application, ensuring that students are well-equipped to handle real-world medical challenges.

Despite the benefits, the implementation of AI in medical education is not without challenges, and the technical difficulties in developing AI applications and assessing their effectiveness pose significant barriers (Chan and Zary 2019). Moreover, the ethical implications of AI use in education, such as data privacy and the potential for bias, require careful consideration and the development of robust ethical frameworks (Knopp et al. 2023; Barreiro-Ares et al. 2023).

The future of medical education in an AI-driven world is one of both opportunity and risk, as AI has the potential to revolutionize the way medical knowledge is acquired, retained, and applied, but it also necessitates a reevaluation of traditional educational models (Knopp et al. 2023). Educators must be prepared to adapt to these changes, incorporating AI into their teaching methodologies and curricula to ensure that future medical professionals are proficient in using AI tools and know how to overcome its limitations. (Masters 2019; Weidener and Fischer 2024a, b).

Interdisciplinary collaboration is essential in this transformative process and by working together, educators, technologists, and healthcare professionals can develop AI applications that address the complex needs of medical education and practice (Knopp et al. 2023). This collaboration will help ensure that AI technologies are implemented responsibly and effectively, enhancing educational quality and clinical outcomes (Latif et al. 2024).

In conclusion, AI's transformative impact on medical education is undeniable and it offers unprecedented opportunities to enhance learning, improve educational outcomes, and prepare students for the technology-driven future of healthcare. However, realizing these benefits requires overcoming significant challenges, including technical, ethical, and educational barriers. By addressing these challenges and fostering collaboration, the medical education community can harness the full potential of AI, ensuring a more effective and equitable educational experience for all and ultimately, better care for our patients.

References

Abd-Alrazaq A, AlSaad R, Alhuwail D, Ahmed A, Healy P, Latifi S, Aziz S, Damseh R, Alrazak S, Sheikh J (2023) Large language models in medical education: opportunities, challenges, and future directions. JMIR Med Educ 9. https://doi.org/10.2196/48291

Abdellatif H, Mushaiqri M, Albalushi H, Al-Zaabi A, Roychoudhury S, Das S (2022) Teaching, learning and assessing anatomy with artificial intelligence: the road to a better future. Int J Environ Res Public Health 19. https://doi.org/10.3390/ijerph192114209

Afzal S, Dhamecha T, Gagnon P, Nayak A, Shah A, Carlstedt-Duke J, Pathak S, Mondal S, Gugnani A, Zary N, Chetlur M (2020) AI medical school tutor. Model Implement:133–145. https://doi.org/10.1007/978-3-030-59137-3_13

Ahmad S, Alam M, Rahmat M, Mubarik M, Hyder S (2022) Academic and administrative role of artificial intelligence in education. Sustainability. https://doi.org/10.3390/su14031101

Ali M, Wahab IBA, Huri HZ et al (2024a) Personalised learning in higher education for health sciences: a scoping review protocol. Syst Rev 13:99. https://doi.org/10.1186/s13643-024-02478-4

Ali O, Murray PA, Momin M, Dwivedi YK, Malik T (2024b) The effects of artificial intelligence applications in educational settings: challenges and strategies. Technol Forecast Soc Change. 0040-1625. 199:123076. https://doi.org/10.1016/j.techfore.2023.123076

Arango-Ibañez J, Posso-Nuñez J, Díaz-Solórzano J, Cruz-Suárez G (2023) Evidence-based learning strategies in medicine using AI. JMIR Med Educ 10. https://doi.org/10.2196/54507

Balcioglu H, Bilge U, Unluoglu I (2015) A historical perspective of medical education. J Educ Sci Environ Health 1(2):111–114

Barreiro-Ares A, Morales-Santiago A, Sendra-Portero F, Souto-Bayarri M (2023) Impact of the rise of artificial intelligence in radiology: what do students think? Int J Environ Res Public Health 20. https://doi.org/10.3390/ijerph20021589

Bohler F, Aggarwal N, Peters G, Taranikanti V (2024) Future implications of artificial intelligence in medical education. Cureus 16. https://doi.org/10.7759/cureus.51859

Bojic I, Mammadova M, Ang C, Teo W, Diordieva C, Pienkowska A, Gašević D, Car J (2023) Empowering health care education through learning analytics: in-depth scoping review. J Med Internet Res 25. https://doi.org/10.2196/41671

Buja LM (2019) Medical education today: all that glitters is not gold. BMC Med Educ 19:110. https://doi.org/10.1186/s12909-019-1535-9

Cardenas L, Castaño L, Guzman C, Alvarez J (2022) Personalised learning model for academic leveling and improvement in higher education. Australas J Educ Technol. https://doi.org/10.14742/ajet.7084

Castro G, Chiappe A, Rodríguez D, Sepulveda F (2024) Harnessing AI for education 4.0: drivers of personalized learning. Electron J e-Learn. https://doi.org/10.34190/ejel.22.5.3467

Challa KT, Sayed A, Acharya Y (2021) Modern techniques of teaching and learning in medical education: a descriptive literature review. MedEdPublish 10:18. https://doi.org/10.15694/mep.2021.000018.1. PMID: 38486533; PMCID: PMC10939590

Chan K, Zary N (2019) Applications and challenges of implementing artificial intelligence in medical education: integrative review. JMIR Med Educ 5(1):e13930. https://mededu.jmir.org/2019/1/e13930. https://doi.org/10.2196/13930

Chan T, Sebok-Syer S, Thoma B, Wise A, Sherbino J, Pusic M (2018) Learning analytics in medical education assessment: the past, the present, and the future. AEM Educ Train 2:178–187. https://doi.org/10.1002/aet2.10087

Chang C-Y, Hwang G-J (2018) Trends of mobile technology-enhanced medical education: a review of journal publications from 1998 to 2016. Int J Mobile Learn Org 12:373–393

Chen CH, Mullen AJ (2020) COVID-19 can catalyze the modernization of medical education. JMIR Med Educ 6(1):e19725. https://doi.org/10.2196/19725. PMID: 32501809; PMCID: PMC7294998

Chowdhury PN, Vaish A, Puri B, Vaishya R (2024) Medical education technology: past, present and future. Apollo Med 21(4):374–380. https://doi.org/10.1177/09760016241256202

Della Monica M, Mauri R, Scarano F, Lonardo F, Scarano G (2013) Genetic drift: the Salernitan school of medicine: women, men, and children. A syndromological review of the oldest medical school in the western world. Am J Med Genet A 161A(4):809–816. https://doi.org/10.1002/ajmg.a.35742. Epub 2013 Feb 26

Dignum V (2021) The role and challenges of education for responsible AI. Lond Rev Educ 19(1). https://doi.org/10.14324/LRE.19.1.01

D'Souza R, Mathew M, Mishra V, Surapaneni K (2024) Twelve tips for addressing ethical concerns in the implementation of artificial intelligence in medical education. Med Educ Online 29. https://doi.org/10.1080/10872981.2024.2330250

Duffy TP (2011) The Flexner Report--100 years later. Yale J Biol Med 84(3):269–276. PMID: 21966046; PMCID: PMC3178858

Ejaz H, McGrath H, Wong B, Guise A, Vercauteren T, Shapey J (2022) Artificial intelligence and medical education: a global mixed-methods study of medical students' perspectives. Digit Health 8. https://doi.org/10.1177/20552076221089099

Elendu C, Amaechi DC, Okatta AU, Amaechi EC, Elendu TC, Ezeh CP, Elendu ID (2024) The impact of simulation-based training in medical education: a review. Medicine (Baltimore) 103(27):e38813. https://doi.org/10.1097/MD.0000000000038813. PMID: 38968472; PMCID: PMC11224887

Farhud DD, Zokaei S (2021) Ethical issues of artificial intelligence in medicine and healthcare. Iran J Public Health 50(11):i–v. https://doi.org/10.18502/ijph.v50i11.7600. PMID: 35223619; PMCID: PMC8826344

Fatima S, Sheikh N, Osama A (2024) Authentic assessment in medical education: exploring AI integration and student-as-partners collaboration. Postgrad Med J. https://doi.org/10.1093/postmj/qgae088

Fazlollahi A, Bakhaidar M, Alsayegh A, Yilmaz R, Winkler-Schwartz A, Mirchi N, Langleben I, Ledwos N, Sabbagh A, Bajunaid K, Harley J, Del Maestro R (2022) Effect of artificial intelligence tutoring vs expert instruction on learning simulated surgical skills among medical students. JAMA Netw Open 5. https://doi.org/10.1001/jamanetworkopen.2021.49008

Frank JR, Snell LS, Cate OT, Holmboe ES, Carraccio C, Swing SR, Harris P, Glasgow NJ, Campbell C, Dath D, Harden RM, Iobst W, Long DM, Mungroo R, Richardson DL, Sherbino J, Silver I, Taber S, Talbot M, Harris KA (2010) Competency-based medical education: theory to practice. Med Teach 32(8):638–645. https://doi.org/10.3109/0142159X.2010.501190

Ghorashi N, Ismail A, Ghosh P, Sidawy A, Javan R (2023) AI-powered chatbots in medical education: potential applications and implications. Cureus 15. https://doi.org/10.7759/cureus.43271

Gifford K, Thoreson L, Burke A, Lockspeiser T, Lockwood L, Reed S, Schumacher D, Mahan J (2020) Describing overarching curricular goals for individualized education. Teach Learn Med 33:282–291. https://doi.org/10.1080/10401334.2020.1835665

Gordon M, Daniel M, Ajiboye A, Uraiby H, Xu N, Bartlett R, Hanson J, Haas M, Spadafore M, Grafton-Clarke C, Gasiea R, Michie C, Corral J, Kwan B, Dolmans D, Thammasitboon S (2024) A scoping review of artificial intelligence in medical education: BEME Guide No. 84. Med Teach 46:446–470. https://doi.org/10.1080/0142159X.2024.2314198

Grunhut J, Marques O, Wyatt A (2021) Needs, challenges, and applications of artificial intelligence in medical education curriculum. JMIR Med Educ 8. https://doi.org/10.2196/preprints.35587

Guo A, Li J (2023) Harnessing the power of ChatGPT in medical education. Med Teach 45:1063–1063. https://doi.org/10.1080/0142159X.2023.2198094

Gwee MC (2009) Problem-based learning: a strategic learning system design for the education of healthcare professionals in the 21st century. Kaohsiung J Med

Sci 25(5):231–239. https://doi.org/10.1016/S1607--551X(09)70067-1. PMID: 19502143

Katznelson G, Gerke S (2021) The need for health AI ethics in medical school education. Adv Health Sci Educ 26:1447–1458. https://doi.org/10.1007/s10459-021-10040-3

Kerimbayev N, Umirzakova Z, Shadiev R et al (2023) A student-centered approach using modern technologies in distance learning: a systematic review of the literature. Smart Learn Environ 10:61. https://doi.org/10.1186/s40561-023-00280-8

Kleisiaris CF, Sfakianakis C, Papathanasiou IV (2014) Health care practices in ancient Greece: the Hippocratic ideal. J Med Ethics Hist Med (7):6. PMID: 25512827; PMCID: PMC4263393

Knopp MI, Warm EJ, Weber D, Kelleher M, Kinnear B, Schumacher DJ, Santen SA, Mendonça E (2023) Turner L AI-enabled medical education: threads of change, promising futures, and risky realities across four potential future worlds. JMIR Med Educ 9:e50373. https://doi.org/10.2196/50373

Kononowicz A, Woodham L, Edelbring S, Stathakarou N, Davies D, Saxena N, Car L, Carlstedt-Duke J, Car J, Zary N (2019) Virtual patient simulations in health professions education: systematic review and meta-analysis by the digital health education collaboration. J Med Internet Res 21. https://doi.org/10.2196/14676

Kosiol J, Silvester T, Cooper H, Alford S, Fraser L (2024) Revolutionising health and social care: innovative solutions for a brighter tomorrow - a systematic review of the literature. BMC Health Serv Res 24(1):809. https://doi.org/10.1186/s12913-024-11099-5. PMID: 38997711; PMCID: PMC11241933

Krive J, Isola M, Chang L, Patel T, Anderson M, Sreedhar R (2023) Grounded in reality: artificial intelligence in medical education. JAMIA Open 6. https://doi.org/10.1093/jamiaopen/ooad037

Kuehn BM (2018) Virtual and augmented reality put a twist on medical education. JAMA 319(8):756–758. https://doi.org/10.1001/jama.2017.20800

Wasib Bin Latif, , Ida Md Yasin, Mohammed Julfikar Ali, Md. Nazrul Islam, Md. Shak Forid (2024). "Transforming applied medical sciences: the impact of AI, VR, and AR on research, education technology, and clinical practices", J Angiother 8(9):1–s

Lee H (2023) The rise of ChatGPT: exploring its potential in medical education. Anat Sci Educ 17:926–931. https://doi.org/10.1002/ase.2270

Lee J, Wu A, Li D, Kulasegaram K (2021) Artificial intelligence in undergraduate medical education: a scoping review. Acad Med 96:S62–S70. https://doi.org/10.1097/ACM.0000000000004291

Lentz A, Siy P, Carraccio M (2021) AI-ssessment: towards assessment as a sociotechnical system for learning. Acad Med 96(7S):S87–S88. https://doi.org/10.1097/ACM.0000000000004104

Lim JY, Ong SYK, Ng CYH, Chan KLE, Wu SYEA, So WZ, Tey GJC, Lam YX, Gao NLX, Lim YX, Tay RYK, Leong ITY, Rahman NDA, Chiam M, Lim C, Phua GLG, Murugam V, Ong EK, Krishna LKR (2023) A systematic scoping review of reflective writing in medical education. BMC Med Educ 23(1):12. https://doi.org/10.1186/s12909-022-03924-4. PMID: 36624494; PMCID: PMC9830881

Liu M, Kang J, Zou W, Lee H, Pan Z, Corliss S (2017) Using data to understand how to better design adaptive learning. Technol Knowl Learn 22:271–298. https://doi.org/10.1007/s10758-017-9326-z

Lozano A, Fleming S, Chiang C, Shah N (2023) Clinfo.ai: an open-source retrieval-augmented large language model system for answering medical questions using scientific literature. Pacific Symposium on Biocomputing Pacific Symposium on Biocomputing 29:8–23. https://doi.org/10.48550/arXiv.2310.16146

Lu H, Alhaskawi A, Dong Y, Zou X, Zhou H, Ezzi S, Kota V, Abdulla M, Abdalbary S (2024) Patient autonomy in medical education: navigating ethical challenges in the age of artificial intelligence. Inquiry 61. https://doi.org/10.1177/00469580241266364

Magnisalis I, Demetriadis S, Karakostas A (2011) Adaptive and intelligent systems for collaborative learning support: a review of the field. IEEE Trans Learn Technol 4:5–20. https://doi.org/10.1109/TLT.2011.2

Majumder MAA, Haque M, Razzaque MS (2023) Editorial: trends and challenges of medical education in the changing academic and public health environment of the 21st century. Front Commun 8:1153764. https://doi.org/10.3389/fcomm.2023.1153764

Mann KV (2011) Theoretical perspectives in medical education: past experience and future possibilities. Med Educ 45(1):60–68. https://doi.org/10.1111/j.1365-2923.2010.03757.x

Masters K (2019) Artificial intelligence in medical education. Med Teach 41:976–980. https://doi.org/10.1080/0142159X.2019.1595557

Mavroudi A, Giannakos M, Krogstie J (2018) Supporting adaptive learning pathways through the use of learning analytics: developments, challenges and future opportunities. Interact Learn Environ 26:206–220. https://doi.org/10.1080/10494820.2017.1292531

McCoy L, Pettit RK, Lewis JH, Bennett T, Carrasco N, Brysacz S, Makin IR, S., Hutman, Ryan and Schwartz, Frederic N.. (2015) Developing technology-enhanced active learning for medical education: challenges, solutions, and future directions. J Osteop Med 115(4):202–211. https://doi.org/10.7556/jaoa.2015.042

McCoy L, Nagaraj S, Morgado F, Harish V, Das S, Celi L (2020) What do medical students actually need to know about artificial intelligence? NPJ Digit Med 3. https://doi.org/10.1038/s41746-020-0294-7

McLean A (2024) Constructing knowledge: the role of AI in medical learning. J Am Med Inform Assoc. https://doi.org/10.1093/jamia/ocae124

Mennella C, Maniscalco U, De Pietro G, Esposito M (2024) Ethical and regulatory challenges of AI technologies in healthcare: a narrative review. Heliyon 10(4):e26297. https://doi.org/10.1016/j.heliyon.2024.e26297. PMID: 38384518; PMCID: PMC10879008

Menon A, Gaglani S, Haynes R, Tackett S (2017) Using "big data" to guide implementation of a web and mobile adaptive learning platform for medical students. Med Teach 39:975–980. https://doi.org/10.1080/0142159X.2017.1324949

Mir MM, Mir GM, Raina NT, Mir SM, Mir SM, Miskeen E, Alharthi MH, Alamri MMS (2023) Application of artificial intelligence in medical education: current scenario and future perspectives. J Adv Med Educ Prof 11(3):133–140. https://doi.org/10.30476/JAMP.2023.98655.1803. PMID: 37469385; PMCID: PMC10352669

Mizumoto A, Eguchi M (2023) Exploring the potential of using an AI language model for automated essay scoring. Res Methods Appl Linguist 2(2):100050, ISSN 2772-7661. https://doi.org/10.1016/j.rmal.2023.100050

Moldt J, Festl-Wietek T, Fuhl W, Zabel S, Claassen M, Wagner S, Nieselt K, Herrmann-Werner A (2024) Assessing AI awareness and identifying essential competencies: insights from key stakeholders in integrating AI into medical education. JMIR Med Educ 10. https://doi.org/10.2196/58355

Mondal H, Marndi G, Behera J, Mondal S (2023) ChatGPT for teachers: practical examples for utilizing artificial intelligence for educational purposes. Indian J Vasc Endovasc Surg 10:200–205. https://doi.org/10.4103/ijves.ijves_37_23

Nagi F, Salih R, Alzubaidi M, Shah H, Alam T, Shah Z, Househ M (2023) Applications of artificial intelligence (AI) in medical education: a scoping review. Stud Health Technol Inform 305:648–651. https://doi.org/10.3233/SHTI230581

Narayanan S, Ramakrishnan R, Durairaj E, Das A (2023) Artificial intelligence revolutionizing the field of medical education. Cureus 15(11):e49604. https://doi.org/10.7759/cureus.49604. PMID: 38161821; PMCID: PMC10755136

Norman G (2012) Medical education: past, present and future. Perspect Med Educ 1:6–14. https://doi.org/10.1007/s40037-012-0002-7

O'Doherty D, Dromey M, Lougheed J et al (2018) Barriers and solutions to online learning in medical education—an integrative review. BMC Med Educ 18:130. https://doi.org/10.1186/s12909-018-1240-0

Obi CO, Onosogbe M, Ehimen AG, Olamide O, Toluwalase TV, Esther O, Joshua DO, Aborode AT (2021) Comparison of the integrated organ/systems-based curriculum with the traditional subjects-based medical curriculum: short communication. Ann Med Surg (Lond) 73:103116. https://doi.org/10.1016/j.amsu.2021.103116. PMID: 35079353; PMCID: PMC8767261

Papapanou M, Routsi E, Tsamakis K, Fotis L, Marinos G, Lidoriki I, Karamanou M, Papaioannou TG, Tsiptsios D, Smyrnis N, Rizos E, Schizas D (2022) Medical education challenges and innovations during COVID-19 pandemic. Postgrad Med J 98(1159):321–327. https://doi.org/10.1136/postgradmedj-2021-140032

Paranjape K, Schinkel M, Nannan Panday R, Car J, Nanayakkara P (2019) Introducing artificial intelligence training in medical education. JMIR Med Educ 5(2):e16048. https://doi.org/10.2196/16048

Patiño A, Peñafiel J (2023) Artificial intelligence tutoring versus tutoring with experts in learning the preclinical and clinical areas of medicine. In: Proceedings of the 21th LACCEI International Multi-Conference for Engineering, Education and Technology (LACCEI 2023): "Leadership in Education and Innovation in Engineering in the Framework of Global Transformations: Integration and Alliances for Integral Development". https://doi.org/10.18687/laccei2023.1.1.1504

Piumatti G, Guttormsen S, Zurbuchen B et al (2021) Trajectories of learning approaches during a full medical curriculum: impact on clinical learning outcomes. BMC Med Educ 21:370. https://doi.org/10.1186/s12909-021-02809-2

Preiksaitis C, Rose C (2023) Opportunities, challenges, and future directions of generative artificial intelligence in medical education: scoping review. JMIR Med Educ 9. https://doi.org/10.2196/48785

Renz A, Hilbig R (2020) Prerequisites for artificial intelligence in further education: identification of drivers, barriers, and business models of educational technology companies. Int J Educ Technol High Educ 17. https://doi.org/10.1186/s41239-020-00193-3

Sandars J, Patel R (2018) Using personalized teaching and learning to improve clinical performance. Br J Hosp Med 79(2):102–105. https://doi.org/10.12968/hmed.2018.79.2.102

Sapci AH (2020) Artificial intelligence education and tools for medical and health informatics students: systematic review. JMIR Med Educ 6(1):e19285. https://doi.org/10.2196/19285

Saqr M (2015) Learning analytics and medical education. Int J Health Sci 9(4):V–VI. https://doi.org/10.12816/0031225

Sato SN, Condes Moreno E, Rubio-Zarapuz A, Dalamitros AA, Yañez-Sepulveda R, Tornero-Aguilera JF, Clemente-Suárez VJ (2024) Navigating the new normal: adapting online and distance learning in the post-pandemic era. Educ Sci 14:19. https://doi.org/10.3390/educsci14010019

Sense F, Velde M, Rijn H (2021) Predicting university students' exam performance using a model-based adaptive fact-learning system. J Learn Anal 8:155–169. https://doi.org/10.18608/jla.2021.6590

Skrzypek A, Szeliga M, Szopa M, Nowakowski M (2016) Personalized education in medical teaching. Gen Prof Educ 2016:34–38

Sparrow R, Hatherley J, Oakley J, Bain C (2024) Should the use of adaptive machine learning systems in medicine be classified as research? Am J Bioeth:1–12. https://doi.org/10.1080/15265161.2024.2337429

Stambuk-Castellano M, Carrera A, Tubbs R, Alario-Hoyos C, Verdú E, Iwanaga J, Reina F (2024) Personalized strategies for academic success in learning anatomy: exploring metacognitive and technological adaptation in medical students. Clin Anat 37:472–483. https://doi.org/10.1002/ca.24155

Stamer T, Steinhäuser J, Flägel K (2022) Artificial intelligence supporting the training of communication skills in the education of health care professions: scoping review. J Med Internet Res 25. https://doi.org/10.2196/43311

Sundaram A, Subramaniam H, Hamid S, Nor A (2024) An adaptive data-driven architecture for mental health care applications. PeerJ 12. https://doi.org/10.7717/peerj.17133

Taylor SJ, Wilson DJ (2007) The Human Tissue Act (2004), anatomical examination and the importance of body donation in Northern Ireland. Ulster Med J 76(3):124–126. PMID: 17853635; PMCID: PMC2075576

Tetzlaff L, Schmiedek F, Brod G (2020) Developing personalized education: a dynamic framework. Educ Psychol Rev 33:863–882. https://doi.org/10.1007/s10648-020-09570-w

Thomae A, Witt C, Barth J (2024) Integration of ChatGPT into a course for medical students: explorative study on teaching scenarios, students' perception, and applications. JMIR Med Educ 10. https://doi.org/10.2196/50545

Tokuç B, Varol G (2023) Medical education in the era of advancing technology. Balkan Med J 40(6):395–399

Tolentino R, Baradaran A, Gore G, Pluye P, Abbasgholizadeh-Rahimi S (2024) Curriculum frameworks and educational programs in AI for medical students, residents, and practicing physicians: scoping review. JMIR Med Educ 10. https://doi.org/10.2196/54793

Tolsgaard M, Pusic M, Sebok-Syer S, Gin B, Svendsen M, Syer M, Brydges R, Cuddy M, Boscardin C (2023) The fundamentals of Artificial Intelligence in medical education research: AMEE Guide No. 156. Med Teach 45:565–573. https://doi.org/10.1080/0142159X.2023.2180340

Turner L, Hashimoto D, Vasisht S, Schaye V (2023) Demystifying AI: current state and future role in medical education assessment. Acad Med 99:S42–S47. https://doi.org/10.1097/ACM.0000000000005598

Varma J, Fernando S, Ting B, Aamir S, Sivaprakasam R (2023) The global use of artificial intelligence in the undergraduate medical curriculum: a systematic review. Cureus 15. https://doi.org/10.7759/cureus.39701

Walkington C, Bernacki ML (2020) Appraising research on personalized learning: definitions, theoretical alignment, advancements, and future directions. J Res Technol Educ 52(3):235–252. https://doi.org/10.1080/15391523.2020.1747757

Wang S, Yang L, Li M, Zhang X, Tai X (2023) Medical education and artificial intelligence: web of science–based bibliometric analysis (2013–2022). JMIR Med Educ 10. https://doi.org/10.2196/51411

Wang S, Yi Z, Bin Z, Liu G, Jinyu Z, Zheng Y, Zequn Z, Yuan L, Feng R (2024) Enhancing self-directed learning with custom GPT AI facilitation among medical students: a randomized controlled trial. Med Teach:1–8. https://doi.org/10.1080/0142159X.2024.2413023

Weidener L, Fischer M (2023) Teaching AI ethics in medical education: a scoping review of current literature and practices. Perspect Med Educ 12:399–410. https://doi.org/10.5334/pme.954

Weidener L, Fischer M (2024a) Artificial intelligence in medicine: cross-sectional study among medical students on application, education, and ethical aspects. JMIR Med Educ 10. https://doi.org/10.2196/51247

Weidener L, Fischer M (2024b) Proposing a principle-based approach for teaching AI ethics in medical education. JMIR Med Educ 10. https://doi.org/10.2196/55368

Wu D, Xiang Y, Wu X, Yu T, Huang X, Zou Y, Liu Z, Lin H (2020) Artificial intelligence-tutoring problem-based learning in ophthalmology clerkship. Ann Transl Med 8. https://doi.org/10.21037/ATM.2019.12.15

Zampieri F, ElMaghawry M, Zanatta A, Thiene G (2015) Andreas Vesalius: celebrating 500 years of dissecting nature. Glob Cardiol Sci Pract 2015(5):66. https://doi.org/10.5339/gcsp.2015.66. PMID: 28127546; PMCID: PMC4762440

Zawacki-Richter O, Marín V, Bond M, Gouverneur F (2019) Systematic review of research on artificial intelligence applications in higher education—where are the educators? Int J Educ Technol High Educ 16. https://doi.org/10.1186/s41239-019-0171-0

Zhang L, Basham JD, Yang S (2020) Understanding the implementation of personalized learning: a research synthesis. Educ Res Rev 31:100339, ISSN 1747-938X. https://doi.org/10.1016/j.edurev.2020.100339

Zhui L, Li F, Xuehu W, Fu Q, Wei R (2024) Ethical considerations and fundamental principles of large language models in medical education: viewpoint. J Med Internet Res 26. https://doi.org/10.2196/60083

Artificial Intelligence in Surgical Simulation Training

7

Abdullah Tahir, Anam Jawaid, Aws Al-Omari, Arian Arjomandi Rad, and Peyman Sardari Nia

Abstract

This chapter outlines how artificial intelligence (AI) is reshaping surgical simulation training. It begins by tracing the evolution of surgical education from apprenticeship and cadaveric practice to high-fidelity, risk-free simulation. AI-driven technologies—machine learning, computer vision, and haptics—now power immersive VR/AR environments that adapt to each learner, deliver real-time objective feedback, and generate personalised learning pathways. Evidence shows these systems accelerate skill acquisition, heighten trainee confidence, and ultimately reduce operative errors. At the same time, the chapter acknowledges technical, ethical, financial, and regulatory hurdles that must be addressed for equitable global adoption. Looking ahead, deeper neural networks, cloud-based analytics, and convergence with 3-D printing and surgical robotics promise to democratise, standardise, and continually update surgical curricula worldwide. By integrating AI responsibly, surgical educators can cultivate a workforce ready for the complexities of modern, technology-enabled healthcare.

A. Tahir (✉)
Department of Trauma and Orthopaedic Surgery, University Hospitals of North Midlands, Stoke-On-Trent, UK
e-mail: abdullah.tahir3@nhs.net

A. Jawaid
Department of Trauma and Orthopaedic Surgery, The Dudley Group NHS Foundation Trust, Dudley, UK

A. Al-Omari
Department of Neurosurgery, Oxford University Hospital NHS Trust, Oxford, UK

A. Arjomandi Rad
Department of Cardiothoracic Surgery, Maastricht University Medical Center, Maastricht, The Netherlands

Department of Cardiothoracic Surgery, John Radcliffe Hospital, Oxford University Hospitals NHS Foundation Trust, Oxford, UK

P. S. Nia
Department of Cardiothoracic Surgery, Maastricht University Medical Center, Maastricht, The Netherlands

Keywords

Artificial intelligence · Surgical simulation · Medical education

7.1 Overview of Surgical Simulation Training

7.1.1 Evolution of Surgical Education and the Emergence of Simulation-Based Training

Surgical education has a rich history that dates back to ancient civilisations, where surgical

J. Malawana et al. (eds.), *Artificial Intelligence in Healthcare and Biomedical Visualization*, Biomedical Visualization 10, https://doi.org/10.1007/978-3-032-06520-9_7

knowledge was often passed down through apprenticeships and oral traditions (Zargaran et al. 2013). Aspiring surgeons would learn by observing experienced practitioners, then progress to assisting, and eventually performing procedures themselves. This mentor-apprentice model, whilst foundational to early medical education models (Vaugh 2000), lacked standardisation or formal assessment of competence, leading to variability in quality of surgical skill and performance (Sachdeva 2021).

The twenty-first century marked a significant shift in models of medical education, with the introduction of structured programs and clear curricula formalising both junior and senior training (Scalese et al. 2007). Institutions placed emphasis not only on technical proficiencies, easily taught with previous mentorship models but also on the scientific underpinnings of surgical practice. Following this, the emergence of simulation-based training in the latter part of the century represented a truly transformative development, not just in surgical education, but across the field of education as a whole (Elendu et al. 2024).

Simulation-based training arose from the need to enhance educational outcomes while minimising risks to patients. High-profile reports on medical errors and patient safety concerns underscored the limitations of traditional training methods. Whilst previously a cornerstone of surgical education, the 'see one, do one, teach one' philosophy relied heavily on experiential learning with real patients (Vozenilek et al. 2004); this gave students unpredictable and non-standardised cases, and further exposed the patient cohort to a basal level of risk (Rodriguez-Paz et al. 2009). Simulation offered a solution by providing a safe space for repeated practice, error correction, and mastery learning without endangering patient welfare (Zahiri et al. 2015).

Initial forays into simulation involved basic task trainers and anatomical models, which allowed trainees to practice fundamental skills in a controlled environment. The advent of computer technology and virtual reality in the 1990s propelled simulation forward, enabling the creation of sophisticated models that could mimic complex surgical procedures with high fidelity (Soloway and Bielaczyc 1994). This education model unlocked the ability to perfect surgical technique in an entirely risk-negated environment, with the option for endless iteration if desired by the student. Accrediting bodies and professional organisations began to recognise the value of simulation-based training in honing surgical technique and skill without any risk to patients, rather optimising their care, leading to its integration into surgical curricula worldwide (Satava 2008).

7.1.2 Importance of Simulation in Enhancing Surgical Skills and Patient Safety

Simulation training is widely recognised as an indispensable, fundamental tool in modern surgical education, offering numerous benefits that enhance both surgical skills and patient safety. One of the primary advantages is the opportunity for deliberate practice (Higgins et al. 2020). Trainees can repetitively perform procedures, receive immediate feedback, and refine their techniques without the pressure of an operating room setting. This iterative learning process is crucial for developing proficiency and confidence (Palter and Grantcharov 2014).

Furthermore, simulation cases can be changed to maximise exposure to a variety of clinical presentations, including rare or high-risk scenarios that one may not see in actual clinical practice, or encounter them only rarely were it not for simulation-based training (Feins et al. 2017). This comprehensive exposure ensures that training surgeons are better prepared to handle a wide range of clinical challenges as they continue to progress through training. Simulation also facilitates the development of non-technical skills essential for safe surgical practice, such as teamwork, communication, and decision-making under pressure (Bearman et al. 2012). These skills are often difficult to teach or measure through conventional means, but can be effectively challenged, and subsequently assessed and cultivated through simulated scenarios and crisis management exercises.

When looking at patient safety, simulation plays a critical role in reducing the incidence of medical errors (Meling and Meling 2020). By allowing surgeons to hone their skills in a risk-free environment, simulation decreases the likelihood of complications arising from inexperience or unfamiliarity with procedures. Studies have demonstrated that simulation-trained surgeons perform more efficiently and with fewer errors compared to those trained exclusively through traditional methods (Aydın et al. 2021). Adverse effects experienced by the patient population, caused by training surgeons practicing procedures for the first time or with inadequate experience, are eliminated (Boyle et al. 2019).

Moreover, simulation serves as a valuable assessment tool; it allows for the standardisation of training experiences (Pietersen et al. 2021). All trainees can be exposed to a consistent set of scenarios, with parity of training and assessment across the trainee cohort. Objective evaluation of a trainee's performance is possible through metrics collected during simulation exercises, enabling educators to identify areas of strength and those requiring improvement (Pangal et al. 2021). This metrics-driven approach, uniform across all trainees, supports personalised learning plans and ensures that objective competency standards are met before advancing to patient care.

Ultimately, incorporating simulation into surgical training aligns with the broader combined healthcare goal of prioritising patient safety alongside quality of care. As surgical procedures become increasingly complex, the need for highly skilled and adaptable surgeons grows. Simulation-based education equips surgeons with the necessary skills and confidence to meet these demands, ultimately leading to better patient outcomes and advancing the field of surgery.

7.2 Introduction to AI in Healthcare

7.2.1 Definition and Basic Concepts of AI

Artificial Intelligence (AI) is a branch of computer science that aims to develop software capable of performing tasks that typically require human intervention. These tasks include: learning from experience, pattern recognition, understanding natural language, problem-solving, and decision-making (Jutel et al. 2023). While the concept of AI spans multiple theoretical and practical domains, it is often categorised into two main domains (Jones et al. 2018):

1. *Narrow AI (Weak AI)*: These refer to systems designed to perform a specific task within a limited context, e.g. voice recognition, image classification, or navigation. This system works optimally within a defined function and lacks self-awareness or a general understanding of the world.
2. *General AI (Strong AI)*: refers to a system with the capability to understand, learn, and apply knowledge across a wide range of tasks at a level comparable to human cognitive abilities. At present, strong AI remains theoretical, with significant research still underway.

Underpinning AI are several key subfields and methods that are currently utilised within medicine and surgical specialities (Jones et al. 2018).

1. *Machine Learning (ML)*: A method where algorithms identify patterns and make decisions or predictions based on data. Supervised, unsupervised, and reinforcement learning are common ML paradigms used in diagnostic tools, predictive analytics, and surgical outcome forecasting. Within this, a subcategory of machine learning, Deep Learning (DL) has emerged. This multifaceted, layered tool utilises deep artificial neural networks. Since its inception, deep learning excels when tasked with image recognition, natural language processing, and facilitating advanced applications like automated report generation or image-guided interventions. This tool has often been used to report and analyse radiological images (Janiesch et al. 2021).
2. *Computer Vision*: This enables machines to process visual information, such as medical imaging data or live video feeds in surgical procedures. It underpins the development of real-time monitoring tools and software used intra-operatively, e.g. that rely on anatomical recognition (Kennedy-Metz et al. 2021).

3. *Natural Language Processing (NLP)*: This branch bridges the gap between computer and human language, utilised in numerous day-to-day hospital functions such as note transcription or generating automated procedural reports (Kim et al. 2022).

The application of these AI concepts in surgery transforms how surgeons are trained, how procedures are planned, and how real-time support is provided in the operating room. Looking at an educational setting and surgical simulation, these same concepts are integrated within simulation models to enhance learning experiences by creating realistic, adaptive, and immersive environments.

7.2.2 Historical Context of AI Application Within Medicine

The earliest traceable roots of AI in healthcare date back to the 1950s and 1960s, aligning closely with the birth of AI as a field (Kaul et al. 2020). Researchers at that time focused on the utilisation of AI expert systems, seeking to encode medical knowledge into rule-based programs in order to support, and ultimately substitute, clinical deduction. Though these initial advancements were not tailored to surgery specifically, they began the age of AI integration within healthcare, evidencing how computational logic could assist clinicians in a plethora of ways. Some such examples include:

1. *Early Expert Systems (1970s–1980s)*: MYCIN, which was developed at Stanford University in the 1970s, demonstrated the potential of AI in aiding clinical decision-making for infectious diseases. It attempted to diagnose patients based on symptoms and initial investigations (Meena 2016).
2. *Rise of Knowledge-Based Systems (Late 1980s–1990s)*: Evolving from the initial, rudimentary AI-based systems, more sophisticated knowledge-based software emerged across various medical specialties. Within surgery, robotic devices and computer-assisted procedures were explored, forming the foundations of robotic surgery today (Hussain et al. 2022).
3. *Integration of Machine Learning (2000s)*: Systems were employed to process large datasets, including medical imaging and patient records, utilising abilities in algorithm-recognition and data-handling. AI-driven methods began to be employed for outcome prediction, surgical planning, and early forms of simulation-based training. Although basic, these simulation-based tools set the groundwork for evolution into the virtual reality (VR) and augmented reality (AR) software and devices we use in practice today (Ağır 2024).
4. *Modern Era of Deep Learning and Big Data (2010s—Present)*: Combining developments in performance computing with newly created deep learning architectures has fuelled the incorporation of AI innovation within healthcare (Esteva et al. 2021). Looking within the domain of surgery, the potential for AI-integration has been exponential: real-time tissue recognition, demarcation of safe surgical zones, predictive analytics for operative risks, and intra-operative data processing (Rahmadian et al. 2024). Looking within education, AI-powered surgical simulators continued to evolve from primitive, rule-based, non-adaptive platforms to dynamic and interactive systems, capable of tailoring even the smallest details to the needs of each specific user.

Through this evolution, one can observe a clear trajectory: from rule-based, expert systems to adaptive approaches that form the foundation of contemporary surgical simulation platforms. Today, AI underpins many aspects of surgical training, from automated performance assessment to personalising learning pathways, increasing the safety, efficiency, and ultimately rigour of surgical education.

In the subsequent sections, we will explore how these AI-driven methodologies converge with advanced simulation technologies to create immersive, high-fidelity training tools that accelerate surgical skill acquisition, thereby improving patient outcomes.

7.3 Rationale for Integrating AI into Surgical Simulation

7.3.1 Complexities of Modern Surgical Procedures

Contemporary surgical practice across multiple disciplines has evolved to incorporate a plethora of surgical techniques, including minimally invasive procedures such as keyhole operations (Basil and Wang 2019), robotic-assisted procedures, and other unique techniques such as endovascular interventions (Tsui et al. 2013). The increasing complexity of these procedures has correlated with a demand for surgeons to develop a niche skill set beyond traditional manual dexterity. In addition to this, an understanding of device mechanics and digital tools is required. However, there are pitfalls to this that cannot be overlooked as a result of having more advanced technology at the surgeon's disposal. Traditional didactic training and conventional simulation models are struggling to keep pace with the rapid evolution of modern procedures (Velez 2022). Thus, by adopting novel AI technologies, simulation practice may offer a fairer reflection of the variability and intricacy encountered by surgeons in real-life practice (Martin et al. 2019). This will inevitably allow trainees to be better equipped for the forthcoming challenges in daily practice.

7.3.2 Limitations of Current Traditional Simulation Models

Traditional surgical simulation typically relies on physical models (Dunkin et al. 2007), cadaveric specimens, or, more recently, the inclusion of standardised virtual reality (VR) platforms (Satava 1993). Whilst these methodologies have considerably advanced surgical education and patient safety, several inherent challenges limit their efficacy:

1. *Resource Intensiveness*: High-fidelity simulation models and cadaver labs require significant financial investment and maintenance. Cadaveric specimens must be carefully preserved, and physical simulators often need continuous updates & servicing to remain relevant. The physical simulation equipment can be extremely expensive in itself, limiting the quantity that institutions can purchase. These costs can restrict access, limiting opportunities for widespread training (Jones and Baraza 2020).
2. *Variability and Limited Feedback*: Cadaveric tissue can vary in quality, whilst mannequin-based simulators may not accurately replicate the dynamic anatomical and physiological changes that occur during real procedures (Song and Jo 2021). This reduces fidelity to real-life surgery and can slow down the process of mastering new skills, or a mismatch in application of classroom-taught skills to real-life procedures (Wilson et al. 2022). Trainees, therefore, often rely on subjective feedback from instructors, which varies hugely depending on instructor's experience. Consequently, pinpointing objective skill deficits and providing tailored guidance can be challenging.
3. *Static Learning Environment*: Many traditional simulations offer a predetermined sequence of events and complications, reducing the potential for adaptive learning and increasing pattern recognition-based performance. As trainee competence improves, traditional models lack the ability to tailor their cases/presentations accordingly, meaning that trainee performance can quickly outperform the simulation model after some rounds of iterative practice (Cardoso et al. 2023). This can inadvertently cultivate repetitive, rote practice rather than fostering a deep understanding of unpredictable operative scenarios and discourage flexibility in the mindset of the student (Feins et al. 2017).

By incorporating AI-driven solutions, these constraints can be systematically addressed. AI can analyse performance data and respond dynamically to learner inputs, creating an immersive experience. Moreover, the scalability and adaptability of AI-based platforms enable more frequent practice and widespread uptake of teaching resources when compared to traditional learning methods (Park et al. 2022). This approach balances the development of necessary competencies in a resource-efficient manner.

7.3.2.1 Enhancing Learning Outcomes with AI

The integration of AI into surgical simulation heralds a landmark shift in how surgeons acquire and refine their technical and clinical decision-making skills. AI-driven simulations offer the potential to overcome these limitations and significantly boost the effectiveness of surgical training in several key ways:

1. *Personalised Learning Pathways*: AI algorithms can track a trainee's performance across multiple sessions, identifying unique strengths and weaknesses. Based on these insights, the simulation environment can automatically adjust difficulty levels and introduce targeted exercises. This personalised approach accelerates skill acquisition by offering deliberate practice where it is needed most (Mariani et al. 2020).
2. *Real-Time Performance Assessment*: Modern simulation platforms capture detailed data, such as instrument path trajectories or applied forces. AI tools then provide immediate, objective feedback, highlighting errors or inefficiencies in technique and suggesting corrective measures, which can be implemented by students instantaneously (Jorna et al. 2025). This continuous feedback loop promotes mastery through iterative improvement and rapid correction of poor technique (Yilmaz et al. 2021).
3. *Enhanced Realism and Predictive Modelling*: AI-enabled simulations can incorporate patient-specific anatomical data and predictive models of tissue behaviour, delivering a level of realism and complexity unmatched by traditional methods (Rangarajan et al. 2020). By simulating variations in anatomy or pathological conditions, trainees are better prepared for the wide range of scenarios encountered in clinical practice.
4. *Adaptive Scenario Generation*: AI-driven systems can dynamically introduce complications or unexpected events based on the trainee's actions, effectively simulating the chaotic and unpredictable nature of the operating room (Mariani et al. 2020). This adaptability fosters the development of critical decision-making skills under pressure, ultimately leading to improved patient outcomes. Such variation and incorporation of uncertainty is unparalleled by traditional simulation models.

By leveraging AI to address the complexities of modern surgical procedures and tackle the inherent limitations of existing simulation models, training programs can substantially enhance the proficiency, preparedness, and confidence of the next generation of surgeons. Ultimately, this leads to safer, more precise surgical care and improved patient outcomes worldwide.

7.4 Applications of AI in Surgical Simulation

7.4.1 AI-Driven Virtual Reality (VR) and Augmented Reality (AR)

7.4.1.1 Development of Immersive Training Environments

Artificial intelligence (AI) has significantly advanced the capabilities of VR and AR platforms in surgical education by enabling more realistic, interactive, and adaptive learning experiences. Techniques such as 3D reconstruction and automated image processing allow the creation of detailed anatomical models via AI systems, closely mimicking real patient physiology (Ryan et al. 2024). These immersive environments expose trainees to complex physical relationships, allowing them to develop spatial awareness and depth perception even in simulated procedures. By continuously adapting the virtual environment to a learner's performance, AI ensures that trainees encounter an appropriate level of challenge and variability, similar to real-world operative conditions.

7.4.1.2 Examples of AI-Enhanced VR/AR Surgical Simulators

Several cutting-edge simulators integrate AI-driven components to dynamically respond to user inputs and surgical actions. For instance, some VR systems can track the trajectory and force application of surgical instruments in real-time, utilising advanced analytics to provide immediate feedback on technique and efficiency (Park et al. 2022). In AR-based applications, AI assists with overlaying critical information, such as anatomical landmarks or risk zones, onto a user's field of view during simulation, helping refine decision-making and precision. These intelligent simulators not only replicate the technical aspects of surgery but also further facilitate communication and teamwork by mimicking the collaborative nature of an operating room (Ağır 2024).

7.4.2 Machine Learning Algorithms for Procedural Training

7.4.2.1 Adaptive Learning Systems That Personalise Training Experiences

Machine learning (ML) algorithms form the backbone of many AI-driven simulation systems by analysing vast amounts of performance data to identify individual learning patterns. Through supervised or reinforcement learning models, these systems can predict when a trainee is ready to progress to more advanced tasks or when they need additional practice on foundational skills. This personalised approach ensures that learners spend time where it matters most, addressing specific deficiencies in technique or decision-making, thus maximising both efficiency and effectiveness in skill development.

7.4.2.2 Real-Time Feedback and Assessment Powered by Machine Learning

A core advantage of AI-integrated simulators is their ability to offer immediate *and* objective feedback. ML-driven software can measure hand movements, grip forces, or even biometric indicators, comparing them against proficiency benchmarks derived from expert surgeons (Bissonnette et al. 2019). Discrepancies are flagged in real-time, prompting users to adjust and refine their technique on the spot. By quantifying performance metrics and correlating them with clinical outcomes, these systems guide evidence-based improvements in technique and taught surgical skills. Trainees can additionally practice unsupervised by a human supervisor, as the simulation software can assess and provide feedback simultaneously, opening the doors for round-the-clock, student-led surgical simulation training (Li et al. 2020).

7.4.3 AI in Haptic Feedback Systems

7.4.3.1 Enhancing Tactile Sensation for Better Skill Transfer

Haptic technology has long been recognised for its potential to bridge the gap between virtual training and real surgical touch. When paired with AI, haptic feedback systems can go beyond basic force replication, adapting the tactile response based on the user's actions and the simulated tissue properties (Tymkiv et al. 2024). This level of sophistication helps trainees develop crucial tactile perception, such as identifying tissue textures, discerning appropriate force thresholds, and refining fine motor control; factors that directly influence operative precision and patient safety (Sung et al. 2020).

7.4.3.2 Integration of AI to Simulate Realistic Tissue Responses

By leveraging machine learning models trained on real surgical data, AI-enabled haptics can accurately replicate the variability and elasticity of different tissue types (Schleer et al. 2020). As the trainee manipulates instruments, the simulator adjusts resistance and vibration to reflect realistic tissue reactions, including responses to cutting, suturing, or retraction. This dynamic interaction helps surgeons develop a nuanced understanding of tissue handling, reinforcing good surgical habits and encouraging a gentler approach (Enayati et al. 2016).

7.4.4 Personalised Training Programs

7.4.4.1 AI's Role in Customising Training to Individual Learning Curves

Every surgeon in training possesses a unique set of strengths, weaknesses, and learning styles; AI-powered systems map a trainee's progress over time, monitoring improvement in both technical performance and cognitive decision-making (Fazlollahi et al. 2022). By comparing individual performance data to aggregated benchmarks, the software identifies areas needing targeted practice and tailors subsequent training modules accordingly. This personalised pathway accelerates competency gains, reducing the time and resources required for mastery.

7.4.4.2 Predictive Analytics for Identifying Areas Needing Improvement

Beyond adaptive scheduling and personalised task selection, AI excels at forecasting future performance gaps before they significantly impact patient outcomes. By analysing historical patterns of individual learners and contrasting them against large-scale datasets, predictive analytics can estimate the likelihood of errors or complications, helping educators intervene proactively (Dixon et al. 2024).

In harnessing the power of AI, from immersive VR/AR environments and machine learning algorithms to advanced haptic feedback systems, surgical education is entering a new era. The ability to personalise training, offer real-time and evidence-based feedback, and replicate the complexities of the operating room in a risk-free setting positions AI at the forefront of enhancing surgical simulation training.

7.5 Benefits of AI in Surgical Simulation Training

7.5.1 Improved Competency and Confidence

7.5.1.1 Evidence of Enhanced Surgical Proficiency Through AI-Assisted Training

AI-driven simulation platforms have demonstrated measurable improvements in surgical proficiency by combining realistic scenarios with personalised feedback. Studies comparing traditional training methods to AI-enhanced modules often show faster skill acquisition and greater retention of complex procedures (Mirchi et al. 2020). By clearly identifying a trainee's areas of objective weakness and offering targeted remediation, these systems streamline the learning process whilst also ensuring robust foundational skills acquisition.

7.5.1.2 Reduction in Surgical Errors and Improved Patient Outcomes

The ultimate goal of advanced surgical education is to reduce complications and optimise patient safety via surgical mastery. Through repeated exposure to high-risk scenarios in a controlled environment, AI-powered simulators help trainees recognise and respond to potential errors before they occur in real-world settings. As a result, surgeons trained with AI support tend to exhibit fewer operative mistakes, better intraoperative decision-making, and improved patient outcomes, reinforcing the value of adopting AI technologies across training programs (Park et al. 2022).

7.5.2 Objective Performance Assessment

7.5.2.1 Data-Driven Evaluation Metrics

Traditional assessments often rely on expert observation and subjective scoring. In contrast, AI-enabled simulators collect detailed performance metrics, such as movement accuracy, force application, and time efficiency (MacDonald et al. 2003). Educators can therefore establish objective benchmarks and provide learners with quantifiable feedback (Toale et al. 2022). This evidence-based approach promotes parity of global assessment, and on a personal level, helps to identify performance gaps, encouraging targeted and meaningful improvements in technique for each trainee.

7.5.2.2 AI's Role in Unbiased Skill Assessment

Human evaluations, while valuable, can be subject to biases, both conscious and unconscious. AI-powered analytics reduce the influence of these biases by using consistent criteria to measure performance (Ciaschi and Barone 2024). By standardising the process of skill assessment, AI not only ensures fairness but also facilitates comparative analyses across different learners, institutions, and training programs (Pedrett et al. 2022). This unbiased evaluation model helps create a level playing field in skill learning and development.

7.5.3 Scalability and Accessibility

7.5.3.1 Democratising Surgical Education Globally

AI-driven simulation allows surgical training to transcend geographical and economic barriers. With the flexibility to deploy these platforms via cloud-based services or portable hardware, institutions in resource-limited settings can access sophisticated, high-fidelity training experiences (Malhotra et al. 2023). Not only this, but software is becoming less reliant on specialised physical machines or equipment, again increasing accessibility to training for institutions that may not otherwise be able to purchase high-cost infrastructure that lacks versatility, such as many traditional simulation training models. This democratisation ensures that aspiring surgeons worldwide have the opportunity to develop and refine their skills, contributing to a more uniformly trained surgical workforce and improved global health outcomes (Jaraczewski et al. 2023).

7.5.3.2 Remote Training Possibilities and Resource Optimisation

Beyond physical simulation labs, AI-powered platforms can support remote learning, enabling trainees to practice essential skills from virtually anywhere (Kılıç 2025). This expands educational reach and reduces the logistical constraints often associated with traditional training. Additionally, as AI-driven simulators collect extensive performance data, training programs can better manage resources—looking on a larger scale, can channel funds and instructor time into the areas and individuals that need it most.

7.5.4 Continuous Learning and Skill Maintenance

7.5.4.1 Lifelong Learning Opportunities for Surgeons Through AI

Surgical competence is not a static target; procedures evolve, new technologies emerge, and best practices are refined. AI-based simulators address this need for continuous learning by offering modules that automatically update to reflect advancements in surgical techniques and standards of care. Surgeons can revisit the platform to practice newly introduced procedures or reinforce existing proficiencies, ensuring their skills remain current and adaptable to clinical innovations.

Even experienced surgeons benefit from periodic skills assessments and refresher training, particularly for complex or high-risk procedures. AI-augmented simulation platforms create individualised learning plans that adapt to a surgeon's progress, allowing professionals to stay at the forefront of emerging techniques (Aggarwal

2023). This commitment to lifelong learning fosters a culture of continual improvement in surgical practice, ultimately resulting in higher standards of patient care and safety.

By offering objective assessments, expanding global access, and supporting continuous professional development, AI solutions have become indispensable in advancing the quality and efficiency of surgical education.

7.6 Challenges and Limitations

7.6.1 Technical Barriers

7.6.1.1 Computational Requirements and System Integration Issues

AI-driven surgical simulation platforms often require substantial computing power to process complex data in real-time. Tasks such as rendering high-fidelity anatomical models, providing instant performance feedback, and running predictive algorithms can strain hardware resources, necessitating advanced processors, graphics, and numerous other technical components (Zuhair et al. 2024). These demands can complicate system integration into existing hospital or academic infrastructures, leading to technical bottlenecks or compatibility challenges (Dawoodbhoy et al. 2021). Moreover, maintaining and updating sophisticated AI systems can become an ongoing burden, both time and financial, underscoring the need for dedicated technical support.

7.6.1.2 Data Privacy and Security Concerns

Many AI simulation systems rely on vast amounts of user data to personalise training experiences and refine algorithms. This raises issues regarding the storage, transmission, and protection of sensitive information, particularly when trainee performance data is linked to real patient data for educational purposes (Kuwaiti et al. 2023). Ensuring compliance with data protection regulations (e.g. HIPAA, GDPR) becomes paramount, requiring robust encryption, strict access controls, and transparent data use policies (Sadeghi et al. 2024). Breaches in data security or misuse of learner performance metrics can undermine confidence in AI-based training solutions and expose institutions to legal and reputational risks (Esmaeilzadeh 2024). Not only this, but any breaches in data will undermine patient confidence in contributing to medical education, emphasising that this is a path to tread on steadily when balancing educational progression with our duty towards our patients.

7.6.2 Ethical and Legal Considerations

7.6.2.1 Accountability in AI-Driven Training Outcomes

As AI takes on more roles in surgical education—analysing performance, providing feedback, and even guiding curriculum decisions- questions arise regarding accountability for trainee outcomes. If an algorithm misclassifies a learner's competency level or provides faulty guidance, it may contribute to suboptimal training and potential harm once the trainee transitions to clinical practice. Therefore, clarifying liability and establishing frameworks for AI oversight is paramount (Cobianchi et al. 2022). Responsibility must initially be shared appropriately between developers, institutions and end-users. Transparent explanations of algorithmic decision-making can help educators and regulatory bodies understand the basis for AI-derived recommendations, but also empower them to apply their own experience and clinical expertise to override or provide additional feedback when required (Satapathy et al. 2023). This approach can help support the gradual integration of initial AI models into education (Rao et al. 2024).

7.6.2.2 Regulatory Hurdles and Compliance with Medical Standards

Medical education and patient safety are heavily regulated domains, requiring rigorous validation and adherence to established standards (Ferreres 2024). AI-based simulators must demonstrate consistent reliability, accuracy, and efficacy to gain acceptance from national health and education bodies. Achieving and maintaining regulatory approval can be time-consuming and costly, adding another layer of complexity to implementing new AI solutions. Moreover, frequent software updates and evolving AI algorithms can trigger the need for repeated assessments and licensing, further increasing administrative burdens.

7.6.3 Cost and Resource Constraints

7.6.3.1 High Initial Investment for AI Technologies

Whilst AI promises to revolutionise surgical education, the initial costs for hardware, software licensing, and specialised staff training can be prohibitive (Bjerrum et al. 2018). Simulation centres will need to invest substantial resources initially to acquire high-performance computing devices, VR/AR equipment, haptic feedback interfaces, and sophisticated data analytics tools. Additionally, ongoing expenses for software updates, maintenance, and technical support add to the financial burden associated with such technologies, impacting the adoption of AI-driven simulation in smaller institutions heavily, again contributing to the very disparity such technologies should be used to tackle.

7.6.3.2 Disparities in Access Due to Economic Factors

Due to financial limitations, there may be an exacerbation of pre-existing inequalities when attempting to adopt AI on a global scale (Abahuje et al. 2024). High-income countries and institutions are better equipped to adopt novel AI solutions, whilst centres from low-income countries may struggle to secure the necessary funding to implement AI technologies. As a result, trainees from the latter will remain dependent on traditional simulation methods, which could potentially increase the gap in training opportunities. Addressing inequalities in training on a global scale has been a perennial issue, but by circumventing these issues with robust infrastructure and appropriate funding, training using AI technology can become a reality (Kirsch et al. 2023).

7.6.4 Acceptance Among Educators and Trainees

7.6.4.1 Resistance to Adopting New Technologies

Shifting from established training methods to AI-powered systems can spark scepticism or resistance among educators accustomed to traditional models, with many adopting a mindset of 'why fix something if it is not broken'. In some instances, educators may question the validity or reliability of AI-generated feedback compared to human expert evaluations (Cobianchi et al. 2022). Similarly, trainees might be hesitant to trust an algorithm's assessment of their skills or to practice extensively in virtual environments instead of hands-on clinical settings (Grunhut et al. 2021).

Overcoming these cultural and professional barriers demands comprehensive audience engagement and clear demonstrations of AI's advantages in enhancing learning outcomes. In order to facilitate this, continued established research on AI models of education is required, combined with an unwavering acceptance of the new dawn of medicine and reality that we are entering, in which AI is the future; the question is not 'do we incorporate AI into training?', but rather 'how?' (Gumbs et al. 2021).

7.6.4.2 Need for Training Educators on AI Systems

Implementing AI successfully in surgical simulation relies on more than the technology itself; instructors who can effectively interpret and apply AI-generated data dictate the bridging between the AI-naive audience and such software. Many educators require additional training to understand algorithmic outputs, troubleshoot technical problems, and integrate AI-driven insights into curricula (Knopp et al. 2023). Institutions will be required to invest in faculty development programs; without this, even the most advanced simulation technologies will not achieve their full educational potential, and outcomes for students will be poor (Wood et al. 2021).

Although AI holds immense promise for transforming surgical education, these challenges serve as warning to the heavy need for careful planning, robust infrastructure, and strong user support. By addressing technical, financial, and ethical barriers, institutions and developers must work together to ensure that AI-driven simulation achieves its fullest potential.

7.7 Future Directions

7.7.1 Advancements in AI Technologies

7.7.1.1 Potential of Deep Learning and Neural Networks in Simulation

Deep learning, powered by intricate neural network architectures, holds immense promise for elevating surgical simulation to unprecedented levels of realism and nuance. By processing vast amounts of data, ranging from high-resolution imaging to real-time biomechanical feedback, deep learning models can better predict tissue behaviour, adapt simulations to trainee performance, and refine operative recommendations. As these algorithms become more sophisticated, they may enable hyper-personalised training modules that rapidly detect and address individual learning gaps, further improving the quality and speed of skill acquisition (Weyers et al. 2024). The volumes of data we can feed to the software have no bounds; therefore, the potential for machine learning in other realms, such as human stress, communication, and other soft skills (Rosendal et al. 2023), could expand the breadth of training feedback even more so in the future.

7.7.1.2 AI and Robotics Convergence in Surgical Training

Another significant development lies in the convergence of AI with surgical robots. Robotic-assisted procedures have already transformed modern surgical practice, with many countries now using the technology. Robotic-assisted procedures yield greater precision, dexterity, and visualisation when performing procedures (Panesar et al. 2019). Incorporating AI into these systems allows real-time feedback, automatic instrument position, and predictive analyses intraoperatively. This interaction may allow for the production of even more advanced surgical robots where the machine behaviour is refined to benefit patient outcomes.

7.7.2 Integration with Other Emerging Technologies

7.7.2.1 Synergies with 3D Printing and Biofabrication

Patient-specific anatomical models are now being revolutionised by 3D printing and biofabrication (Ikhsan et al. 2024). The combination of this with AI simulation has allowed for highly realistic practice scenarios, which can be tailored specifically for individual patient anatomies (Sokmen et al. 2024). Through this approach, there is potential for trainees to practice, for example, complex reconstructive procedures on an individualised 3D printed map of the patient's anatomy, all whilst obtaining feedback from the AI software. The ceiling of this is yet to be determined—there is even potential for 3D printing to produce specimens that mimic living physiology, offering a high-fidelity learning experience. Ultimately, this will bridge the gap between simulation training and operating on real patients.

7.7.2.2 Cloud Computing and Big Data Analytics in Training

Cloud-based infrastructures and data analytics are propagating the dissemination of AI-driven simulations. By utilising training modules and performance metrics in secure online environments, institutions worldwide can now access the latest simulation platforms and share anonymised learner data on a large scale. Data algorithms analyse huge datasets to reveal patterns, refine performance benchmarks, and drive the evolution of the simulation curriculum. This collaborative approach ensures that trainees benefit from the collective insights of a global surgical community (Shi et al. 2024).

7.7.3 Global Collaboration and Standardisation

7.7.3.1 International Efforts to Standardise AI-Based Training

As AI becomes more deeply integrated into surgical education, the need for standardised guidelines and accreditation frameworks is paramount. National and international bodies are increasingly working together to create consensus on core competencies, data-sharing protocols, and ethical guidelines. These collaborative efforts aim to ensure that AI tools meet universally accepted quality and safety standards, promoting global consistency in training outcomes as well as a recognised objective standard of safe and expected surgical practice (Shi et al. 2024).

7.7.3.2 Sharing of Best Practices and Collaborative Platforms

Establishing open-access platforms for sharing AI-driven simulations, performance data, and research findings fosters transparency and collective growth. Surgical educators from different regions can contribute localised case studies and proven teaching methodologies. These knowledge-exchange networks catalyse innovation by allowing institutions with limited resources to adopt successful models developed by more experienced or well-equipped centres but also allow for a huge amalgamation of global data which AI software can digest and utilise.

7.7.4 Impact on Surgical Education and Healthcare Delivery

7.7.4.1 Transforming Curricula to Include AI Competencies

As AI technologies become integral to the surgical landscape, educational programs must evolve accordingly. In the future, education platforms and curricula will likely expand to include core AI competencies, ranging from interpreting algorithmic feedback to understanding ethical considerations in machine-driven decision-making (Grunhut et al. 2021). By integrating these competencies early in training, future generations of surgeons will be equipped to leverage AI effectively throughout their careers, whilst also remaining vigilant about its limitations and potential risks.

7.7.4.2 Long-Term Implications for Patient Care and Surgical Innovation

The growing convergence of AI, advanced simulation, and emerging technologies heralds a paradigm shift in both surgical practice and healthcare delivery (Ağır 2024). AI's ongoing integration within surgical education promises not only improved competence and safety but also the potential to redefine the very boundaries of surgical possibility (Guerrero et al. 2022). In the long term, surgeons trained in AI-supported environments may demonstrate greater precision, lower complication rates, and higher adaptability to novel operative methods or techniques (Nanda et al. 2024).

Ultimately, by focusing on deeper neural network integration, embracing synergistic use with cutting-edge technologies and fostering remote collaboration, AI-driven surgical simulation will continue to shape the future of operative training. This trajectory envisions a new standard of surgical excellence, one in which safe, personalised and efficient training, and therefore care, is accessible to surgeons worldwide.

7.8 Concluding Thoughts

AI-powered simulation tools are transforming surgical education by enhancing skill development through high-fidelity, risk-free training environments. Unlike traditional methods reliant on cadaveric practice and real-world patient interactions, AI-driven platforms offer repeated practice opportunities until proficiency is achieved.

A major benefit of AI-enhanced simulations is real-time feedback and objective performance assessments. Machine learning algorithms track progress, identify areas for improvement and personalise training pathways. Computer vision analyses hand movements and tool usage, while reinforcement learning dynamically adjusts training modules to match a trainee's evolving skill level. These AI-driven enhancements contribute to greater surgical precision, but also greater quality and depth of educational experience. High-fidelity simulations incorporate interactive 3D models, haptic feedback, and augmented reality to deepen understanding of complex procedures. They enable practice for rare and high-risk surgeries, fostering critical thinking, decision-making, and technical dexterity in trainees unmatched by traditional methods.

Despite these advantages, challenges remain in accessibility, cost, and the need for ongoing technological updates. In these initial phases, therefore, AI should complement, not replace, traditional hands-on training and mentorship; human judgment and experience remain indispensable in surgical education, and a necessary adjunct when initially walking this path of traditional and AI integration.

Ultimately, AI-powered simulations are the future of not just surgical, but global education efforts. They offer a personalised yet data-driven approach to training. As technology advances, these tools will become integral to curricula, enhancing training efficiency and patient care. Embracing AI in surgical education ensures that future surgeons are better prepared for the complexities of modern healthcare and that the workforce is trained appropriately alongside technology that will inevitably dominate the future climate of medicine.

References

Abahuje E, Tuyishime E, Alayande B (2024) Global surgical simulation education, current practices, and future directions. Surgery 180:109050. https://doi.org/10.1016/j.surg.2024.109050

Aggarwal D (2023) Exploring the scope of artificial intelligence (AI) for lifelong education through personalised & adaptive learning. J Artif Intell Mach Learn Neur Netw. https://doi.org/10.55529/jaimlnn.41.21.26

Ağır E (2024) Advanced AI and augmented reality (AR) integration in medical and surgical practice. Next Front Life Sci AI. https://doi.org/10.62802/vhzwwb94

Aydın A, Ahmed K, Abe T, Raison N, Van Hemelrijck M, Garmo H, Ahmed H, Mukhtar F, Al-Jabir A, Brunckhorst O, Shinohara N, Zhu W, Zeng G, Sfakianos J, Gupta M, Tewari A, Gözen A, Rassweiler J, Skolarikos A, Kunit T, Knoll T, Moltzahn F, Thalmann G, Powers A, Chew B, Sarıca K, Khan M, Dasgupta P (2021) Effect of simulation-based training on surgical proficiency and patient outcomes: a randomised controlled clinical and educational trial. Eur Urol. https://doi.org/10.1016/j.eururo.2021.10.030

Basil G, Wang M (2019) Trends in outpatient minimally invasive spine surgery. J Spine Surg 5(Suppl 1):S108–S114. https://doi.org/10.21037/JSS.2019.04.17

Bearman M, O'Brien R, Anthony A, Civil I, Flanagan B, Jolly B, Birks D, Langcake M, Molloy E, Nestel D (2012) Learning surgical communication, leadership and teamwork through simulation. J Surg Educ 69(2):201–207. https://doi.org/10.1016/j.jsurg.2011.07.014

Bissonnette V, Mirchi N, Ledwos N, Alsidieri G, Winkler-Schwartz A, Del Maestro R (2019) Artificial intelligence distinguishes surgical training levels in a virtual reality spinal task. J Bone Joint Surg Am 101:e127–e127. https://doi.org/10.2106/JBJS.18.01197

Bjerrum F, Thomsen A, Nayahangan L, Konge L (2018) Surgical simulation: current practices and future perspectives for technical skills training. Medical Teacher 40:668–675. https://doi.org/10.1080/0142159X.2018.1472754

Boyle J, Ghuysen A, D'orio V, De Céniga V, Chakfé N (2019) Time to embrace simulation in vascular surgical training: little things matter. Eur J Vasc Endovasc Surg 58(2):161–162. https://doi.org/10.1016/j.ejvs.2019.07.009

Cardoso S, Suyambu J, Iqbal J, Jaimes D, Amin A, Sikto J, Valderrama M, Aulakh S, Ramana V, Shaukat B, Patel T (2023) Exploring the role of simulation training in improving surgical skills among residents: a narrative review. Cureus 15. https://doi.org/10.7759/cureus.44654

Ciaschi M, Barone M (2024) Exploring the role of Artificial Intelligence in assessing soft skills. In: 2024 19th conference on computer science and intelligence systems (FedCSIS), pp 573–578. https://doi.org/10.15439/2024F2063

Cobianchi L, Verde J, Loftus T, Piccolo D, Mas D, Mascagni P, Vázquez G, Ansaloni L, Marseglia G, Massaro M, Gallix B, Padoy N, Peter A, Kaafarani H (2022) Artificial intelligence and surgery: ethical dilemmas and open issues. J Am Coll Surg 235(2):268–275. https://doi.org/10.1097/XCS.0000000000000242

Dawoodbhoy F, Delaney J, Cecula P, Yu J, Peacock I, Tan J, Cox B (2021) AI in patient flow: applications of artificial intelligence to improve patient flow in NHS acute mental health inpatient units. Heliyon 7. https://doi.org/10.1016/j.heliyon.2021.e06993

Dixon D, Sattar H, Moros N, Kesireddy S, Ahsan H, Lakkimsetti M, Fatima M, Doshi D, Sadhu K, Hassan M (2024) Unveiling the influence of AI predictive analytics on patient outcomes: a comprehensive narrative review. Cureus 16. https://doi.org/10.7759/cureus.59954

Dunkin B, Adrales G, Apelgren K, Mellinger J (2007) Surgical simulation: a current review. Surg Endosc 21:357–366. https://doi.org/10.1007/s00464-006-9072-0

Elendu C, Amaechi D, Okatta A, Amaechi E, Elendu T, Ezeh C, Elendu I (2024) The impact of simulation-based training in medical education: a review. Medicine 103. https://doi.org/10.1097/MD.0000000000038813

Enayati N, De Momi E, Ferrigno G (2016) Haptics in robot-assisted surgery: challenges and benefits. IEEE Rev Biomed Eng 9:49–65. https://doi.org/10.1109/RBME.2016.2538080

Esmaeilzadeh P (2024) Challenges and strategies for wide-scale artificial intelligence (AI) deployment in healthcare practices: a perspective for healthcare organizations. Artif Intell Med 151:102861. https://doi.org/10.1016/j.artmed.2024.102861

Esteva A, Chou K, Yeung S, Naik N, Madani A, Mottaghi A, Liu Y, Topol E, Dean J, Socher R (2021) Deep learning-enabled medical computer vision. NPJ Digit Med 4. https://doi.org/10.1038/s41746-020-00376-2

Fazlollahi A, Bakhaidar M, Alsayegh A, Yilmaz R, Winkler-Schwartz A, Langleben I, Mirchi N, Ledwos N, Harley J, Del Maestro R (2022) 510 Artificial intelligence tutoring compared with expert instruction in neurosurgical simulation training: a randomized controlled trial. Neurosurgery 68:128–129. https://doi.org/10.1227/NEU.0000000000001880_510

Feins R, Burkhart H, Conte J, Coore D, Fann J, Hicks G, Nesbitt J, Ramphal P, Schiro S, Shen R, Sridhar A, Stewart P, Walker J, Mokadam N (2017) Simulation-based training in cardiac surgery. Ann Thorac Surg 103(1):312–321. https://doi.org/10.1016/j.athoracsur.2016.06.062

Ferreres A (2024) Ethical and legal issues regarding artificial intelligence (AI) and management of surgical data. Eur J Surg Oncol:108279. https://doi.org/10.1016/j.ejso.2024.108279

Grunhut J, Marques O, Wyatt A (2021) Needs, challenges, and applications of artificial intelligence in medical education curriculum. JMIR Med Educ 8. https://doi.org/10.2196/preprints.35587

Guerrero D, Asaad M, Rajesh A, Hassan A, Butler C (2022) Advancing surgical education: the use of artificial intelligence in surgical training. Am Surg 89:49–54. https://doi.org/10.1177/00031348221101503

Gumbs A, Frigerio I, Spolverato G, Croner R, Illanes A, Chouillard E, Elyan E (2021) Artificial intelligence surgery: how do we get to autonomous actions in surgery? Sensors (Basel, Switzerland) 21. https://doi.org/10.3390/s21165526

Higgins M, Madan C, Patel R (2020) Deliberate practice in simulation-based surgical skills training: a scoping review. J Surg Educ. https://doi.org/10.1016/j.jsurg.2020.11.008

Hussain S, Brunetti A, Lucarelli G, Memeo R, Bevilacqua V, Buongiorno D (2022) Deep learning based image processing for robot assisted surgery: a systematic literature survey. IEEE Access 10:122627–122657. https://doi.org/10.1109/ACCESS.2022.3223704

Ikhsan R, Rahayu S, Arribathi A, Azizah N (2024) Integrating artificial intelligence with 3D printing technology in healthcare: sustainable solutions for clinical training optimization. ADI J Recent Innov (AJRI). https://doi.org/10.34306/ajri.v6i2.1126

Janiesch C, Zschech P, Heinrich K (2021) Machine learning and deep learning. Electron Mark 31:685–695. https://doi.org/10.1007/s12525-021-00475-2

Jaraczewski T, SenthilKumar G, Ramamurthi A, Nimmer K, Yang X, Kothari A (2023) Teaming with artificial intelligence to support global cancer surgical care. J Surg Oncol 128. https://doi.org/10.1002/jso.27442

Jones D, Baraza W (2020) Comment on: systematic review of the current status of cadaveric simulation for surgical training. Br J Surg 107. https://doi.org/10.1002/bjs.11628

Jones L, Golan D, Hanna S, Ramachandran M (2018) Artificial intelligence, machine learning and the evolution of healthcare. Bone Joint Res 7:223–225. https://doi.org/10.1302/2046-3758.73.BJR-2017-0147.R1

Jorna C, Margallo J, Margallo F (2025) Artificial intelligence applications for learning in robotic surgery. Br J Surg. https://doi.org/10.1093/bjs/znae322.020

Jutel M, Zemelka-Wiącek M, Ordak M, Pfaar O, Eiwegger T, Rechenmacher M, Akdis C (2023) The artificial intelligence (AI) revolution: how important for scientific work and its reliable sharing. Allergy 78. https://doi.org/10.1111/all.15778

Kaul V, Enslin S, Gross S (2020) The history of artificial intelligence in medicine. Gastrointest Endosc. https://doi.org/10.1016/j.gie.2020.06.040

Kennedy-Metz L, Mascagni P, Torralba A, Dias R, Perona P, Shah J, Padoy N, Zenati M (2021) Computer vision in the operating room: opportunities and caveats. IEEE Trans Med Robotics Bionics 3:2–10. https://doi.org/10.1109/TMRB.2020.3040002

Kılıç S (2025) Augmented reality (AR) in medical training: AI-powered simulations for enhanced learning experiences. Next Front Life Sci AI. https://doi.org/10.62802/c6xk2k47

Kim J, Vivas A, Arvind V, Lombardi J, Reidler J, Zuckerman S, Lee N, Vulapalli M, Geng E, Cho B, Morizane K, Cho S, Lehman R, Lenke L, Riew K (2022) Can natural language processing and artificial intelligence automate the generation of billing codes from operative note dictations? Glob Spine J 13:1946–1955. https://doi.org/10.1177/21925682211062831

Kirsch M, Mangham C, Lin Y (2023) GlobalSurgBox: a portable surgical simulator for surgical trainees worldwide. J Surg Educ. https://doi.org/10.1016/j.jsurg.2023.01.012

Knopp M, Warm E, Weber D, Kelleher M, Kinnear B, Schumacher D, Santen S, Mendonca E, Turner L (2023) AI-enabled medical education: threads of change, promising futures, and risky realities across four potential future worlds. JMIR Med Educ 9. https://doi.org/10.2196/50373

Kuwaiti A, Nazer K, Al-Reedy A, Al-Shehri S, Al-Muhanna A, Subbarayalu A, Muhanna D, Al-Muhanna F (2023) A review of the role of artificial intelligence in healthcare. J Personal Med 13. https://doi.org/10.3390/jpm13060951

Li L, Li X, Yang S, Ding S, Jolfaei A, Zheng X (2020) Unsupervised-learning-based continuous depth and motion estimation with monocular endoscopy for virtual reality minimally invasive surgery. IEEE Trans Ind Inform 17:3920–3928. https://doi.org/10.1109/TII.2020.3011067

MacDonald J, Williams R, Rogers D (2003) Self-assessment in simulation-based surgical skills training. Am J Surg 185(4):319–322. https://doi.org/10.1016/S0002-9610(02)01420-4

Malhotra K, Wong B, Lee S, Franco H, Singh C, Silva L, Iraqi H, Sinha A, Burger S, Breedt D, Goyal K, Dagli M, Bawa A (2023) Role of artificial intelligence in global surgery: a review of opportunities and challenges. Cureus 15. https://doi.org/10.7759/cureus.43192

Mariani A, Pellegrini E, De Momi E (2020) Skill-oriented and performance-driven adaptive curricula for training in robot-assisted surgery using simulators: a feasibility study. IEEE Trans Biomed Eng 68:685–694. https://doi.org/10.1109/TBME.2020.3011867

Martin J, Anton N, Timsina L, Whiteside J, Myers E, Stefanidis D (2019) Performance variability during training on simulators is associated with skill transfer. Surgery 165(6):1065–1068. https://doi.org/10.1016/j.surg.2019.01.013

Meena A (2016) Study and analysis of MYCIN expert system. Int J Eng Comput Sci. https://doi.org/10.18535/IJECS/V4I10.41

Meling T, Meling T (2020) The impact of surgical simulation on patient outcomes: a systematic review and meta-analysis. Neurosurg Rev 44:843–854. https://doi.org/10.1007/s10143-020-01314-2

Mirchi N, Bissonnette V, Yilmaz R, Ledwos N, Winkler-Schwartz A, Del Maestro R (2020) The virtual operative assistant: an explainable artificial intelligence tool for simulation-based training in surgery and medicine. PLoS One 15. https://doi.org/10.1371/journal.pone.0229596

Nanda I, Khatua L, Porwal S, Singhal D (2024) Machine learning and computer vision driving precision in robotic surgery. Commun Appl Nonlinear Anal. https://doi.org/10.52783/cana.v32.2272

Palter V, Grantcharov T (2014) Individualized deliberate practice on a virtual reality simulator improves technical performance of surgical novices in the operating room: a randomized controlled trial. Ann Surg 259:443–448. https://doi.org/10.1097/SLA.0000000000000254

Panesar S, Cagle Y, Chander D, Morey J, Fernandez-Miranda J, Kliot M (2019) Artificial intelligence and the future of surgical robotics. Ann Surg. https://doi.org/10.1097/SLA.0000000000003262

Pangal D, Kugener G, Cardinal T, Lechtholz-Zey E, Collet C, Lasky S, Sundaram S, Zhu Y, Roshannai A, Chan J, Sinha A, Hung A, Anandkumar A, Zada G, Donoho D (2021) Use of surgical video-based automated performance metrics to predict blood loss and success of simulated vascular injury control in neurosurgery: a pilot study. J Neurosurg:1–10. https://doi.org/10.3171/2021.10.JNS211064

Park J, Tiefenbach J, Demetriades A (2022) The role of artificial intelligence in surgical simulation. Front Med Technol 4. https://doi.org/10.3389/fmedt.2022.1076755

Pedrett R, Mascagni P, Beldi G, Padoy N, Lavanchy J (2022) Technical skill assessment in minimally invasive surgery using artificial intelligence: a systematic review. Surg Endosc 37:7412–7424. https://doi.org/10.1007/s00464-023-10335-z

Pietersen P, Bjerrum F, Tolsgaard M, Konge L, Andersen S (2021) Standard setting in simulation-based training of surgical procedures. Ann Surg 275:872–882. https://doi.org/10.1097/SLA.0000000000005209

Rahmadian R, Alif M, Abi Q, Ariliusra Z (2024) Artificial intelligence in surgery: role of AI in pre-operative, intra-operative, and post-operative. Surg Gastroenterol Oncol. https://doi.org/10.21614/sgo-672

Rangarajan K, Davis H, Pucher P (2020) Systematic review of virtual haptics in surgical simulation: a valid educational tool? J Surg Educ. https://doi.org/10.1016/j.jsurg.2019.09.006

Rao L, Yang E, Dissanayake S, Cuomo R, Seth I, Rozen W (2024) The use of generative artificial intelligence in surgical education: a narrative review. Plast Aesthet Res. https://doi.org/10.20517/2347-9264.2024.102

Rodriguez-Paz J, Kennedy M, Salas E, Wu A, Sexton J, Hunt E, Pronovost P (2009) Beyond "see one, do one, teach one": toward a different training paradigm. Qual Saf Health Care 18:63–68. https://doi.org/10.1136/qshc.2007.023903

Rosendal A, Sloth S, Rölfing J, Bie M, Jensen R (2023) Technical, non-technical, or both? A scoping review of skills in simulation-based surgical training. J Surg Educ. https://doi.org/10.1016/j.jsurg.2023.02.011

Ryan M, Wang S, Pandya S (2024) Integrating artificial intelligence into the visualization and modeling of three-dimensional anatomy in pediatric surgical patients. J Pediatr Surg. https://doi.org/10.1016/j.jpedsurg.2024.07.014

Sachdeva A (2021) Preceptoring, proctoring, mentoring, and coaching in surgery. J Surg Oncol 124:711–721. https://doi.org/10.1002/jso.26585

Sadeghi Z, Alizadehsani R, Cifci M, Kausar S, Rehman R, Mahanta P, Bora P, Almasri A, Alkhawaldeh R, Hussain S, Alatas B, Shoeibi A, Moosaei H, Hladík M, Nahavandi S, Pardalos P (2024) A review of explainable artificial intelligence in healthcare. Comput Electr Eng 118:109370. https://doi.org/10.1016/j.compeleceng.2024.109370

Satapathy P, Hermis A, Rustagi S, Pradhan K, Padhi B, Sah R (2023) Artificial intelligence in surgical education and training: opportunities, challenges, and ethical considerations – correspondence. Int J Surg (London,

England) 109:1543–1544. https://doi.org/10.1097/JS9.0000000000000387

Satava R (1993) Virtual reality surgical simulator. Surg Endosc 7:203–205. https://doi.org/10.1007/BF00594110

Satava R (2008) Historical review of surgical simulation—a personal perspective. World J Surg 32:141–148. https://doi.org/10.1007/s00268-007-9374-y

Scalese R, Obeso V, Issenberg S (2007) Simulation technology for skills training and competency assessment in medical education. J Gen Intern Med 23:46–49. https://doi.org/10.1007/s11606-007-0283-4

Schleer P, Kaiser P, Drobinsky S, Radermacher K (2020) Augmentation of haptic feedback for teleoperated robotic surgery. Int J Comput Assist Radiol Surg 15:515–529. https://doi.org/10.1007/s11548-020-02118-x

Shi H, Zhang X, Wang J, Fan W, Liu G (2024) Enhancing global surgical education through equitable simulation training: a critical analysis of technological integration and international collaboration. Int J Surg (London, England) 110:8185–8186. https://doi.org/10.1097/JS9.0000000000001792

Sokmen S, Çakmak S, Oksuz I (2024) 3D printing of an artificial intelligence-generated patient-specific coronary artery segmentation in a support bath. Biomed Mater 19. https://doi.org/10.1088/1748-605X/ad3f60

Soloway E, Bielaczyc K (1994) Interactive learning environments: where they've come from & where they're going. In: Conference companion on human factors in computing systems. https://doi.org/10.1145/257089.257386.

Song Y, Jo D (2021) Current and potential use of fresh frozen cadaver in surgical training and anatomical education. Anat Sci Educ 15:957–969. https://doi.org/10.1002/ase.2138

Sung M, Kang B, Kim J, Kim T, Song H (2020) Intelligent haptic virtual simulation for suture surgery. Int J Adv Comput Sci Appl 11. https://doi.org/10.14569/ijacsa.2020.0110208

Toale C, Morris M, Kavanagh D (2022) Perspectives on simulation-based assessment of operative skill in surgical training. Medical Teacher 45:313–320. https://doi.org/10.1080/0142159X.2022.2134001

Tsui C, Klein R, Garabrant M (2013) Minimally invasive surgery: national trends in adoption and future directions for hospital strategy. Surg Endosc 27:2253–2257. https://doi.org/10.1007/s00464-013-2973-9

Tymkiv, P., Klos-Witkowska, A., Bahrii-Zaiats, O., & Kovalyk, S., 2024. Smart prosthetics in surgery: AI-driven tactile feedback using piezoelectric sensors. pp 208–217

Vaugh M (2000) Surgical education in the middle ages. Dynamis 20:283–304

Velez D (2022) Modern didactic formats in surgery: a systematic review. Am Surg 89:1701–1708. https://doi.org/10.1177/00031348221074252

Vozenilek J, Huff J, Reznek M, Gordon J (2004) See one, do one, teach one: advanced technology in medical education. Acad Emerg Med Off J Soc Acad Emerg Med 11(11):1149–1154. https://doi.org/10.1197/J.AEM.2004.08.003

Weyers A, Von Waldenfels G, Gebert P, Henrich W, Hinkson L (2024) Reducing trainee mistakes. Better performance with changing to a high-fidelity simulation system? AJOG Glob Rep 4. https://doi.org/10.1016/j.xagr.2024.100326

Wilson C, Davidson J, Chahine S, Chan E, Stringer L, Quantz M, Saklofske D, Wang P (2022) What is transferred and how much is retained? A simulation study of complex surgical skills. J Surg Res 280:411–420. https://doi.org/10.1016/j.jss.2022.07.040

Wood E, Ange B, Miller D (2021) Are we ready to integrate artificial intelligence literacy into medical school curriculum: students and faculty survey. J Med Educat Curri Develop 8. https://doi.org/10.1177/23821205211024078

Yilmaz R, Winkler-Schwartz A, Reich A, Del Maestro R (2021) SP2.1.1 continuous monitoring and assessment of surgical technical skills using deep learning. Br J Surg. https://doi.org/10.1093/bjs/znab361.022

Zahiri H, Park A, Pugh C, Vassiliou M, Voeller G (2015) "See one, do one, teach one": inadequacies of current methods to train surgeons in hernia repair. Surg Endosc 29:2867–2872. https://doi.org/10.1007/s00464-015-4411-7

Zargaran A, Fazelzadeh A, Mohagheghzadeh A (2013) Surgeons and surgery from ancient Persia (5,000 years of surgical history). World J Surg 37:2002–2004. https://doi.org/10.1007/s00268-013-2055-0

Zuhair V, Babar A, Ali R, Oduoye M, Noor Z, Chris K, Okon I, Rehman L (2024) Exploring the impact of artificial intelligence on global health and enhancing healthcare in developing nations. J Prim Care Community Health 15. https://doi.org/10.1177/21501319241245847

Interstellar Informatics: Visualizing Space Medicine Through Artificial Intelligence

8

Hiba Khan

Abstract

The advent of interstellar exploration necessitates the advancement of space medicine, a field fraught with unique challenges due to the harsh conditions of space. This chapter delves into the pivotal role of artificial intelligence and biomedical visualization in addressing the health needs of astronauts. We begin by outlining the necessity for space medicine and the integral role of AI and visualization technologies in this domain. The chapter then explores the unique challenges of space medicine, including the effects of microgravity, cosmic radiation, and psychosocial stressors, and reviews the current medical technologies employed in space.

A significant focus is placed on artificial intelligence capabilities in monitoring astronaut health through wearable technology, predictive health analytics, and emergency response systems. The visualization of complex medical data in microgravity environments is examined, highlighting the use of virtual and augmented reality, as well as interactive 3D models for educational purposes. We also discuss AI-driven medical procedures, such as telemedicine, robotic surgery, and autonomous health systems, which are crucial for long-duration missions.

Further, this chapter addresses the groundbreaking potential of AI in bioprinting for tissue engineering in space, outlining both the possibilities and the challenges posed by microgravity. The integration of AI into interplanetary telemedicine networks and personalized medicine for astronauts is discussed, along with speculative technologies that promise future advancements in space medicine.

Finally, the chapter considers the ethical and practical implications of deploying AI in space missions, including data privacy, ethical decision-making, and the reliability of AI systems in critical situations. Concluding with a recapitulation of AI's transformative impact on space medicine, the chapter envisions a future where artificial intelligence and space exploration converge to overcome the final frontier of medical challenges.

Keywords

Space medicine · Astronaut health · Personalized medicine · Interplanetary telemedicine

H. Khan (✉)
Medics.Academy and The School of Medicine, University of Central Lancashire, Preston, UK
e-mail: Hiba.khan@medics.academy

J. Malawana et al. (eds.), *Artificial Intelligence in Healthcare and Biomedical Visualization*, Biomedical Visualization 10, https://doi.org/10.1007/978-3-032-06520-9_8

8.1 Introduction

Space medicine, defined as 'the practice of all aspects of preventative medicine including screening, healthcare delivery, maintaining human performance in the extreme environment of space, and preserving the long-term health of space travellers' (Pool 2007), is rapidly evolving in response to humanity's expanding ambitions for interstellar exploration. As we push the boundaries of human presence into deep space, the challenges associated with maintaining astronaut health grow increasingly complex, necessitating innovative approaches to medical care.

Artificial intelligence (AI) and biomedical visualization technologies stand at the forefront of this evolution, offering unprecedented opportunities to address the unique physiological and psychological challenges posed by space environments. This chapter explores the transformative potential of AI-driven solutions in space medicine, highlighting how advanced biomedical visualization can facilitate better understanding, monitoring, and management of astronaut health in microgravity conditions.

The chapter will first outline the historical context and current state of space medicine, identifying key challenges such as microgravity-induced physiological changes, cosmic radiation exposure, and psychosocial stressors associated with prolonged spaceflight. We will then delve deeply into the role AI plays in monitoring and predicting astronaut health through wearable technologies, predictive analytics, and autonomous medical decision-making systems.

Biomedical visualization, particularly through virtual and augmented reality, interactive 3D models, and advanced medical imaging, will be discussed as essential tools for medical training, emergency response, and ongoing health management in space. Furthermore, we will examine groundbreaking developments in AI-assisted medical procedures, including robotic surgery, telemedicine, and bioprinting for tissue regeneration, underscoring their potential for sustaining astronaut health on long-duration missions.

Finally, this chapter will consider critical ethical and practical implications of implementing AI technologies in space healthcare, including data privacy, reliability of autonomous systems, and ethical decision-making frameworks. By exploring these elements, the chapter aims to illustrate a future where AI and biomedical visualization revolutionise space medicine, enabling safe, sustainable human exploration further into space.

8.2 Space Medicine: Unique Challenges and Solutions

8.2.1 Overview of Space Medicine

Though the 'Space Race' began in the 1940s; it was not until the 1950s that aerospace research began to gain prominence through research and investment. During this period, there were multiple unknowns and hypotheses about the effect of microgravity on human physiology, which had only begun to be tested. Early tests took place on high-altitude balloon and aeroplane flights to develop the initial life support systems (Jedrick 2013). Following success in those terrestrial experiments, in April 1961, the Soviet Union's Yuri Gagarin went on humanity's first orbit around Earth and proved that spaceflight of this distance, type, and duration had no immediate adverse effects on the human body (Gagarin 2006). Gagarin spent a total of 108 min in orbit. Less than a month later, National Aeronautics and Space Administration (NASA's) Alan Shepard took a 15-min suborbital flight and became the first American to reach Space (Williams 2001).

Project Mercury was NASA's first man-in-space programme, which lasted five years and comprised 6 manned missions. The aim of the programme was to better understand human capabilities and requirements for survival in Space and the process of safe return to Earth (Link 1965). The missions and their objectives were as follows:

Mission 1: Mercury Redstone 3——Freedom 7 piloted by Astronaut Alan Shepard
Date: 5th May 1961
Objective: To understand human capabilities and survival in the Space environment
Duration: 15 min 28 s

Mission 2: Mercury Redstone 4—Liberty Bell 7 piloted by astronauts Virgil Grissom and John Glenn
Date: 21st July 1961
Objective: To corroborate the observation in Mission 1 that humans were capable of space flight and survival in Space
Duration: 15 min 37 s

Mission 3: Mercury Atlas 6: Friendship 7 piloted by John Glenn.
Date: 20th February 1962
Objective: To place man in Earth's orbit for a prolonged period, accurately track his location and maintain communication until a point where he could be readily found
Duration: 4 h, 55 min, 23 s

Mission 4: Mercury Atlas 7: Aurora 7 piloted by astronaut Scott Carpenter
Date: 24th May 1962
Objective: Repeat mission 3 with a consistent orbit and perform the first experiments in flight
Duration: 4 h 56 min 5 s

Mission 5: Mercury Atlas 8: Sigma 7 piloted by astronaut Walter Schirra
Date: 3rd October 1962
Objective: Evaluate the performance of the manned spacecraft in a six-pass orbital mission and evaluate the effect of prolonged spaceflight on the astronaut and compare the results to those of previous missions
Duration: 9 h 13 min 11 s

Mission 6: Mercury Atlas 9: Faith 7 piloted by astronaut Gordon Cooper
Date: 15th May 1963
Objective: To complete a manned one day mission in orbit
Duration: 1 Day, 10 h, 19 min, 49 s

The work conducted by the Project Mercury team was based on the assumption that the principles of Aviation Medicine could be extended to Space Medicine; however there was concern around the unknowns related to short-term spaceflight. Project Mercury progressed the understanding of human capabilities in space over 1 day duration in orbit (Grimwood 1963).

Following this work, in 1957, after the launch of Sputnik I, US President D. Eisenhower established the President's Scientific Advisory Committee (PSAC) to give Science and Space a voice in higher office. Led by Dr. James Killian (President of the Massachusetts Institute of Technology,) the Committee soon published a White Paper recommending the development of a formal Space Programme, listing the following four key reasons:

(i) The compelling urge of man to explore and to discover
(ii) Defensive considerations
(iii) The factor of national prestige
(iv) The new opportunities for scientific observation and experiment offered by space technology that would add to man's knowledge and understanding of the Earth, the solar system, and the universe (Finan 2023)

Following federal work in the form of a bill, the National Aeronautics and Space Administration (NASA) came into law on July 29, 1958. From this work and the President's Scientific Advisory Committee (PSAC), the Stever Committee working group, named after Guyford Stever, a physicist and science administrator who served as the Director of the Office of Science and Technology Policy (OSTP) under American President Gerald Ford, was set up to concentrate on furthering the biomedical requirements for manned spaceflight. Its remit was 13 technical areas—life sciences programme administration, the effects of acceleration, high intensity radiation in space, cosmic radiation, nuclear propulsion, ionization effects, human information processing and communication, displays, closed-cycle living, balloon simulators, space capsules, crew selection and training, research centres and launch sites (Stever et al. 1989).

At this point, it was widely felt that Space Medicine research groups should first look to aviation and submarine medicine and aim to build more advanced technology on top of existing work.

The NASA Life Sciences Committee and Life Sciences programme were directed to study the immediate medical problems associated with manned spaceflight and anticipate new problems posed by the space environment. The committee was composed of key representatives from the army, navy, air force, Department of Defense, Research,and Medicine.

During World War I, a School of Aviation Medicine at Mineola, Long Island, was set up and was later relocated to Randolph Air Force Base in Texas to be the first aviation, medical research, and education centre in the world. After World War II, Colonel Harry G. Armstrong collaborated with German aeronautical scientists to set up the school, appointing Dr. Hubertus Strughold as the first Professor of Space Medicine in 1949 (Campbell et al. 2013). With his team, he identified two key problems with spaceflight: solar radiation and weightlessness, which research from German aeromedical laboratories helped to solve. In 1950 and 1951, two symposia were held in Texas, which resulted in the publication of 'Physics and Medicine of the Upper Atmosphere'—a collection of boundary-spanning learning from the event as a synthesis of astrophysics, aeronautical engineering, radiobiology, and aviation medicine (Miles 1952).

This post-war period saw aviation research progressing at a faster pace than before. Flights were faster and were pushing the boundaries of altitude to a point where scientists began to focus on outer atmospheric flight experiments. October 1947 marked a historic event where pilot Charles E. Yeager flew the rocket USAF-NACA-X1 faster than the speed of sound (Yeager 1956). Following this, Lieutenant Colonel John P. Stapp became known in the media as 'the fastest man on Earth' in 1954 after travelling at 632 mph in one of his experiments.

In addition to speed, higher altitudes were also being explored. Seven atmospheric layers have been identified to date; closest to Earth is the troposphere, then the stratosphere, mesosphere, thermosphere, ionosphere, the exosphere, and lastly, the magnetosphere.

In 1927, the US army's Captain Gray managed to reach 28,910 feet in a balloon, setting an unofficial world record. In 1931, Germany's Auguste Piccard and Paul Kipfer successfully broke this record by reaching the stratosphere at 51,777 feet in a similar hydrogen balloon. Once survival at this altitude had been achieved, global rivals continued to push for increasingly greater altitudes, culminating in the US's Dr. David G. Simon's 32-hour manned flight on a balloon at 101,516 feet, where he studied the effects of near space altitude on human physiology on what is remembered as the Manhigh II mission in August 1957. Though Dr. Simons had to use a facemask for oxygenation during significant parts of the trip, it was a broadly successful mission from which Colonel John Stapp concluded that 'Human performance in an environment equivalent to space is now known to be possible' (Hall 2017).

8.2.1.1 The Early Age of Space Medicine

Following World War II, limited biological experimentation had been carried out to support manned spaceflight decisions. Until then, testing of weightlessness and the effects of radiation on living organisms had only been conducted at a limited level. One of the first space biology experiments took place in December 1946 with the testing of the effects of upper atmospheric radiation on fungal spores. Sponsored by the National Institutes of Health, lucite cylinders were propelled into the upper atmospheric region; however, the experiment failed due to the cylinders being irrecoverable (McWilliams 1958). Learning from this event, methods were improved to conduct an experiment on recovered seeds and fruit flies to test the effect of altitude using V-2 rockets at the Holloman Air Base in New Mexico the following year, as a cooperative research project between the US Naval Research Laboratory and Harvard Biology Department. The project was successful, as after the cylinders containing the seeds and flies were propelled to 160 km (well above the Karaman line (100 km above Earth)) for a period, they were parachuted down to Earth, and all flies were still alive and in good health (Hanrahan 1952). Reaching this distance above Earth enabled the team to safely conclude that this experiment has been conducted in Space. Following the success of this work, teams across the world began to set their ambitions on sending mammals to Space. This work was pioneered by a team led by Dr. P. James Henry, Head of the Acceleration unit of the biophysic branch of the Aeromedical Laboratory, in collaboration with Captain Simons and his team at Wright Field. Their goal was to send a small monkey into the upper atmosphere in a V-2 rocket, which would require a pressurized capsule that could protect the monkey against the external environment. They developed a pressurized capsule in the nose of the rocket which would hold Albert—an anaesthetized rhesus monkey— to conduct the Albert I Project, which was launched on 18 June 1948 (Beischer and Fregley 1962). This project was fraught with many difficulties. First, even before the launch, the team was unable to detect the monkey's respiratory function through a device failure, so it is unknown whether the monkey even reached the atmosphere alive. Second, the capsule which carried the monkey was cramped and could have in itself been inadequate to sustain life, even for short periods with pressurization. Third, the parachute recovery system the team developed to recover Albert towards the end of the experiment also failed; so though the nose cone did lower down towards Earth, the parachute did not deploy and the speed of collision upon impact on Earth would have also caused Albert's death. Posthumous identification yielded several ways in the experiment failed to sustain Albert. There were early indications that Albert died even before launch from breathing difficulties in the pressurized capsule. A recorder that was successfully recovered from the capsule showed zero physiological activity at any time during the flight, which indicates that either Albert was dead prior to launch or there was a complete failure of all detection devices, including respiratory and electrocardiographic monitoring from the outset. Finally, even if the capsule came back to Earth as it was meant to, the failure of the parachute system meant that Albert would have been killed upon impact on his return (Hanrahan 1952).

The team learnt from this experimental failure, took a year to improve their processes, devices and technology, and launched Albert II into space on 14 June 1949, 133 km above Earth, into its outer atmosphere. Unfortunately, the parachute recovery system failed again, and Albert II died upon impact with Earth on his return. However, until this point, the rest of the experiment had been successful and consistently transmitted both respiratory and electrocardiographic data from Albert II to the command centre, confirming that a monkey had lived throughout an entire flight into the upper atmosphere (Lee 2020).

Subsequent flights were required to iron out technical issues, including rocket performance, parachute deployment, efficacy, and recovery programmes. The fifth V-2 rocket flight with Aeromedical Laboratories was planned to explore the effects of subgravity on mammalian physiology in 1950. This time, an awake mouse was sent into the upper atmosphere with a camera in its capsule, which would take photographs at fixed intervals. The recovery system on this flight failed and the mouse was killed upon impact, however, photographs showed that the mouse conveyed normal muscular coordination' and no preference for certain movements or directions throughout subgravity. This strengthened the research team's understanding of the ability of mammals to withstand the effects of subgravity for short periods (Burgess 2007). Parallel to this, the first successful high altitude balloon flight took place at the Holloman Air Force Base in September 1950, where eight mice reached an altitude of 30 km above Earth and were successfully received back on Earth (Burgess 2007).

After this experiment, testing transferred to the Holloman Air Force Base, where the newly developed high altitude rocket Aerobee set off on its first aeromedical expedition on 18 April 1951 (Joseph 2012). This experiment repeated the V-2 monkey experiments and corroborated the working hypothesis that high altitudes and short periods under subgravity did not alter mammalian physiology. The second of these experiments occurred in September 1951 and sent a monkey and 11 mice up 72 km and was successful in bringing all animals back down to Earth alive, demonstrating an improvement in parachute recovery system function (Angelo 2014). Two hours after landing back on Earth, the monkey died; however, the autopsy revealed that this was not due to the effects of the upper atmosphere, but due to landing shock or heat exhaustion, believed to be due to the delay in recovery of the capsule, which touched down at midday in New Mexico but was not recovered for some time. Two of the eleven mice also died within two hours of return landing, but the cause was not believed to be due to cosmic radiation. One of the mice was sent into the atmosphere after surgical removal of its vestibular systems, but did not seem affected by the loss of gravity. However, the other control mouse seemed to be disturbed by the subgravity portion of the journey, which was indicated through its uncharacteristic clawing of the air.

The third and final aeromedical Aerobee flight was the most successful. The rocket, which took off on 21 May 1952 and flew up to an altitude of 57 km, housed two mice and two monkeys, who landed back on Earth unscathed and were collected from the New Mexico desert without delay (Gebhardt 2016). Mouse A, who was given a rod to cling onto, maintained orientation, tactile ability, and did not show signs of agitation during the subgravity portion of the journey. Mouse B, who did not have anything to hold onto, showed signs of temporary disorientation during the period of complete weightlessness. The two monkeys, one of whom was seated upright and the other who was supine, were also retrieved unharmed by the flight conditions.

On Friday, October 4, 1957, the Soviet Union launched the first artificial satellite into space—Sputnik (Divine 1993). Following this, the USA vowed to accelerate its space programme outcomes and formed the 'Man in Space' task force headed by General Schreiver and included military, civilian, and technology companies. Their aim was to achieve animal test flights by 1959 and send the first man into Space by 1960. In July 1958, President Eisenhower ratified the space agenda as a US priority through the National Aeronautics and Space Act, which enabled the National Aeronautics and Space Administration (NASA) to begin operations in October 1958 (Maltby 1958).

NASA was founded as a US governmental agency for the research and development of activities and vehicles for the exploration of Space. The organization was subdivided into four main mission directorates (Jacob 2008):

1. Aeronautics research—for the development of advanced aerospace technologies.
2. Science—understanding space, our solar system, and the universe.
3. Space Technology—to develop Space Science and exploration technologies.
4. Human exploration and Operations—pertaining to space exploration logistics and operation and crew recruitment, training, and development.

Dr. T Keith Glennan was selected to be NASA's first administrator, appointed by the President of the United States after conferring with the Senate. Dr. T Keith Glennan's background in electrical engineering from Yale University, innovative work in sound motion pictures for the entertainment industry, his tenure as director of the US Navy's underwater sound laboratories, and President of Case Institute of Technology in Cleveland, Ohio, made him suitable for the role. During his three years leading NASA, he focussed on abolishing silo working by amalgamating laboratories, space exploration projects, and satellite projects to unify US Space work under NASA. By the end of his time at NASA, he had secured all the component parts of an organization that would be competitive in both Space and Defense research and development on the world stage (Glennan 1993).

Though the Ames Research Centre (a field centre for NASA) was set up in 1939, its goal was always to be a pioneer in new technologies, innovations, and capabilities related to the Aerospace industry. In 1987, the Ames Research Centre duo Peter Friedland and Henry Lum published the paper Building Intelligent Systems: Artificial Intelligence Research at NASA Ames Research Centre. In the paper, they outline the long-term vision of an intelligent system that 'will have full responsibility for a major functional component of a space station; examples include power, communications, thermal management, and environmental control. It will be responsible for nominal control, acute and chronic failure discovery, diagnosis, and correction, and communications/cooperation with both interested humans (astronauts, ground controllers, scientists) and other intelligent computational systems' (Friedland and Lum 1987).

They went on to discuss the four key abilities of an artificial intelligence system:

1. Reasoning under uncertainty.
2. Ability to learn and improve.
3. Common sense reasoning with the ability to bypass established reasoning mechanisms.
4. Self-understanding—the ability to understand.

They then concluded that the development of these systems can only be achieved if humans master the following artificial intelligence methodologies:

1. Better knowledge acquisition—the tools and ability for the software to develop a knowledge base.
2. Managing and optimizing large knowledge bases.
3. Validation of Intelligence systems.

Since then, the teams at the NASA Ames Research Centre have been progressing this work and developing artificial intelligence methodologies to support astronauts and their teams in space. One of the applications for the work conducted at the NASA Ames Research Centre is in the use of artificial intelligence in Space Medicine (Andrews 1985).

8.2.1.2 Health Risks Associated with Space Travel

There are three key health risks associated with space travel: the effects of microgravity on the human body, exposure to space radiation, and the psychosocial effects of space travel on the mind.

Microgravity

The effects of microgravity on the human body have been well documented (Stratmann 2015; Iwase 2020). The visual, somatosensory, and vestibular systems help us to orient ourselves relative to time, position, and activity. In particular, the vestibular complex: semicircular canals and otoliths detect linear and angular velocity and acceleration that, combined with visual and proprioceptive stimuli, enable human orientation in time and space. Exposure to microgravity can distort the input signals received by our sensory system. The fluid shift hypothesis predicts that the loss of hydrostatic pressure in microgravity leads to a cranial shifting of body fluids from the lower body (McCarthy 2005). The cranial shifting of body fluids leads to facial and upper body oedema, an increase in the intracranial pressure, an increase in the cerebrospinal fluid pressure and the inner ear; thus distorting input and response reactions of the vestibular system and causing space motion sickness. A second hypothesis, called the sensory conflict hypothesis, attributes space motion sickness to a mismatch of actual and anticipated signals received by the vestibular system, particularly the otolith tilt mechanism, which directly contributes to spatial orientation (Previc 2018). Space motion sickness is experienced by 60–80% of space travellers in the first few days of entry into space and consists of the following symptoms: nausea, vomiting, fatigue, loss of appetite, sweating, pallor, increased body temperature, and malaise (Heer and Paloski 2006).

The effect of microgravity on the cardiovascular system begins with the fluid shift from the lower body to the thorax. This increase in thoracic fluid volume causes atrial stretching and cardiac distension within the first twenty-four hours of space flight (Williams 2016). Increased filling results in left ventricular end-diastolic volume increase, with research showing that heart chamber size increases by 20%. Atrial natriuretic peptide was found to increase by 80% in humans after the first day in microgravity (Aubert et al. 2005). Atrial natriuretic peptide (ANP) stimulates vasodilation and promotes glomerular filtration of sodium and water, and increases vascular permeability, thus promoting fluid loss from the intravascular to the extravascular compartments. Blood volume also decreases in microgravity and, under chronic conditions of a week or more, results in the human body adapting to lower stroke volume and, by day 7, facilitating a 50% reduction in ANP. Chronic microgravitational conditions cause other adaptations in the human body, including a reduction in left ventricular volume, stroke volume, ANP, and an increase in renin, aldosterone, vasopressin, and glomerular filtration rate, which leads to reduced urinary excretion and increased sodium retention, resulting in further swelling of the face and upper extremities.

Furthermore, the composition of an astronaut's blood is also affected by microgravity, noted as a reduction in red blood cell mass, plasma volume, and a reduced erythropoietin and reticulocyte count, indicating a slowing of erythropoiesis in space. Though heart rate and blood pressure on Earth and in space have not been significantly different, a constant observation has been the decrease in heart rate in space compared to Earth and a slow recovery after return to earth, believed to be related to an increase in parasympathetic activity triggered by the microgravitational force in space (Aubert et al. 2005).

Microgravity also affects the structure and function of the brain. A decrease in the grey matter of the brain, a reduction in synapses, and degeneration of axonal terminals have been observed (Koppelmans et al. 2016). However, there have been fewer studies on brain function (Hupfeld et al. 2021). Demertzi et al. conducted a study in 2016 on a 44-year-old astronaut after he spent 6 months in space and found evidence of cortical reorganization, impaired motor coordination, and vestibular ataxia post-flight. 'Dual tasking' is the ability to multi-task and is used as a way to measure the effect of an environment or stressor on human management of cognitive load and executive function. Manzey et al. found that motor and memory dual tasking was significantly impaired in space, but recovered to pre-flight baselines after three weeks in space, which indicates an adaptive response (Manzey 1998).

Muscle volume loss is another key physiological impact of spaceflight, with atrophy reaching as high as 10% and occurring by an astronaut's eighth day in space (Lee 2023). The key reasons for muscle atrophy are lack of mechanical use and constraining factors in space. At a molecular level, studies have shown an increased breakdown of myocytes as well as a decrease in protein synthesis relating to the human oxidative stress response in space (Reynolds 2020).

Microgravity is also known to affect the bone health of astronauts. The effect of spaceflight and lack of mechanical loading through bones and joints leads to an increase in Ca^{2+} loss from bones and a resultant increased risk of renal stones and fractures (Goldsmith 1972). Gravity has been shown to influence the long bones of the human body and keep the osteoblastic bone formation and osteoclastic bone resorption in balance, but creates weight and exerts pressure on the skeleton, mediating mechanical impact. A lack of gravity leads to increased bone resorption, which leads to decalcification, bone loss, and the development of osteoporosis (Iwase 2013). This is a significant hazard to an astronaut's health as osteoporosis is not reversible and it confers a significant fracture risk, even after return to Earth (Man et al. 2022).

The effect of microgravity on immune regulation has been shown to manifest through a reduction of T lymphocytes and suppression of T helper cells identified in the blood samples of astronauts post-flight (Makedonas 2018). Similarly, a higher rate of reactivation of latent herpes virus in astronauts compared with controls was also observed, indicating a decrease in cell-mediated immunity during spaceflight (Rooney et al. 2019). Furthermore, studies show that 50% of astronauts experience some form of immunological condition and that the effect of spaceflight on the human body can affect all components of the immune system (Reynolds 2020).

Space Radiation

Radiation is a form of energy that is emitted in the form of electromagnetic waves, rays, or particles. The electromagnetic spectrum shows the range of different types of radiation across different frequencies and how they can present as visible and non-visible. Ionizing radiation is a type of radiation energy that acts by removing electrons from atoms or molecules (Christensen et al. 2014). Space radiation is a form of ionizing radiation from space and has four known sources (Nelson 2016):

1. Galactic cosmic rays
2. The Sun in steady state
3. Short-term solar emissions [solar particle events (SPEs)]
4. Trapped radiation belts (Van Allen belts) around the Earth

Humans on Earth are exposed to constant background radiation that does not pose them significant harm. However, astronauts are exposed to far more radiation in Space and the effects of space radiation on the human body have been described (Chancellor 2014).

A key cellular effect of radiation is the induction of DNA damage through single and double-stranded breaks, as well as damage to bases. Usually, organisms are equipped to conduct cellular repair; however, if the damage exceeds repair capabilities, the organism can switch to cellular senescence or undergo tumorigenesis. This is the mechanism by which higher levels of radiation exposure have been linked to cancer in humans (Furukawa et al. 2020).

The effects related to the different sources of space radiation exposure include; alteration of gene expression, induction of oxidative stress, gastrointestinal tract bacterial translocation and immune system activation, peripheral hematopoietic cell activity and counts, sickness in the form of nausea and vomit known as 'radiation sickness', dysfunction in blood coagulation, skin changes, changes in behaviour, physical and mental fatigue, radiation induced heart disease, visual dysfunction from pressure or pathological changes, mortality and morbidity rates and other long-term effects such as the development of cancer and cataract in future years even if there has been no return to space (Cucinotta 2014; Kennedy 2014; Nelson 2016).

The known radiation exposure experienced by astronauts is 1mSV (millisievert) per day, which is 150 times more than experienced by humans on Earth. Much of Space medicine has been concentrating on the amelioration of these symptoms and the prevention of the more serious biological effects and longer-term consequences of space flight (Ohnishi and Ohnishi 2004).

The effects of radiation on humans can be categorized into acute, intermediate, and late effects (Nelson 2016). Solar particle events, which occur when concentrated solar particles (solar flares or storms) are emitted from the sun, and galactic cosmic rays, which are high-energy particles that travel almost as fast as the speed of light, deliver high doses of radiation in space. Acute radiation sickness, which can induce nausea, vomiting, diarrhoea, and intense fatigability and skin changes, can occur between 4 and 24 h after exposure (Hu 2020). Intermediate effects of radiation include a dysregulation of human immune function, which renders astronauts more susceptible to infections in space through a reduction in cell-mediated immunity (Cucinotta 2003). An exacerbation of bone loss and skeletal architecture is another intermediate effect of space travel. The mechanism by which this is believed to occur is through the effect of the radiation on osteoclastic activity, which is further upregulated due to oxidative damage at molecular levels. Cancer, cataracts, and heart disease are well known as possible results of long-term or repeated exposure to space radiation Kennedy 2014).

Psychosocial Stressors

The known observed and experienced psychological risks associated with space travel have been documented in detail. Dr. Andrew Liu's research at the Massachusetts Institute of Technology documented a significant disruption in astronauts' circadian rhythms (Liu 2023). In a given 24-hour day, astronauts experience 16 sunrises and sunsets at the International Space Station. This, coupled with the artificial blue light that keeps the station lit, disrupts the natural release of melatonin and the human circadian clock (Ramanathan et al. 2018). The circadian system works through the suprachiasmatic nuclei in the brain to regulate human sleep-wake cycles and is stimulated by light and dark (Liu et al. 2007). Circadian rhythm has an integrated effect on almost all metabolic processes in the body. Dysregulation of the normal sleep/wake cycle has been linked with mood changes, impaired cognition and concentration, obesity, impaired glucose tolerance, cancer spread, and increased relative mortality risk, anxiety, depression, and precipitation of psychiatric disorders (Serin and Acar 2019).

The concept of isolation from the world for extended periods of time is an obvious psychosocial stressor. Astronauts now typically spend six months on a space mission and there are key human factors associated with being in a crew, isolated from home, family, and friends for such an extended period of time (Navarro 2023).

Unlike on Earth, confinement to a shuttle where the liveable space can vary but is usually just over 2000 cubic feet shared between 6 crew members makes guaranteed privacy and personal space difficult (Boltz 1998).

Several tests have been conducted to monitor the stress levels of astronauts during space travel. One such experiment was conducted by Stein and Schutler in 1994 with a working hypothesis that increased stress levels during spaceflight would cause increased cytokine release, similar to the human physiological response on Earth. Urinary interleukin-6 (IL-6) levels were measured from four crew members, 11 days before flight, during the 8 days of flight, and 7 days after landing back on Earth. The researchers found an increase in IL-6 and cortisol levels on day 1 of the flight and immediately after landing, signalling an acute phase stress response (Stein and Schulter 1994).

Since then, several other studies have been conducted describing the short and long-term effects of stress on astronauts. The known psychological and human factor stressors of spaceflight have been identified as; isolation, danger from limited rescue options, confinement, hostile external environment, fatigue, boredom, homesickness, loneliness, tension with ground crew, social conflicts, personality differences with crew members, communication demands, sexuality, adaptation to the artificial environment, limited hygiene, poor ventilation, food restrictions and monotony (Smith 2022).

Mood changes and emotional instability, visual phenomena, anxiety, and depression have also been observed through manned space flight missions (Arone et al. 2021).

This is all very important as stress and psychosocial issues have clear negative effects on any given mission. An example of this is when interpersonal tensions amongst the Apollo 13 crew resulted in steps being taken to potentially end the mission early, which would have halted key experiments and cost millions of dollars (Seamans 2005). Luckily, this outcome was narrowly avoided through the amelioration of the situation. Similarly, the team on Skylab 4 achieved such a degree of animosity between crewmates that they demanded a whole day off work to solve their issues. This resulted in a key day in space not being utilized as planned (Johnson 2007). Similarly, during the Saylut mission, the flight crew fell out with the ground crew to such a degree that they did not communicate with ground mission control for 48 h (Smith 2022).

There are also some surprisingly positive psychosocial effects of space travel. In 2007, researchers from the Aerospace Medical Association (AMA) surveyed astronauts and people who lived or spent long periods in harsh environments such as arctic stations or submarines and described the positive effects on wellbeing. The researchers surveyed the individuals before and after they entered and adapted to the harsh conditions and found evidence of reduced stress levels after adaptation and *salutogenesis*—the positive effect of having adapted to harsh conditions (Ihle et al. 2006). The same AMA researchers, Ritsher, Ihle, and Kanas surveyed 39 astronauts after space travel and found that all astronauts were retrospectively positive about their experiences of spaceflight, which led the researchers to conclude that space travel in itself is a meaningful experience that makes an enduring positive impression on astronauts' (Ihle 2003).

8.3 Artificial Intelligence in Monitoring Astronaut Health

8.3.1 Wearable Technology for Health Monitoring

One of the main goals of introducing artificial intelligence into space medicine was the development of an accurate Precision Space Health (PSH) system (Scott 2023). One of the key studies used to develop this was the NASA Twins Study, which monitored a pair of monozygotic twins for a one-year period, where one twin was monitored in space and the other was a control on Earth. The concept behind this study was to observe the effect of space vs Earth on genetically matched subjects. Through this study, they were able to obtain, monitor, and analyse samples of stool, saliva, skin, urine, and blood aboard the International Space Station and conduct regular cognitive and physical assessments on both subjects (Garrett-Bakelman et al. 2019). Since then, wearable technologies for health monitoring in space have been developed and improved. During early missions on Apollo 13, the detection of cardiac rhythm through electrocardiography helped diagnose arrhythmias in astronauts, resulting in treatment before the development of adverse outcomes.

The use of artificial intelligence and technology has come a long way since then and Precision Space Health systems have become more sophisticated.

One key space condition that needed to be overcome was spatial disorientation. Spatial disorientation is the inability of a person to correctly determine their body position in space and has been found to be one of the most common root causes of space and aviation aircraft accidents, accounting for 6–32% of major accidents and 15–26% of fatal accidents (Newman and Faicd 2007). Dr. Vimal et al. at Brandeis University, MA, in the United States, developed a vibrotactile device to help astronauts maintain orientation and proprioception in space. The device was tested on human subjects using a Multi-Axis Rotation system (MARS) device, which would be used to manoeuvre their position and mimic Earth and Space environments. The vibrotactile feedback was set to sense movement and activate at different degrees of deviation away from the balance setting. The researchers found that the vibrotactile feedback devices enhanced stabilization performance. However, performance was not recovered to the same level as performance on Earth due to an internal conflict between vibrotactile orientation and sensory perception. Though delivering training did further improve performance, it was not improved to the level experienced on Earth, and it was therefore suggested that the device be used to further enhance activities where proprioception and manoeuvring are paramount, such as extravehicular activities on planetary surfaces and key manual control tasks (Vimal et al. 2023).

Another key issue was being able to anticipate deterioration and fluctuations in astronaut health during a mission. In 2019, the Canadian Space Health Agency developed the 'Biomonitor smart shirt system,' which is a wearable health monitoring technology for daily use aboard the International Space Station. The 'smart shirt' measures:

- Heart rate and electrical activity of the heart
- Blood pressure
- Respiratory rate and tidal volume
- Skin temperature
- Blood oxygen saturation
- Physical activity levels

The garment itself was designed to be as comfortable as an everyday t-shirt and can be worn at all times, including sleep and during periods of exercise. It was trialled by astronaut David Saint-Jacques and is now part of the Canadian Space Health Study 2023, where this smart system is integrated with the artificial intelligence computing platform Artemis on Earth, where scientists can monitor astronaut health. This integration enables data storage, analysis, and the use of artificial intelligence algorithms to identify patterns, anticipate health deterioration, and attribute risk profiles to individual astronauts before, during, and after spaceflight. The Biomonitor-Artemis integration has also demonstrated benefits to subjects on Earth, including monitoring premature babies in neonatal intensive care, military, firefighters, and to aid sports performance (Canadian Space Agency 2023). The Canadian Space Health Study is currently underway as a collaboration with NASA's Expedition 70 crew of seven astronauts, all wearing the Bio-Monitor for 6 months to further the study of this health monitoring system in Space.

Most recently, the US-based health monitoring company Empatica released its smartwatch for astronauts the EmbracePlus which can store 55 days worth of data in case of connectivity issues and measures:

- Movement
- Sleep cycles
- Temperature
- Cardiac activity
- Respiratory activity
- Electrical activity

The device, which is already used in clinical trials, monitors human health and uses machine learning to carry out a detection function in order to identify illness early (Qu 2024). This, if successful in space, would offer the ability to prevent or treat early signs of illness prior to it causing deterioration of the human condition.

8.3.2 Predictive Health Analytics Using Machine Learning

Due to the invasive and impractical nature of blood draws in space, point-of-care testing is being explored as a method to aid predictive health analytics in space. The Swedish finger-prick blood analyser 'Haemacue', often used on Earth for rapid blood testing, was tested onboard the International Space Station. Crucian et al. tested this analysis method, focussing on white blood cell fluctuations in 2020 and 2021 on one space crew member onboard the International Space Station. Their findings showed that the device was capable of accurately detecting white blood cell levels in their subjects that were in the same range as healthy human subjects on Earth. This was promising, because white blood cell plasma levels changes are one of the earlier indicators of infectious or inflammatory conditions. Therefore, early identification could result in early treatment or prevention of the fulminant condition, which would benefit the crew member, the wider crew, and the mission. Interestingly, practical issues with conducting the test such as difficulty controlling a single drop of blood from a finger prick in microgravity and issues with storage of control solutions were also observed during this study; with the main challenge being the practicality of temporal testing versus the inability to continuously monitor blood plasma in space in order to closely monitor for the earliest observable signs of illness (Crucian et al. 2021). We are now able to use this method and the method of less frequent blood draws for biomedical testing in space (European Space Agency, 2016).

Ong et al. studied continuous glucose monitoring in 26 participants who partook in centrifuge-simulated spaceflight. Their results showed that continuous blood glucose monitoring is possible in spaceflight conditions as well as generally reliable with monitor results, aside from four false low blood glucose results during the experiment. Further feasibility studies would be needed to conclude the acceptability and reliability of the technology in space, where additional stressors could affect monitoring and results (Ong et al. 2022a, b). Achievement of continuous blood monitoring in astronauts would further advance space medicine to be able to detect the earliest signs of illness. This could not only benefit human ambitions for space travel and exploration, but also improve life and prevent the advancement of disease on Earth, through early detection and precision-based targeted treatment.

The next step after being able to successfully monitor vital signs and conduct continuous biomedical tests in a spaceflight setting would be to develop a method of constant analysis, identification, and stratification of abnormal findings.

In 2013, Wang et al. from Hong Kong proposed a machine learning framework for disease prediction during spaceflight (Wang et al. 2013). Machine learning is a type of artificial intelligence methodology where software synthesizes past data using statistics, probability, and improvement techniques to identify and apply patterns and predictions to current data sets. There are two approaches to machine learning: supervised and unsupervised learning. Supervised learning uses labelled training data so there is a view of what the 'correct answer' looks like. Examples of supervised learning include artificial neural networks, mixture Gaussian models, support vector machines, and decision trees.

Unsupervised learning does not use labelled training data and can be used to achieve three things:

1. Clustering—to discover patterns in sets of data
2. To ascertain the distribution of data
3. Projection and visualization of data

Prognostics and Health Management is a methodology that aims to predict when a system component will start to deteriorate. Aerospace medicine concepts are predicated on similar principles of aiming to predict health alterations in the context of space scenarios.

Wang et al. (2013) proposed using a machine learning framework to use physiological monitoring data for disease prediction amongst crew members. The machine learning method through which this would occur is through the support vector machine classification process used to distinguish healthy and deteriorating vital signs, which are continuously measured throughout the flight.

The research team then went on to use this methodology on the EEG data of 19 patients after 'learning' through an established data set related to epilepsy and seizures. They found that the machine was able to correctly predict every seizure in 16 out of 19 patients and concluded that this model could be useful for disease prediction during space missions (Wang 2014).

8.3.3 AI in Emergency Response and Decision Making

Though a significant part of Space Medicine aims to detect and prevent disease, it is essential that astronauts are equipped to deal with medical emergencies in space, should they arise.

The medical issues that have arisen on spaceflight include: viral upper respiratory tract infections (Apollo 7), urinary tract infection (Apollo 13), ocular fibreglass irritation (Apollo 10), and in many cases, radiation sickness (Summers 2005). Though deaths in space have occurred, these have been due to engineering or mechanical failures and not due to medical emergencies (Mallak 2018).

Currently, the medical requirement for a manned mission to the Moon is not obligated to be entirely medically equipped for any treatment plan, only to be able to stabilize a medical emergency for long enough for return to Earth. However, as the human race expands its horizons to flying for longer durations and colonizing other planets like Mars, arrangements must be made to ensure the delivery of safe medical care in the deep space environment.

NASA's Human Research Programme has documented 30 possible health risks associated with the space environment under five main categories: (1) Space radiation; (2) altered gravitational fields; (3) hostile/closed environments; (4) isolation/confinement, and (5) distance from Earth. Following extensive research and modelling, they have risk stratified the conditions with the highest likelihood and adverse impact to be as follows; (1) the effects of space radiation on health—chiefly cancer, cardiovascular disease, and cognitive conditions (2) spaceflight-associated neuro-ocular syndrome, (3) deterioration in behavioural health and performance, and (4) inadequate food and nutrition. The focus is now on overcoming these high-risk conditions from a prevention and management position (Patel et al. 2020).

Radiation sickness and the carcinogenic effect of repeated or significant radiation exposure are well documented (National Research Council 2012). However, radiation can also cause and exacerbate non-cancerous conditions on Earth and in Space. Studies have shown that radiation confers a higher risk of myocardial infarction or stroke (Sylvester et al. 2018). Furthermore, research has shown that radiation exposure from a Mars mission is more likely to precipitate death from cardiac rather than cancerous disease. Current research is being conducted to optimize prediction and risk stratification prior to astronaut selection, followed by prevention and identification of precipitants in space and emergency medical stabilization and treatment (Lowery 2025).

Central Nervous System disease is also a high risk because it can cause alterations in neurocognitive function. Impaired cognition and neurological status can seriously affect missions with both performance and the ability to carry out crucial flight duties en route.

Spaceflight Associated Neuro-ocular syndrome (SANS) encompasses a spectrum of signs and symptoms, including optic disc swelling, chorioretinal folds, globe flattening, and shifts in refractive error, manifesting as visual distortion, reduced visual acuity, and in some cases a shortening of the ocular axial length (Lee 2018). SANS affects 70% of crew members on space missions that are 30 days or longer, and pathogenesis has not yet been confirmed. Aetiological theories include ocular venous congestion, an increase in intraocular pressure, and anatomical variability leading to genetic susceptibility in different subjects. Research on the pathogenesis and effective prevention and management of SANS has been prioritized by NASA. This will include development of diagnostic devices for use in space to aid decision-making with regard to management of the condition and whether or not to continue a mission (Martin Paez 2020).

Deterioration in performance due to the effect of Space on psychological health is also a key concern. The two key concerns related to performance are the deterioration in crew mental health leading to suboptimal performance, and the development of a psychiatric disorder rendering the entire mission at risk. Radiation exposure, isolation, extended confinement, disrupted circadian rhythm, homesickness, and additional space-related stressors all contribute negatively to psychological health. Though the development of a psychiatric condition is less of a risk, emergency medical management of the condition should be possible if required.

Another critical situation astronauts could find themselves in is experiencing inadequate food and nutrition. The minimum requirement is to meet the nutritional needs of and therefore prevent nutritional deficiencies in astronauts. However, it is key to note that poor nutrition, even if basic requirements are met, can lead to overall worsening astronaut health in the longer term as it has been linked to cancer, cardiovascular disease, and osteoporosis (Dakkumadugula et al. 2023). In order to support astronaut health, a preflight assessment is always conducted to ascertain astronaut vitamin, mineral, and electrolyte levels, haematology and bone markers, and renal stone risk profile. In addition, dietary intake monitoring, body weight measurements to identify bone loss velocity, and vision tests are conducted whilst in-flight. However, much more work needs to be done to optimize in-flight nutrition as well as identify the nutritional intake and activities that astronauts should undertake between flights to further benefit their health whilst in space. In addition, more sophisticated monitoring of nutritional signs, symptoms, and biochemical changes needs to be developed to better take care of astronauts and crew members (Patel et al. 2020).

So far, no guidelines for managing emergency health conditions and acute deterioration in health in microgravity exist, which is also necessary when planning for longer missions.

8.3.3.1 Medical Emergencies in Space

The cardiovascular effects of space include the development of ectopic beats and minor dysrhythmias, which are well tolerated by the healthy flight crew who are rigorously selected for optimal ability to cope with spaceflight. With the advent of space tourism, the health profile of humans in space will include less physically conditioned astronauts and, therefore, more significant cardiovascular issues are anticipated. These would be arrhythmias leading to cardiac arrest, myocardial infarction, and venous thromboembolic disease. In 2020, Hinkelbein et al. put together an international aerospace medicine working group to determine the most appropriate management of cardiac arrest in space. The team created a guideline which determined that in the basic life support process, the chest compression method of choice should be the Evetts-Russomano method (Hinkelbein et al. 2020).

However, in an event requiring advanced life support, the patient should be secured into the crew medical restraint system and the handstand method should be used.

They also concluded that the most appropriate airway device should be the supraglottic airway device and airway management should only be performed if two rescuers are present. The International Space Station is equipped with electrocardiogram (ECG) capability, cardiac defibrillation devices, vascular access equipment, the ability to give intravenous fluid infusions, conduct bladder catheterization, and nasogastric tube placement facilities, which have all been conducted in microgravity for experimental purposes (McCuaig and Houtchens 1992).

Biochemically, the immune system is dampened by microgravity and spaceflight stressors. Infections were one of the earliest diagnosed medical conditions in space (Mermel 2013). During the Apollo 11 flight, all of the crew suffered from the symptoms of a viral upper respiratory tract infection, which led to a two-week preflight quarantine becoming part of subsequent flight protocols (Gohd 2020). The effect of this measure was noticed instantly with a significant reduction in reported infection symptoms from the Apollo 13 flight onwards. Though only minor infections such as gingivitis, boils, and styes have been reported in space, long-haul flights pose a higher risk of the life-threatening consequences of infection, such as systemic inflammatory response syndrome, sepsis, and septic shock.

Another high-risk condition could be the development of symptomatic renal calculi (kidney stones). Spaceflight itself increases the risk of developing calculi during increased urinary calcium through an upregulation of bone remodelling in the microgravitational environment (De Santo et al. 2005). Renal colic can be extremely painful and can lead to renal tract infections, septicaemia, and renal failure. It is therefore essential that the condition is promptly identified and managed in space. Management of renal stones can be non-invasive or invasive, depending on the size of the obstructing stone. Treatment may include shockwave lithotripsy, ureteroscopy, percutaneous nephrolithotomy, or nephrolithotripsy.

Emergency Surgery

Surgery has not yet been performed during spaceflight; however, the likelihood of surgical procedures during spaceflight increases with the duration of space flight, interplanetary missions and space tourism. Emergencies being considered currently with respect to their surgical requirements include penetrating trauma, blunt trauma or fractures from injuries and falls, abscess drainage, appendectomy, and cholecystectomy. The first animal laparotomy in space was carried out in 1967 (Laroshenko et al. 1967). It revealed key technical and logistical issues required to develop the necessary conditions to be able to perform surgery safely in space. These include: restraint of the patient and surgeon to ensure precision, managing the weightlessness of the instruments, maintaining aseptic technique, and adequate waste disposal. Consideration also must be taken to mitigate intra-operative issues such as the effect of weightlessness on the abdominal viscera during laparotomy. On Earth, it can be difficult to prevent the bowels from blocking key surgical work; however, in Space, mitigations need to be put in place to prevent the bowels and other organs from floating up and out of the abdominal incision and prevent the life-threatening effects of perforation. Currently, the International Space Station is only equipped for minor surgical procedures with the goal of stabilization and transportation back to Earth for astronauts who experience more serious illness (Stewart et al. 2007). The use of artificial intelligence could help to improve the identification of management of these life-threatening conditions.

8.4 Biomedical Visualization in Microgravity

8.4.1 Medical Imaging in Microgravity

The first test of in-flight imaging was echocardiography and was first performed in 1982 onboard the Salyut-6 and Soyuz-T6/Salyut-7 flights in a joint Soviet-French research study (Sargsyan 2008). Subsequently, validation of abdominal ultrasound and feasibility studies on various machines, including Philips and Aeris, were successfully conducted. Currently, ultrasound is the most viable imaging modality in space. This is due to operational adaptations such as the ability for there to be remote guidance from medical teams on Earth whilst carrying out the imaging, the development of wearable ultrasound machines that mitigate the effects of microgravity and the use of artificial intelligence (Scott et al. 2021a, b). Tele-ultrasound is the use of ultrasound by non-medical crew members to diagnose and treat medical conditions with the assistance of physicians on Earth through telecommunication (Haney 2020). Though successful for a range of ailments including renal calculi, limitations include the ultrasound's inability to diagnose cerebral conditions, bone conditions, or lung and bowel pathology. The next step currently being researched is the use of artificial intelligence and namely deep learning to carry out diagnostic functions, which would result in less need for remote physician assistance. This technology is currently being used on Earth, for example, in differentiating between benign and malignant thyroid nodules with 83% accuracy using machine learning methodology as well as the segmentation of breast tissue images in 3D breast ultrasound imaging in order to diagnose breast cancers (Xu et al. 2019; Ma et al. 2020).

Several studies into the utility of other imaging modalities, such as Magnetic Resonance Imaging (MRI) aboard the International Space Station, have also been conducted. The benefits of MRI would be to monitor bone and mass strength whilst in Space in order to identify developing conditions early (Sarty and Obenaus 2012). One of the drawbacks of MRI is the time patients are required to spend in the scanner in order to yield an accurate image; however, artificial intelligence is supporting the acceleration of scan time on Earth. Chen et al. from Imperial College University, London, have explored the possibility of a shortened MRI acquisition time through deep learning based compressed sensing MRI (Chen et al. 2022). Compressed sensing uses a mathematical framework to reconstruct data and is a form of artificial intelligence that is currently being tested on animal models.

Computed tomography (CT) scans are also not currently used in space due to the size of the machine and a rotating gantry would exert an equal and opposite torque on the spacecraft. The development of a lightweight, immobile, modular scanner may be a way to enable CT scans in space (Cramer et al. 2018). X-ray technology has also not yet embedded itself in the International Space Station. However, UK company Adaptix is developing a mobile 3D-X Ray device with the aim of creating a suitcase-sized machine with a cost price similar to the equivalent 2D X-ray delivery on Earth (UK Space Agency, 2023). There are currently several artificial intelligence technologies that enable accurate interpretation of X-rays. A collaborative study between Warwick, King's College London, and several NHS sites funded by the Wellcome Trust used a large language model to analyse 2.8 million X-rays and was found to be able to interpret X-ray imaging just as or more accurately than radiologists (King's College London 2023). It is clear that once X-ray capability has been established in space, it will only be a matter of time until artificial intelligence adjuncts are deployed with it. Though there are many promising studies taking place, ultrasound imaging is currently the only medical imaging method available at the International Space Station.

8.4.2 Virtual and Augmented Reality Applications

Virtual (VR) and augmented reality (AR) are increasingly being explored as a way to accelerate the implementation of medical care in space. Virtual and augmented reality applications are already being used in space for research purposes. Currently, control of robotic arms using VR inputs relaying haptics, motion, and simulated touch is paving the way for smoother ergonomic operations on spacecraft workstations and Moon missions. This technology is already being used on Earth to carry out robotic surgery, which can improve outcomes for patients. The Japan Aerospace Exploration Agency (JAXA) has been testing the use of AR in assisting astronauts to carry out the maintenance and repair functions on spacecraft, with the aim being to carry out repairs without any support from Earth. Microsoft tested a similar concept through the AR-enabled Hololens, which is an eyewear headset that would allow transmission of the image the astronaut was seeing to a team nearby. The team would also be able to guide the astronaut to make repairs through a blackboard-style system that would, in turn, appear in the astronaut's vision. These innovations will enable longer missions where communication to Earth may not be reliable. Further research is being conducted using both VR and AR to better understand the astronaut experience of time and space, depth perception, grip and sensation; all key aspects of administering emergency medical care or carrying out surgery in space. From a health perspective, immersive exercise tests that incorporate the VR environment are being tested as part of an effort to make exercise more appealing in space and on Earth (NASA 2024).

In the realm of biomedical visualization, Ong et al. (2022a, b) are working on a NASA-funded study guiding the development of a compact virtual reality visual assessment device to monitor ocular structure and function during spaceflight. The aim of this was to aid early identification of Spaceflight Associated Neuro-Ocular Syndrome (SANS), which presents as optic disc oedema, posterior globe flattening, total and retinal nerve layer thickening, optic nerve sheath distension, chorioretinal folds, retinal cotton wool spots, and hyperopic refractive shift. The virtual reality-based device would be adapted from devices currently used on Earth and measure visual acuity, contrast sensitivity, dynamic visual acuity, eye-tracking technology, and metamorphopsia assessment, and use machine learning to enhance diagnostic capability in space. The machine learning methodologies proposed by Ong and the team include supervised machine learning for retinal vessel segmentation and unsupervised machine learning for denoizing retinal fundus images in order to improve image quality. In addition, a generative adversarial network (GAN) was used to generate fluorescein angiography images from colour fundus photographs. The technology will need to be adapted for space travel with special attention to weight limitations, testing time requirements and maximizing diagnostic potential to minimize communication with medical experts on Earth. Ong et al. created a computer-aided design of the hardware device, which is significantly more compact and mobile than the larger machines used on Earth. The research team is also enthusiastic about the application and impact of this technology, particularly the combination of the compact hardware and the advanced software on its ability to support diagnosis of key ophthalmic conditions in low and middle-income countries on Earth (Ong et al. 2022a, b).

Though VR and AR advances in Space Medicine are relatively modest, key research is being conducted in order to better utilize these artificial intelligence technologies in space. It is clear that any travel far from Earth would necessitate artificial intelligence support.

8.5 Artificial Intelligence-Driven Medical Procedures in Space

Artificial intelligence has the potential to radically redefine, improve, and accelerate the prospect and delivery of medical procedures in space. Key areas where the long-term development of artificial intelligence is being explored include: telemedicine and robotic surgery, autonomous health systems, and the role of AI in psychological health.

8.5.1 Telemedicine and Robotic Surgery

The concept of telemedicine is the passage of diagnostic, procedural, and therapeutic medical information between doctor and patient or among doctor, patient, and a lay intermediary without needing to travel. Early telemedicine included voice communication via telephone and radio; however, the rapid advancements in information technology and satellite communications have enabled space agencies across the globe to explore the possibilities of developing telemedicine for space travel. Through the work of the European Space Agency on the Olympus Utilization Programme in 1996, satellite broadband (384 kbit/s to 2 Mbit/s) was tested to send medical images back to Earth for review by the medical team and for video conferencing between Earth and the International Space Station. The speed and quality of image transfer and video conference were deemed acceptable. The next phase of this work was to directly link the X-ray machine and cameras in the operating theatre to the system, which would enable remote assistance (European Space Agency, 2003). Since then, further advances have been made, including the connection of wearable technologies to the satellite broadband system, enabling real-time transfer of data to Earth and the ability for the medical team on Earth to monitor the vital signs and other health data to be able to identify any deterioration in health much earlier (Pathak and Wagh 2023).

Currently, communication between the International Space Station and NASA mission control in Houston, Texas, occurs almost in real-time. Before the launch of any mission, training is delivered to astronauts on all medical devices and technology available to them in space. Some astronauts may undergo 40 h of additional paramedic training to become a designated crew medical officer whilst onboard. During this training, they learn to take histories and perform clinical examinations related to common in-flight conditions such as space-sickness, musculoskeletal pain and skin irritation. Following this, through telehealth satellite communication, they will liaise with the medical mission crew on Earth to confirm management plans and treat the crew member with medication or a procedure using the onboard medical kit.

Furthermore, part of pre-flight medical training involves simulation of emergency scenarios, such as a crew member choking, with the idea that for these emergency situations, astronauts would be able to refer to easy-to-access algorithms and draw upon their knowledge and skills from training. This is in contrast to less critical medical conditions, where the astronauts can log into a videoconference with the doctors at mission control on Earth. Through the videoconferencing method, these expert clinicians will be able to evaluate the patient and recommend treatment. Though this method of application of telemedicine has been heralded as successful, longer missions constitute communication delays of minutes to hours, which would make telemedicine in its current form unsuitable for this sort of flight plan (Menon et al. 2017).

More recently, Vincent Vidal and his team at the French Radiology Society have developed the ‘Mars IR Toolbox’, a device that is incorporated with ultrasound to conduct minimally invasive surgery in order to manage emergency conditions in Space. A team of 18 space engineers and interventional radiologists is working together on this. The aim of the toolbox is to be able to treat eleven acute and potentially deadly conditions that may develop in space: pneumothorax, urinary retention, haematoma, pleural effusion, cardiac tamponade, abscess, cholecystitis, renal colic, and ascites. This work is particularly important with regard to distance travel. We know that the delay in communication transmission between Earth and Mars is approximately 45 min. Therefore, real-time medical support from the Earth team will not be possible once humans venture further (Vidal and Luciani 2023).

As part of the Asclépios III project in the summer of 2023, the device was tested by six astronauts in the Lunar South Pole environment set up in Sasso San Gottardo, Switzerland. Prior to the mission, the astronauts were trained in ultrasound-guided drainage on a plastic abdomen and successfully carried out this procedure in simulated lunar conditions. The next part of experimental actualization will involve conducting this procedure in zero gravity conditions to demonstrate feasibility. In anticipation of this, certain features of the toolkit have been developed, such as a valve on the drain to prevent liquid spread, lightweight and easily movable devices, automated guidance systems, and an autonomous power source. If successful, this toolkit would be applicable to situations on Earth where healthcare accessibility is a problem, such as during humanitarian crises and military operations (Euronews 2023).

Space medicine research teams are now exploring the potential of telesurgery—teleoperated surgical robots operated by surgeons on Earth on astronauts in Space through satellite broadband links. This concept is not too far from inception. The US Department of Defense is currently working on the 'Trauma Pod'—an artificial intelligence, holistic diagnostic and treatment vehicle that would be able to travel to remote areas to deliver lifesaving care on the battlefield (Garcia et al. 2009). The Trauma Pod is equipped with X-ray, ultrasound, and CT scanners and can take vital signs, samples, and conduct imaging, and is equipped to deliver lifesaving surgery, such as vascular surgery from serious bleed injuries on the battlefield through tele-connection with a surgeon and medical team who are based at a safer site away from the risky war zone areas. Phase I of three has now been completed with a prototype robot built that was able to safely and successfully carry out the surgical procedures of bowel closure and shunt placement following major iliac vessel injury on a phantom human model (Garcia et al. 2009). Phase II will focus on reducing the weight and size of components and instruments to make the Trauma Pod more mobile, as well as optimizing instrumentation. Finally, Phase III will combine all elements into an unmanned autonomous vehicle for testing and deployment. It is estimated that the Trauma Pod will be in use within the next 10 years, and the artificial intelligence and technology demonstrated will serve as the basis for robotic telesurgery in Space.

The integration of artificial intelligence into robotic surgery has not yet been deployed; however autonomous robotic surgical devices are being developed. Currently, the makeup of any robotic surgery device consists of a visualizing system, slave arms, and a master controller. Most surgeries are conducted in the same room or in the vicinity of the operating table with the human surgeon guiding the arm through the controller whilst watching the surgical field. The most popular commercial devices include: the Da Vinci System by American technology company Intuitive Surgical Inc., and the Zeus Telesurgical System also by an American company Computer Motion Inc. These systems mostly support laparoscopic procedures to make them even more minimally invasive, with higher precision and offer better visualization. Other operations that successfully use robotic surgery include prostatectomies, heart valve repairs, renal surgery, and neurosurgery. Scientists at the University of Washington Biorobotics Lab have developed a 22 kg portable robot, which they have named Raven. Raven has two slave arms that have been adapted to hold surgical tools. Designed to be assembled by non-engineers, the robot surgeon has also been adapted for long-distance remote control manipulation. The German Aerospace Centre Institute of Robotics and Mechatronics has built lightweight robotic arms for use in space. They are currently developing the MIROsurge robot arms, which weigh only 10 kg and have been lauded for its ability to manage high loads with great accuracy. A research team at the University of Nebraska, US, has developed the first self-assembling robots that can be controlled with external magnets. This technology is promising when considering autonomous requirements related to almost any activity on longer space missions. The European Union Seventh Framework programme ARAKNES project is an international research collaboration aimed at developing autonomous robots capable of performing surgery in the endolumen for use in Space (Menciassi 2009). This is developing the autonomous capability of robots. Another international research project demonstrated the feasibility of long-distance telesurgery through an intercontinental telesurgery project, which demonstrated success in carrying out basic surgical tasks across continents. In 2001, the first transatlantic robotic cholecystectomy was conducted on a 68-year-old woman in Strasbourg whilst the surgeon controlled the robotic arms from over 7000 km away in New York. The procedure was successful and there were no complications; however, the distance rendered the procedure a momentous day in history. Since then, longer distance experiments have taken place, as well as underwater in the ocean.

Though the first surgical experiments in space were conducted by Russian astronauts in 1967, the first animal to survive post-procedure did not occur until 1998. The 1967 Russian experiment was a laparotomy on rabbits, whereas the 1998 experiment was an endoscopic experiment conducted on rats. The first experiment on humans occurred on the European Space Agency Airbus A-300 in 2006 and was a cyst removal procedure from a patient's arm. Following this, NASA carried out its first zero-gravity robotic surgery in space in 2007. Surgical tasks using robotics have also been demonstrated in Space through knot tying and suturing experiments in the weightless environment of Space onboard a DC-9 aircraft (Haidegger et al. 2011).

Significant advances in space robotic surgery have not been made due to the various technical limitations. The primary issue relates to the communication lag time between the Spacecraft and Earth, which would compromise effective telesurgical treatment. Another issue is the development of an advanced robotic machine with demonstrated acceptability and successful feasibility studies with regard to outcomes and reliability. It is estimated that it may take another 10 years to develop technology of this calibre. Therefore, currently, the gold standard option seems to be having a flight surgeon onboard a longer mission with access to telementoring from a master surgeon on Earth and assistance from a surgical robot that can optimize in space motion scaling, suturing, spatial, and speed movements during surgery.

8.6 AI and Bioprinting for Tissue Engineering in Space

Advances in the use of artificial intelligence in bioprinting for tissue engineering in space are another part of human capability requirements for long-duration space travel.

Tissue engineering itself is the manufacturing of new tissues and organ systems for the regeneration and replacement of components of the human body and is a key frontier of medicine. The concept of patient-derived tissue engineering is a favourable concept in both Earth and Space medicine due to the scarcity of organ and tissue availability within the timeframes they are needed and the frequent possibility of transplant rejection.

8.6.1 The Potential of Bioprinting Organs and Tissues

There are several different methods of bioprinting organs and tissues; however, the basic concept remains the same. A pre-processing preparatory phase is required, where 3D models are designed by computer software such as CAD or CAM. The designs are then rendered to 2D layered images of varying thickness prior to printing. Step 2 is a processing step that involves printing of the tissues with the pre-selected ink and materials using additive manufacturing. Additive manufacturing is the process of creating a 3D object by building it one layer at a time. Step 3 is called post-processing and is the maturation of the printed material in a bioreaction and/or finishing activities such as removing support or excess material, washing and curing, sanding, polishing, painting, or colouring (Agarwal et al. 2020). These are:

1. Sterolithography (SLA)—which uses a computer-controlled laser beam that operates via a layered approach to form the required structure by hardening a liquid polymer once it is in contact with the laser. This method is used for high-accuracy elements requiring features as small as 0.07 mm.

2. Selective Laser Sintering (SLS)—a powder-based additive assembly approach that uses a laser beam to melt and fuse powder elements, then stack them using a layered approach. This method is used for creating parts requiring flexibility and durability.
3. Fused deposition modelling (FDM)—uses continuous filaments of thermoplastics to heat and deposit plastic layers using a moving printer head in order to create 3D printed objects. This method is the quickest and most cost-effective method of 3D printing, but the final product lacks tensile strength.
4. Digital Light Process (DLP)—uses micro electro-mechanical technology through a digital micromirror device to project a light source to create intricate resin-based design products. It is often used for low-volume production and is known to be one of the fastest methods of 3D printing.
5. Multi Jet Fusion (MJF)—uses an infrared energy source combined with a fusing agent to produce each layer of the build from nylon powder. Because of its method, MJF is known for its consistent mechanical properties and improved surface finish.
6. Polyjet—layers photopolymer resins using UV light and inkjet heads to create the 3D product. It is known for its ability to create flexible features and complex parts and can create objects across a spectrum of durabilities.
7. Direct Metal Laser Sintering (DMLS)—is a computer-controlled 3D printing process that uses a high-power laser beam to melt and fuse layers of metallic powder to form a metal object. It can create accurate metal end-use parts, but production takes approximately 7 days.
8. Electron Beam Melting (EBM)—is a computer-aided 3D printing process that uses electron beams guided by a magnetic field to melt powdered metal into layers that create the object.

Bioprinting is the use of 3D printing technology with materials that are made up of or support viable living cells (Daly 2021). The concept of bioprinting organs and tissues is a relatively new but rapidly evolving research area. Common biomaterials include synthetic polymers such as polylactic acid (PLA), Poly-D-L-lactic acid, Acrylonitrile Butadiene Styrene, Polyethylene Glycol, Polyether Ether Ketone, Poly-glycolic acid, Poly Caprolactone, Polybutylene Terephthalate, Polyurethane, Poly-vinyl alcohol, and Polylactic-co-glycolic acid (Vanaei et al. 2021). Bioprinting can be conducted using a scaffold-based or scaffold-free method. In the scaffold-based method, the biomaterial needs a matrix on which it forms its cellular layers. The matrix should try to mimic the extracellular matrix and is usually a hydrogel, nanofibers, or a film—a 3D construct on which the printer can print biomaterial onto. The scaffold-free method is the direct deposition of cells in a structured pattern. This method uses a higher concentration of cells and it is therefore expected that an extracellular matrix will form organically (Agarwal et al. 2020).

The three common techniques used in bioprinting are:

1. Inkjet bioprinting dispenses droplets of dilute solutions driven by thermal, piezoelectric, or microvalve processes (Rider et al. 2018). This method is useful in printing accurately; however, the dilute nature of the solutions used can be a limitation to creating a durable 3D object.
2. Fused deposition modelling (FDM) is a popular method of bioprinting that uses thermoplastics as a support for bioinks.
3. Extrusion-based bioprinting works by extruding bioinks onto a building substrate using either pneumatic force from pressurized air or gas or mechanical force through a piston or screw. This method is widely used due to its ability to incorporate a wide range of bioprinting materials and its capacity for high cell density deposition.

Other methods, such as stereolithography, laser-assisted bioprinting, vat polymerization, magnetic bioprinting, acoustic bioprinting, and bioplotting, are also used in tissue engineering.

On Earth, bioprinting is being explored and developed for a variety of purposes. Early studies using 3D bioprinting techniques to bioprint skin in order to treat murine subjects with full-thickness excisional wounds have demonstrated success. Albanna et al. printed skin to treat the full-thickness wounds of 36 mice and found that the skin construct provided epithelial coverage after 1 week and later organized into fully formed skin and integrated with the rest of the mouse skin surface. This work was then validated on porcine models, which took longer to organize but incorporated the bioprinted skin graft nonetheless (Albanna et al. 2019). Though work is very promising with regards to diabetes care, the emergency battlefield setting and burns patients, there are also many potential applications in space medicine, in particular long long-duration missions.

Bioprinting has also demonstrated feasibility on Earth in muscle tissue engineering, in particular demonstration of printing of the musculotendon unit, which demonstrates an acceptable elasticity. It has also been used to print viable neural tissue, lung tissue, and cartilaginous tissues. Extrusion-based printing has also been used to successfully develop pancreatic tissue. Arguably, the most exciting bioprinting advancements in tissue engineering have been in the application to cancer diagnosis and treatment. Bioprinting methods have been used in developing chemo-resistant cells, in vivo bone regeneration methods to support treatment of cortical bone cancers, and simulating breast and ovarian cancer pathophysiology for research. However, key limitations in this area still persist and are: inconsistent results in maintaining structure resolution, conserving cell viability, long fabrication time, temperature volatility, and durability (Vanaei et al. 2021).

More recently, the use of artificial intelligence in bioprinting has been considered. Artificial intelligence is currently being explored with respect to the monitoring of material quality, printed structure resolution, and integrity, and for prediction and optimization of the process at key quality control checkpoints (Lee 2023). Research teams have incorporated artificial intelligence into bioprinting mostly to optimize process efficiency and end product quality. Examples of this include the use of machine learning to detect defects in the print material through neural networks (Yu and Jiang 2020), predicting the accuracy and success rate of scaffolds (Shin et al. 2022), adjusting printing parameters through machine learning and evaluating the printability of gelatin methacrylate and hyaluronic acid methacrylate bioinks using Bayesian optimization (Shin et al. 2022). The future of the implementation of artificial intelligence in the bioprinting process is aimed at increasing performance and reducing the need for human interference at each of the three phases: preparation, bioprinting, and the post-bioprinting process (Bhardwaj et al. 2023).

The ability to use artificial intelligence to bioprint in space would be a significant step forward for space medicine. Currently, work towards this vision includes assessing the feasibility of bioprinting in the microgravitational environment. Key considerations include: the fabrication and change in structure of printed tissues in microgravity, the deposition of bioink, the effect of printing onto a receiving surface, particulate shear rates, and the resultant properties of any bioprinted tissue or organ. Sarabi et al. (2023) also considered the effect of microgravity on tissue growth, integration, and wound healing in the context of bioprinting for application in space. Regeneration studies on flatworms (Planaria) with the separation of their body parts in space found differing results on Earth and onboard the International Space Station, with one phenotype regenerating two heads in space. As suggested, the use of bioprinted materials as grafts in space needs further investigation due to the unpredictable nature of healing and regeneration with xenografts in microgravity due to its effects on blood flow, stem cell differentiation, and gene regulation (Rezapour 2023). However, Warth et al. at the Centre for Translational Bone, Joint and Soft Tissue Research in Dresden, Germany, have developed a handheld bioprinter for in situ wound treatment in space. The device consists of a dispenser, guide wheels, and two bioink cartridges containing the bioink, which is composed of fluorescent Polymethylmethacrylate (PMMA) micro-particles, which are used to stimulate cells. In February 2022, astronaut Matthias Maurer successfully tested the handheld bioprint onboard the International Space Station, depositing a printed plaster-like covering for skin wounds using bioink. The hope for this work is to eventually print bio-plasters incorporating a patient's own skin cells in order to grow grafts and stimulate the growth of skin and other tissues. This could in the future also result in personalized wound care options for patients (Warth et al. 2024).

Simultaneous activity in this research area has also been demonstrated aboard the International Space Station, where the use of magnetic fields to assemble three-dimensional tissue constructs was successfully conducted. The study involved tissue spheres fabricated from human chondrocytes in Kazakhstan being mixed with thermoreversible hydrogel and loaded onto a magnetic bioassembler bioprinter organ. Bioassembly was found to occur similarly to the pre-flight simulation, and chondrocytes were seen to maintain their viability and physiological activity (Parfenov et al. 2020). Though these advances are being made, there is sector acknowledgement that there is still a long way to go with regard to using artificial intelligence in bioprinting processes in space. The Biomanufacturing in Space Symposium is an annual academic conference that aims to further biomanufacturing capabilities in space and advance regenerative medicine and space medicine. This symposium was the first step in prioritizing this area of research through public-private partnerships and developing a roadmap to biomanufacturing in space (Sharma et al. 2022). The roadmap itself involves four key phases;

1. Business foundation development.
2. Research identification, prioritization, and development.
3. Technology translation, approval, and application, and.
4. Technology manufacturing and commercialization.

Though currently in its early phases, the application of artificial intelligence in bioprinting processes in space could support safer and more sustainable long-term travel and exploration in space.

8.7 The Future of Space Medicine and Artificial Intelligence

The future for the role of artificial intelligence in space medicine is extremely promising.

8.7.1 AI'S Role in Personalized Medicine for Astronauts

One of the more predictable roles for artificial intelligence is in personalized medical care for astronauts. Personalized medicine is the process of tailoring medical decisions and management to an individual person. Personalized medicine is currently used in genomics and genetics testing, cancer treatment, rare disease management, biological therapies, and in preventative medicine through personalized risk stratification. Pavez et al. (2021) observed that several factors require consideration when exploring the use of personalized medicine in space. These are gender, physical status, nutrition, their current and potential environment, their individual immune response, pharmacokinetics and pharmacodynamics, their individual tissue repair response, age, ageing process, genetics and epigenetics, and the duration of the mission. The research team also acknowledged that other key variations in certain individual responses to space stressors need to be accounted for when developing personalized medicine for astronauts. Individual variation in skin response to space travel was considered to be one of these variations, namely, delayed epidermal proliferation, decreased hydration and increased elasticity, and transepidermal water loss, which affects some astronauts worse than others. They explored the use of bioengineering and, in particular, bioprinting using a patient's own skin cells to enable successful reconstructive skin grafting in space as a precision-based medicine approach to management away from Earth (Pavez Loriè et al. 2021).

As discussed previously in this chapter, the effects of space radiation can vary. However, individual factors such as age, genetic susceptibility, current inflammatory state, and comorbidities have an impact on individual radiosensitivity and therefore acceptable radiation levels can be slightly different for different individuals and subsets of populations. Currently, research is being conducted on ascertaining certain radiation biomarkers (Durante 2005) as well as radiation risk stratification profiles to support more personalized radiation protection plans for astronauts and space travellers (Locke 2016). A further complication in this area that has occurred is the appreciation that space activity has now evolved such that astronauts are conducting more extravehicular activity than previously. This means that radiation sensitivity measures and radiation risk determination need to be planned and suitable for work on planetary surfaces rather than spaceflight alone. As we become more accustomed to traveling to Mars and working on the Moon, this will become more important to astronaut health and illness prevention.

Furthermore, each individual has a similar immune system that can mount a unique immune response determined by environmental, physiological, and psychological factors. Research has shown there to be different levels and types of immune response to spaceflight, and personalized medicine promises the advent of continuous immune biomarker detection to simultaneously identify, predict, and manage human immune reactions in space (Pavez Loriè 2021). In addition, pre-mission screening and treatment such as vaccines for viruses and dietary supplementation of glutathione, as well as personalized exercise advice, have also been shown to modulate individual immune responses in space and better prepare astronauts ahead of their missions (Pavez Loriè et al. 2021).

Another area where artificial intelligence could be used in the future of space medicine is in the use of medicines by astronauts in space. Studies have shown a variation in pharmacokinetics, which are believed to be due to the space environment, including the effects of radiation and microgravity (Kast et al. 2017). Changes to gastrointestinal tract transit time, microcirculatory pressure, fluid shifts, and renal function all contribute to differing pharmacokinetics in individual astronauts in space. The future could utilize artificial intelligence to understand individual pharmacogenetic variation with drug metabolizing enzymes, transporters, receptors, and ion channels in order to suggest optimal drug dosage and delivery form. Current challenges lie in the translation of pharmacogenetic variation into drug type and dosage recommendations. It is predicted that an artificial intelligence-powered clinical decision support system will need to be developed in order to bridge this gap (Russell 2023). Though this seems distant, the speed of advances in artificial intelligence in recent years may indicate that the development of such a support system isn't as distant as we may think.

Artificial intelligence-enabled personalized space medicine will need to integrate and analyse several inputs, including the specifics around particular space environments, the length of the mission, clinical profiling, and biological profiling, in order to deliver evidence-based personalized care recommendations to astronauts in space (Pavez Loriè et al. 2021).

8.7.2 Integrating AI into Interplanetary Telemedicine Networks

Considerations into the application of artificial intelligence in the future of space medicine are most developed around the interplanetary telemedicine networks. Seibert et al. explore NASA's plan to develop the Next Generation Relay Programme, a plan that links communication among the Earth, Moon and Mars through the Tracking and Data Relay Satellite system that has currently been put in place around the Earth and Moon (Seibert et al. 2019). Through the NASA Biologic Analog Science Associated with Lava Terrains BASALT Programme, further work is being conducted to simulate the human approach to extending the astronauts' regular work to Mars (Beaton et al. 2020). This research's applications to telecommunications in space medicine found that any communication link must be constant, the communications work would be expensive and extensive, and would likely require further satellite technology around Mars, which could take 10–30 years to achieve. The role of artificial intelligence in this work would be around the maintenance and running of the communication link to enable connections between physician experts on Earth with astronaut teams in outer and/or deep space.

8.7.3 Speculative Technologies and Frontier Advancements

As part of its Technology Roadmap, NASA has been working on the development of an autonomous medical support system through the Earth Independent Medical Operations Project. The concept behind this is that this device will use artificial intelligence to amalgamate crew health data, the environment, and point-of-care tests to support the crew medical officer in managing arising conditions in space with minimal support from Earth. Currently, no such device has been developed; however, research is being conducted in order to work towards the aim of autonomous healthcare management in space (NASA, 2023).

Several sector experts have posited future uses of artificial intelligence in space medicine. Though the future goal of artificial intelligence in space medicine will be to accurately identify, diagnose, and recommend treatments for routine medical conditions in support of astronauts working in deep space, artificial intelligence also has significant potential in the ability to predict future health problems of individual astronauts, as well as forecast when they will manifest. This would be incredibly beneficial for space exploration as it would provide teams with the ability to plan their crew members for different-length missions, anticipate the need for medical treatments onboard specific flights, and most importantly, prevent astronauts from unnecessary harm related to spaceflight. Though this chapter has discussed the many artificial intelligence research streams that are being conducted towards this aim, such as biosensors, the use of virtual and augmented reality, telemedicine, and wearable technology, there are several challenges to overcome in order to reach the collective vision. These are;

(i) The impact of interplanetary transmission delays for telecommunication.
(ii) There is limited training data on astronauts to be able to train artificial intelligence algorithms for use in space.
(iii) Research in space is usually retrospective rather than prospective, which limits artificial intelligence development around the identification and prediction of conditions at the early stages.
(iv) Current technology is not yet as sophisticated as human intelligence and needs to improve in order to be deployed meaningfully in space.

Another speculative technology that could utilize artificial intelligence in space would be the use of blockchain technology to safeguard space health records. Blockchain technology is an innovative database that is a decentralized, distributed ledger that stores and records ownership of digital assets and data and can facilitate levels of access. In the context of healthcare and medicine, blockchain technology has been successfully used to store patient health records, in clinical trials, remote patient monitoring, tracking pharmaceuticals, determining the authenticity of medical devices, data security, and genomic sequencing. With the example of patient health records, patients can determine levels of access for different healthcare providers and be sure that their data will be secure. Shinde et al. 2024 explored the use of blockchain technology to address key challenges in the development of artificial intelligence, namely, in improving the quality of input data sets and improving the reliability of data through ensuring data security and privacy. The use of blockchain AI has the potential to rapidly progress the ability for artificial intelligence modalities to access and synthesize accurate data in order to learn and make better predictions and decisions. Integrating remote patient monitoring data through blockchain technology with machine learning applications could enable superior diagnostic capabilities. If this technology were available in space, it would help astronauts to diagnose and treat medical conditions more accurately and with less reliance on telecommunication with Earth, thus enabling safer deep space exploration.

The route to the future of space medicine currently being planned and explored includes; advancements in telemedicine and remote biomedical health monitoring for remote diagnosis and in-flight treatment, counteracting the physical deconditioning associated with spaceflight through diet, exercise programmes and pharmacological treatment, developing radiation mitigation strategies such as radiation shielding, environmental controls and biological radiation countermeasures, advancements in bioengineering and regenerative medicine in order to facilitate medically self-sufficient spaceflights with regards to personalized medicine and treatments and psychological support programmes to maintain mental health and wellbeing and prevent deteriorations in mental health during space missions. However, the foreseeable future of artificial intelligence in space medicine is currently predicted to be centred around the development of autonomous health systems and robotics, data analytics and decision support, medical imaging and real-time diagnosis, personalized medicine, telemedicine, and robotic surgery, and their integration into astronauts' daily life during longer missions away from Earth (Chelladurai et al. 2024). Looking further into the future, artificial intelligence could be used to establish and run interconnected medical centres across the Earth, Moon, and Mars, scope and identify medical materials on other planets and for the accurate prediction and selection of astronauts who will be least affected by and most likely to be successful living in space, thus facilitating the formation of the first human space colony.

8.7.4 Ethical Considerations

With the advancements of artificial intelligence in space medicine and its potential for the future, there are also key ethical considerations to be made.

One of the first is data security. Whilst data is central to any artificial intelligence learning system, use of any and all data is carefully restricted by the General Data Protection Regulation, which states that any and all identifiable data, including satellite images, counts as personal data. With an increasing number of public and private organizations making use of artificial intelligence and satellite technology as image sources, key data on all of us is quickly becoming accessible from multiple sources without our direct permission. In addition, whole genome sequencing will likely be a prerequisite for space travel in the future; however, how an astronaut's genomic data is held and used will need to be considered. As artificial intelligence becomes more sophisticated, issues around data privacy, lack of transparency, repurposing of data and rights around access, correction, and erasure will need to be addressed (Gal et al. 2020).

Discrimination is another ethical issue that must be addressed as soon as possible. Artificial intelligence has already shown signs of clear bias in relation to its use in the healthcare sector, and as an adaptive learning model, it is susceptible to developing biases over time. For example, a mortality prediction tool developed using data consisting of most of a certain population may discriminate against that population over others and predict worse outcomes. This may be of significance in the context of space medicine, where there is little room for error. Furthermore, automation bias can occur where the artificial intelligence space medicine support tool's advice is followed without holistic clinical judgement and never questioned, which can also be quite dangerous for the patient. Finally, the artificial intelligence model will be programmed with a desired goal or outcome, and due to a lack of regulation, this programming could easily favour the goal of the space mission rather than the individual patient, which is another form of bias that could lead to discrimination (DeCamp and Lindvall 2020).

Furthermore, the integration of artificial intelligence in space medicine risks compromising the astronaut-doctor relationship and the strong ethical framework this concept is based on. The Hippocratic basis of medicine, most compromised by the use of artificial intelligence in space medicine, is confidentiality and patient-centred care. The relationship now becomes the patient-artificial intelligence–doctor relationship instead, bringing with it questions about informed consent, accountability, and responsibility if misdiagnosis by the technology resulted in a poor outcome. This also has legal implications related to whether artificial intelligence engineers or industry leaders need to be regulated in order to deploy this technology in good faith. Moreover, crew confidence and fidelity will be essential to the success of artificial intelligence in space medicine. As artificial intelligence evolves from predictive diagnosis to interpretation and recommendation, the crew who will ultimately be reliant on its use must be confident in its ability and aware of its limitations (Waisberg et al. 2022). Scott et al. posited that in order to develop crew confidence and fidelity, the crew, flight medical staff, and wider staff team should be trained comprehensively on how a particular artificial intelligence system was selected, how it continues to be evaluated, its deployment limitations and biases, as well as how and when to use it. Once a technology has been used by different crews successfully for several missions, there will be more willingness to use similar or more advanced artificial intelligence support tools (Scott et al. 2021a, b).

Considering the ethical principle of beneficence, the use of artificial intelligence in dealing with emergency medical events with multiple casualties in space far away from Earth and without a flight surgeon onboard, highlights a grey area with regard to what would be the right or wrong course of action. Acting in the greater good of the mission would likely be most beneficial to the sponsoring organization; however, if a doctor was first at the scene, the priority would be the patients in front of them. Much consideration needs to go into the ethical development of these autonomous medical systems as well as the education of the teams using them (Waisberg et al. 2022).

8.8 Conclusion

This chapter has explored the transformative potential of AI and biomedical visualization in advancing space medicine. As humanity embarks on the era of interstellar exploration, the health, well-being, and medical safety of astronauts become paramount. AI, with its capabilities in monitoring, predictive analytics, and autonomous decision-making, emerges as a potential route to addressing the unique challenges posed by space environments.

This chapter explored the history of space medicine and discussed the necessity for space medicine to advance in order to keep up with the human ambitions of deep space exploration. We examined the health risks associated with space travel, including microgravity, cosmic radiation, and psychosocial stressors, and reviewed the current medical technologies utilized in space missions. Our exploration of AI's role in astronaut health monitoring highlighted the importance of wearable technology, machine learning-driven predictive analytics, and AI-assisted emergency responses.

The visualization of complex medical data in microgravity through virtual and augmented reality, as well as interactive 3D models, was shown to be crucial for effective medical education and decision-making. We discussed AI-driven medical procedures, such as telemedicine and robotic surgery, which are essential for long-duration missions, and the potential of autonomous health systems to provide continuous care.

Bioprinting, facilitated by AI, represents a frontier in space medicine, offering the promise of organ and tissue engineering in microgravity. Whilst the challenges are significant, the advancements in this area could revolutionize medical treatment for astronauts.

Looking towards the future, the integration of AI into interplanetary telemedicine networks and personalized medicine will be vital for the success of deep space missions. We also speculated on emerging technologies that could further enhance space medicine.

We have also considered the ethical and practical considerations of implementing AI in space, such as data privacy, ethical decision-making, and the reliability of AI systems.

In summary, the convergence of AI, biomedical visualization, and space exploration presents a promising future where the health challenges of space travel can be effectively managed. The journey ahead is filled with potential, and the advancements discussed in this chapter are just the beginning of what is possible in the realm of space medicine. As we continue to push the boundaries of exploration, AI will undoubtedly play a critical role in ensuring the safety and health of those who venture beyond our planet.

References

Adaptix (2023) X-ray technology from space, UK Space Agency blog. Available at: https://space.blog.gov.uk/2023/07/05/x-ray-technology-from-space/. Accessed 20 June 2024

Agarwal S, Saha S, Balla VK, Pal A, Barui A, Bodhak S (2020) Current developments in 3D bioprinting for tissue and organ regeneration—a review. Front Mech Eng 6:589171

Albanna M, Binder KW, Murphy SV, Kim J, Qasem SA, Zhao W, Tan J, El-Amin IB, Dice DD, Marco J, Green J (2019) In situ bioprinting of autologous skin cells accelerates wound healing of extensive excisional full-thickness wounds. Sci Rep 9(1):1856

Andrews AE (1985 August) AI at Ames: artificial intelligence research and application at NASA Ames Research Center, Moffett Field, California, February 1985. In NASA, Washington, Proceedings: Computer Science and Data Systems Technical Symposium, Volume 1

Angelo JA (2014) Human spaceflight. Infobase Publishing

Arone A, Ivaldi T, Loganovsky K, Palermo S, Parra E, Flamini W, Marazziti D (2021) The burden of space exploration on the mental health of astronauts: a narrative review. Clin Neuropsychiatry 18(5):237

Asclepios III Mission (2023) Asclepios. Available at: https://asclepios.ch/asclepios-iii-3/. Accessed 20 June 2024

Aubert AE, Beckers F, Verheyden B (2005) Cardiovascular function and basics of physiology in microgravity. Acta Cardiol 60(2):129–151

Autonomous Medical Operations (2023) Autonomous medical operations | SBIR.gov. Available at: https://www.sbir.gov/node/2291855. Accessed 08 June 2024

Beaton KH, Chappell SP, Menzies A, Luo V, Kim-Castet SY, Newman D, Hoffman J, Norheim J, Anandapadmanaban E, Abercrombie SP, Nawotniak SEK (2020) Mission enhancing capabilities for science-driven exploration extravehicular activity derived from the NASA BASALT research program. Planet Space Sci 193:105003

Beischer DE, Fregly AR (1962) Animals and man in space: a chronology and annotated bibliography, through the year 1960, vol 5. US Naval School of Aviation Medicine, US Naval Aviation Medical Center

Bhardwaj N, Sood M, Gill SS (2023) Artificial intelligence-empowered 3D bioprinting. In: AI for big data-based engineering applications from security perspectives. CRC Press, pp 1–20

Bioprint first aid handheld bioprinter (2021) ESA. Available at: https://www.esa.int/ESA_Multimedia/Images/2021/12/Bioprint_First_Aid_handheld_bioprinter. Accessed 20 June 2024

Blood draw in space (2016) ESA. Available at: https://www.esa.int/ESA_Multimedia/Images/2016/03/Blood_draw_in_space. Accessed 20 June 2024

Boltz FW (1998) Space shuttle family: shuttle II, mini shuttle, and micro shuttles. J Spacecr Rocket 35(6):852–855

Burgess C, Dubbs C (2007) Animals in space: from research rockets to the space shuttle. Springer Science & Business Media

Campbell M, Harsch V (2013) Hubertus Strughold: life and work in the fields of space medicine. BoD–Books on Demand

Canadian Space Agency (2023) The Space Health Study: using space flight to improve how we monitor health on Earth, Canadian Space Agency. Available at: https://www.asc-csa.gc.ca/eng/sciences/space-flight-improve-monitor-health-earth.asp. Accessed 11 Feb 2024

Chancellor JC, Scott GB, Sutton JP (2014) Space radiation: the number one risk to astronaut health beyond low earth orbit. Life 4(3):491–510

Chelladurai SK, Natarajan A, Rathinam P, Saravanan SB, Rajendiran S, Pandian PP, Tamizhanban D (2024) A review on current innovation in space medicine. J Pharma Insight Res 2(2):128–135

Chen Y, Schönlieb CB, Liò P, Leiner T, Dragotti PL, Wang G, Rueckert D, Firmin D, Yang G (2022) AI-based reconstruction for fast MRI—a systematic review and meta-analysis. Proc IEEE 110(2):224–245

Christensen DM, Iddins CJ, Sugarman SL (2014) Ionizing radiation injuries and illnesses. Emerg Med Clin 32(1):245–265

Cordis. europa.eu (2013) Array of robots augmenting the kinematics of endoluminal surgery: Araknes project: Fact sheet: FP7: CORDIS: European Commission, CORDIS. Available at: https://cordis.europa.eu/project/id/224565. Accessed 20 June 2024

Cramer A, Hecla J, Wu D, Lai X, Boers T, Yang K, Moulton T, Kenyon S, Arzoumanian Z, Krull W, Gendreau K (2018) Stationary computed tomography for space and other resource-constrained environments. Sci Rep 8(1):14195

Crucian B, Valentine R, Calaway K, Miller R, Rubins K, Hopkins M, Salas Z, Krieger S, Makedonas G, Nelman-Gonzalez M, McMonigal K (2021) Spaceflight validation of technology for point-of-care monitoring of peripheral blood WBC and differential in astronauts during space missions. Life Sci Space Res 31:29–33

Cucinotta FA (2014) Space radiation risks for astronauts on multiple international Space Station missions. PLoS One 9(4):e96099

Cucinotta FA, Wu H, Shavers MR, George K (2003) Radiation dosimetry and biophysical models of space radiation effects. Gravit Space Biol 16(2):11–19

Dakkumadugula A, Pankaj L, Alqahtani AS, Ullah R, Ercisli S, Murugan R (2023) Space nutrition and the biochemical changes caused in astronauts health due to space flight: a review. Food Chemistry: X 20:100875

Daly AC, Prendergast ME, Hughes AJ, Burdick JA (2021) Bioprinting for the biologist. Cell 184(1):18–32

De Santo NG, Cirillo M, Valenti G, Perna A, Anastasio P, Drummer C (2005) Renal function in space: the link between osteoporosis, hypercalciuria, and aquaporins. J Ren Nutr 15(1):183–188

DeCamp M, Lindvall C (2020) Latent bias and the implementation of artificial intelligence in medicine. J Am Med Inform Assoc 27(12):2020–2023

Demertzi A, Van Ombergen A, Tomilovskaya E, Jeurissen B, Pechenkova E, Di Perri C, Litvinova L, Amico E, Rumshiskaya A, Rukavishnikov I, Sijbers J (2016) Cortical reorganization in an astronaut's brain after long-duration spaceflight. Brain Struct Funct 221:2873–2876

Divine RA (1993) The sputnik challenge. Oxford University Press

Durante M (2005) Biomarkers of space radiation risk. Radiat Res 164(4):467–473

Expedition 70 2024. NASA. Available at: https://www.nasa.gov/mission/expedition-70/#crewcargo. Accessed 20 June 2024

Finan WF III (2023) The Budget Bureau's Administrative Doctrine and the Creation of an Independent NASA, 1958. Fed Hist 15:29

Friedland P, Lum H (1987) Building intelligent systems: artificial intelligence research at NASA. Ames Research Center

Furukawa, S., Nagamatsu, A., Nenoi, M., Fujimori, A., Kakinuma, S., Katsube, T., Wang, B., Tsuruoka, C., Shirai, T., Nakamura, A.J. and Sakaue-Sawano, A., 2020. Space radiation biology for "Living in space". BioMed Research International, 2020

Gagarin Y (2006) Man in space–the development of the manned capsule. Spacecraft Technology: The Early Years 23(33):231

Gal GA, Santos C, Rapp L, Markovich R, van der Torre L (2020) Artificial intelligence in space. arXiv preprint arXiv:2006.12362

Garcia P, Rosen J, Kapoor C, Noakes M, Elbert G, Treat M, Ganous T, Hanson M, Manak J, Hasser C, Rohler D (2009) Trauma pod: a semi-automated telerobotic surgical system. Int J Med Robot Comput Assist Surg 5(2):136–146

Garrett-Bakelman FE, Darshi M, Green SJ, Gur RC, Lin L, Macias BR, McKenna MJ, Meydan C, Mishra T, Nasrini J, Piening BD (2019) The NASA twins study: a multidimensional analysis of a year-long human spaceflight. Science 364(6436):eaau8650

Gebhardt C (2016) Aerobee-19: 65 years after animal flight that paved the way for Project Mercury. https://www.nasaspaceflight.com/2016/09/aerobee-19-65-years-animal-flight-project-mercury/#:~:text=Eight%20months%20and%20one%20day,successfully%20parachuting%20back%20to%20Earth

Glennan TK, Hunley JD (1993) The birth of NASA: the diary of T. Keith Glennan (No. NASA-SP-4105)

Gohd C (2020) What quarantine is like for an astronaut, Space.com. Available at: https://www.space.com/what-is-quarantine-like-for-astronauts-coronavirus.html. Accessed 20 June 2024

Goldsmith RS (1972) Calcium metabolism under stress and in response. Life Sci Space Res 10:87–101

Gómez X, Sanon S, Zambrano K, Asquel S, Bassantes M, Morales JE, Otáñez G, Pomaquero C, Villarroel S, Zurita A, Calvache C (2021) Key points for the development of antioxidant cocktails to prevent cellular stress and damage caused by reactive oxygen species (ROS) during manned space missions. npj Microgravity 7(1):35

Grimwood JM (1963) Project mercury: a chronology, vol 4001. Office of Scientific and Technical Information, National Aeronautics and Space Administration

Haidegger T, Sándor J, Benyó Z (2011) Surgery in space: the future of robotic telesurgery. Surg Endosc 25:681–690

Hall L (2017) Early human factors studies for spaceflight at the aeromedical field laboratory at Holloman Air Force Base. Aerosp Med Hum Perform 88(6):608–609

Haney NM, Urman A, Waseem T, Cagle Y, Morey JM (2020) AI's role in deep space. J Med Artif Intell 3

Hanrahan JS (1952) The beginnings of research in space biology at the Air Force Missile Development Centre. Holloman Air Force Base, New Mexico, pp 1946–1952

Heer M, Paloski WH (2006) Space motion sickness: incidence, etiology, and countermeasures. Auton Neurosci 129(1–2):77–79

Hinkelbein J, Kerkhoff S, Adler C, Ahlbäck A, Braunecker S, Burgard D, Cirillo F, De Robertis E, Glaser E, Haidl

TK, Hodkinson P (2020) Cardiopulmonary resuscitation (CPR) during spaceflight-a guideline for CPR in microgravity from the German Society of Aerospace Medicine (DGLRM) and the European Society of Aerospace Medicine Space Medicine Group (ESAM-SMG). Scand J Trauma Resusc Emerg Med 28:1–18

How NASA uses telemedicine to care for astronauts in Space (2017) Harvard Business Review. Available at: https://hbr.org/2017/07/how-nasa-uses-telemedicine-to-care-for-astronauts-in-space. Accessed 20 June 2024

Hu S, Barzilla JE, Semones E (2020) Acute radiation risk assessment and mitigation strategies in near future exploration spaceflights. Life Sci Space Res 24:25–33

Human research roadmap (no date) NASA. Available at: https://humanresearchroadmap.nasa.gov/. Accessed 20 June 2024

Hupfeld KE, McGregor HR, Reuter-Lorenz PA, Seidler RD (2021) Microgravity effects on the human brain and behavior: dysfunction and adaptive plasticity. Neurosci Biobehav Rev 122:176–189

Iaroshenko GL, Terent'ev VG, Mokrov MN (1967) Peculiarities of surgical intervention under conditions of weightlessness. Voenno-meditsinskii Zhurnal 10:69–70

Ihle E (2003, September) Exploring the positive effects of being in space. In 54th International Astronautical Congress of the International Astronautical Federation, the International Academy of Astronautics, and the International Institute of Space Law (pp. G-4)

Ihle EC, Ritsher JB, Kanas N (2006) Positive psychological outcomes of spaceflight: an empirical study. Aviat Space Environ Med 77(2):93–101

Iwase S, Nishimura N, Mano T (2013) Osteoporosis in spaceflight. In: Topics in osteoporosis. IntechOpen, London, pp 259–279

Iwase S, Nishimura N, Tanaka K, Mano T (2020) Effects of microgravity on human physiology. In Beyond LEO-human health issues for deep space exploration, IntechOpen

Jacob E (2008) UNIVERSE Britannica illustrated science library

Jedrick R (2013) A brief history of flight medicine. [Online] available at: https://www.goflightmedicine.com/history-of-flight-medicine. Last Accessed 19 Apr 2025

Johnson MP (2007) Skylab: the human side of a scientific mission. University of North Texas

Joseph T (2012) Holloman Air Force Base. Arcadia Publishing

Kast J, Yu Y, Seubert CN, Wotring VE, Derendorf H (2017) Drugs in space: pharmacokinetics and pharmacodynamics in astronauts. Eur J Pharm Sci 109:S2–S8

Kennedy AR (2014) Biological effects of space radiation and development of effective countermeasures. Life Sci Space Res 1:10–43

King's College London (2023) AI trained on X-rays can diagnose medical issues as accurately as doctors, King's College London. Available at: https://www.kcl.ac.uk/news/ai-trained-on-x-rays-can-diagnose-medical-issues-as-accurately-as-doctors. Accessed 20 June 2024

Koppelmans V, Bloomberg JJ, Mulavara AP, Seidler RD (2016) Brain structural plasticity with spaceflight. npj Microgravity 2(1):2

Lee H (2023) Engineering in vitro models: bioprinting of organoids with artificial intelligence. Cyborg Bionic Syst 4:0018

Lee AG, Mader TH, Gibson CR, Brunstetter TJ, Tarver WJ (2018) Space flight-associated neuro-ocular syndrome (SANS). Eye 32(7):1164–1167

Lee WC, Kim KS, Kwon YH (2020) Review of the history of animals that helped human life and safety for aerospace medical research and space exploration. Korean J Aerosp Environ Med 30(1):18–24

Lee PH, Chung M, Ren Z, Mair DB, Kim DH (2022) Factors mediating spaceflight-induced skeletal muscle atrophy. Am J Phys Cell Phys 322(3):C567–C580

Link MM (1965) Space medicine in project mercury. Scientific and Technical Information Division, National Aeronautics and Space Administration

Liu AC, Lewis WG, Kay SA (2007) Mammalian circadian signaling networks and therapeutic targets. Nat Chem Biol 3(10):630–639

Liu AM, Galvan-Garza RC, Flynn-Evans EE, Rueger M, Natapoff A, Lockley SW, Oman CM (2023) Effects of caffeine and blue-enriched light on spare visual attention during simulated space teleoperation. npj Microgravity 9(1):94

Locke PA, Weil MM (2016) Personalized cancer risk assessments for space radiation exposures. Front Oncol 6:38

Lowery C, Heft N, Beger S, Stewart LH (2025) Emergency medicine in spaceflight. In: Precision medicine for long and safe permanence of humans in space. Academic Press, pp 179–206

Ma X, Xi B, Zhang Y, Zhu L, Sui X, Tian G, Yang J (2020) A machine learning-based diagnosis of thyroid cancer using thyroid nodules ultrasound images. Curr Bioinforma 15(4):349–358

Makedonas G, Chouker A, Mehta S, Simpson R, Stowe R, Sams C, Pierson D, Crucian B (2018) Mechanistic clues to overcome spaceflight-induced immune dysregulation. Curr Pathobiol Rep 6:185–192

Mallak CT (2018) Death on orbit: extreme environmental conditions and the deaths of American astronauts. Academic Forensic Pathol 8(1):112–118

Maltby WR (1958) National aeronautics and space act of 1958 patent provisions. Geo Wash L Rev 27:49

Man J, Graham T, Squires-Donelly G, Laslett AL (2022) The effects of microgravity on bone structure and function. npj Microgravity 8(1):9

Manzey D, Lorenz B, Poljakov V (1998) Mental performance in extreme environments: results from a performance monitoring study during a 438-day spaceflight. Ergonomics 41(4):537–559

Martin Paez Y, Mudie LI, Subramanian PS (2020) Spaceflight associated neuro-ocular syndrome

(SANS): A systematic review and future directions. Eye and Brain 12:105–117

McCarthy ID (2005) Fluid shifts due to microgravity and their effects on bone: a review of current knowledge. Ann Biomed Eng 33:95–103

McCuaig KE, Houtchens BA (1992) Management of trauma and emergency surgery in space. J Trauma Acute Care Surg 33(4):610–626

McWilliams G (1958) History off research in Space Biology and Biodynamics. Available at: https://discover.dtic.mil/technical-reports/. Accessed: 20 April 2025

Medical-grade smartwatch can monitor astronauts, patients 2024. NASA. Available at: https://spinoff.nasa.gov/Medical-Grade_Smartwatch_Can_Monitor_Astronauts_Patients. Accessed: 20 June 2024

Menciassi A, Dario P (2009, September) Miniaturized robotic devices for endoluminal diagnosis and surgery: A single-module and a multiple-module approach. In: In 2009 Annual International Conference of the IEEE Engineering in Medicine and Biology Society. IEEE, pp 6842–6845

Menon A, Gray LC, Fatehi F, Darssan D, Bird D, Bennetts D, Russell AW (2017) A comparison of characteristics of patients seen in a tertiary hospital diabetes telehealth service versus specialist face-to-faceoutpatients. J Telemed Telecare, 23(10):842–849

Mermel LA (2013) Infection prevention and control during prolonged human space travel. Clin Infect Dis 56(1):123–130

Miles WR (1952) Physics and Medicine of the Upper Atmosphere: A Study of the Aeropause. Proceedings of a Symposium on the Physics and Medicine of the Upper Atmosphere held at San Antonio, Texas, November 6–9, 1951. Clayton S. White and Otis O. Benson. Jr., Eds. Albuquerque: Univ. New Mexico Press, 1952. (For theLovelace Foundation for Medical Education and Research.) 611 pp. Illus. $10.00. Sci 116(3024):670–670

NASA. The birth of NASA. 2024. The diary of t. keith glennan. Available at: https://history.nasa.gov/SP-4105.pdf. Accessed: 20 June 2024

National Research Council, Division on Engineering, Physical Sciences, Space Studies Board and Committee for Evaluation of Space Radiation Cancer Risk Model, 2012. Technical evaluation of the NASA model for cancer risk to astronauts due to space radiation

Navarro Morales DC, Kuldavletova O, Quarck G, Denise P, Clément G (2023) Time perception in astronauts on board the International Space Station. npj Microgravity 9(1):6

Nelson GA (2016) Space radiation and human exposures, a primer. Radiat Res 185(4):349–358

Newman DG, Faicd A (2007) An overview of spatial disorientation as a factor in aviation accidents and incidents, vol 2007. Australian Transport Safety Bureau, Canberra City

Nine ways we use AR and VR on the International Space Station (2024) NASA. Available at: https://www.nasa.gov/missions/station/nine-ways-we-use-ar-and-vr-on-the-international-space-station/. Accessed: 20 June 2024

Ohnishi K, Ohnishi T (2004) The biological effects of space radiation during long stays in space. Biol Sci Space 18(4):201–205

Ong J, Tavakkoli A, Zaman N, Kamran SA, Waisberg E, Gautam N, Lee AG (2022a) Terrestrial health applications of visual assessment technology and machine learning in spaceflight associated neuro-ocular syndrome. npj Microgravity 8(1):37

Ong KM, Rossitto JJ, Ray K, Dufurrena QA, Blue RS (2022b) Blood glucose alterations and continuous glucose monitoring in centrifuge-simulated spaceflight. Aerosp Med Hum Perform 93(9):688–695

Parfenov VA, Khesuani YD, Petrov SV, Karalkin PA, Koudan EV, Nezhurina EK, Pereira FD, Krokhmal AA, Gryadunova AA, Bulanova EA, Vakhrushev IV (2020) Magnetic levitational bioassembly of 3D tissue construct in space. Sci Adv 6(29):eaba4174

Patel ZS, Brunstetter TJ, Tarver WJ, Whitmire AM, Zwart SR, Smith SM, Huff JL (2020) Red risks for a journey to the red planet: the highest priority human health risks for a mission to Mars. npj Microgravity 6(1):33

Pathak MA, Wagh R (2023) Revolutionising healthcare access. The transformative role of space technology in telemedicine and telehealth. Chelonian Research Foundation 18(2):2008–2017

Pavez Loriè E, Baatout S, Choukér A, Buchheim JI, Baselet B, Dello Russo C, Wotring V, Monici M, Morbidelli L, Gagliardi D, Stingl JC, Surdo L, Yip VLM (2021) The future of personalized medicine in space: from observations to countermeasures. Front Bioeng Biotechnol 9:739747

Pool SL, Davis JR (2007) Space medicine roots: a historical perspective for the current direction. Aviat Space Environ Med 78:A3–A4

Previc FH (2018) Intravestibular balance and motion sickness. Aerosp Med Hum Perform 89(2):130–140

Qu Y (2024) Validation study of the Empatica EmbracePlus wristband for measuring Electrodermal activity utilizing a virtual reality protocol (Master's thesis, University of Twente)

Ramanathan C, Kathale ND, Liu D, Lee C, Freeman DA, Hogenesch JB, Cao R, Liu AC (2018) mTOR signaling regulates central and peripheral circadian clock function. PLoS Genet 14(5):e1007369

Reynolds RJ (ed) (2020) Beyond LEO: human health issues for deep space exploration. BoD–Books on Demand

Rezapour Sarabi M, Yetisen AK, Tasoglu S (2023) Bioprinting in microgravity. ACS Biomater Sci Eng 9(6):3074–3083

Rider P, Kačarević ŽP, Alkildani S, Retnasingh S, Barbeck M (2018) Bioprinting of tissue engineering scaffolds. J Tissue Eng 9:2041731418802090

Rooney BV, Crucian BE, Pierson DL, Laudenslager ML, Mehta SK (2019) Herpes virus reactivation in astro-

nauts during spaceflight and its application on earth. Front Microbiol 10:432964
Russell BK, Burian BK, Hilmers DC, Beard BL, Martin K, Pletcher DL, Easter B, Lehnhardt K, Levin D (2023) The value of a spaceflight clinical decision support system for earth-independent medical operations. npj Microgravity 9(1):46
Sargsyan AE (2008) Medical imaging. In: Principles of clinical medicine for space flight. Springer, New York, pp 181–207
Sarty GE, Obenaus A (2012) Magnetic resonance imaging of astronauts on the international space station and into the solar system. Can Aeronaut Space J 58(1):60–68
Scientists train astronauts to Solve Health Emergencies in Space. 2023. euronews. Available at: https://www.euronews.com/next/2023/10/19/scientists-test-new-procedures-to-solve-health-emergencies-in-space. Accessed 20 June 2024
Scientists train astronauts to Solve Health Emergencies in Space (no date) euronews. Available at: https://www.euronews.com/next/2023/10/19/scientists-test-new-procedures-to-solve-health-emergencies-in-space. Accessed 20 June 2024
Scott JM, Downs M, Martin DS, Hougland E, Sarmiento L, Arzeno N, Pettit DR, Ploutz-Snyder R, Cunningham D, Jones LW, Do R (2021a) Teleguided self-ultrasound scanning for longitudinal monitoring of muscle mass during spaceflight. IScience 24(4):102344
Scott RT, Antonsen EL, Sanders LM, Hastings JJ, Park SM, Mackintosh G, Reynolds RJ, Hoarfrost AL, Sawyer A, Greene CS, Glicksberg BS (2021b) Beyond low earth orbit: biomonitoring, artificial intelligence, and precision space health. arXiv preprint arXiv:2112.12554
Scott RT, Sanders LM, Antonsen EL, Hastings JJ, Park SM, Mackintosh G, Reynolds RJ, Hoarfrost AL, Sawyer A, Greene CS, Glicksberg BS (2023) Biomonitoring and precision health in deep space supported by artificial intelligence. Nature Machine Intelligence 5(3):196–207
Seamans RC (2005) Project Apollo: the tough decisions, vol No. 37. Government Printing Office
Seibert MA, Lim DS, Miller MJ, Santiago-Materese D, Downs MT (2019) Developing future deep-space telecommunication architectures: a historical look at the benefits of analog research on the development of solar system internetworking for future human spaceflight. Astrobiology 19(3):462–477
Serin Y, Acar Tek N (2019) Effect of circadian rhythm on metabolic processes and the regulation of energy balance. Ann Nutr Metab 74(4):322–330
Sharma A, Clemens RA, Garcia O, Taylor DL, Wagner NL, Shepard KA, Gupta A, Malany S, Grodzinsky AJ, Kearns-Jonker M, Mair DB (2022) Biomanufacturing in low Earth orbit for regenerative medicine. Stem Cell Reports 17(1):1–13
Shin J, Lee Y, Li Z, Hu J, Park SS, Kim K (2022) Optimized 3D bioprinting technology based on machine learning: A review of recent trends and advances. Micromachines 13(3):363
Shinde R, Patil S, Kotecha K, Potdar V, Selvachandran G, Abraham A (2024) Securing AI-based healthcare systems using blockchain technology: A state-of-the-art systematic literature review and future research directions. Trans Emerg Telecommun Technol 35(1):e4884
Smith LM (2022) The psychology and mental health of the spaceflight environment: A scoping review. Acta Astronaut 201:496–512
Stein TP, Schluter MD (1994) Excretion of IL-6 by astronauts during spaceflight. Am J Physiol-Endocrinol Metabol 266(3):E448–E452
Stever HG, Adams LJ, Anders WA, Bement AL Jr, Charyk JV, Cooper RN, Cooper RS, David EE Jr, Logsdon JM, Ostriker JP, Phillips SC (1989) Towards a new era in space: realigning US policies to new realities. Space Policy 5(3):237–255
Stewart LH, Trunkey D, Rebagliati GS (2007) Emergency medicine in space. J Emerg Med 32(1):45–54
Stratmann HG (2015) Microgravity and the human body. In: Using medicine in science fiction: the SF writer's guide to human biology. Springer International Publishing, Cham, pp 121–150
Summers RL, Johnston SL, Marshburn TH, Williams DR (2005) Emergencies in space. Ann Emerg Med 46(2):177–184
Sylvester CB, Abe JI, Patel ZS, Grande-Allen KJ (2018) Radiation-induced cardiovascular disease: mechanisms and importance of linear energy transfer. Front Cardiovasc Med 5:5
Telemedicine—ESA (2003). Available at: https://www.esa.int/esapub/bulletin/bullet114/chapter6_bul114.pdf. Accessed 20 June 2024
Vanaei S, Parizi MS, Salemizadehparizi F, Vanaei HR (2021) An overview on materials and techniques in 3D bioprinting toward biomedical application. Eng Regener 2:1–18
Vidal V, Boyer L, Luciani A (2023) Bringing interventional radiology to Mars! Cardiovasc Intervent Radiol 46(4):425–427
Vimal VP, Panic AS, Lackner JR, DiZio P (2023) Vibrotactile feedback as a countermeasure for spatial disorientation. Front Physiol 14:1249962
Waisberg E, Ong J, Paladugu P, Kamran SA, Zaman N, Lee AG, Tavakkoli A (2022) Challenges of artificial intelligence in space medicine. Space: Science & Technology
Wang N, Lyu MR (2014) Extracting and selecting distinctive EEG features for efficient epileptic seizure prediction. IEEE J Biomed Health Inform 19(5):1648–1659
Wang N, Lyu MR, Yang C (2013, March) A machine learning framework for space medicine predictive diagnostics with physiological signals. In: In 2013 IEEE Aerospace Conference. IEEE, pp 1–12
Warth N, Berg M, Schumacher L, Boehme M, Windisch J, Gelinsky M (2024) Bioprint FirstAid: a handheld bioprinter for first aid utilization on space exploration missions. Acta Astronaut 215:194–204
White CS, Benson OO (eds) (1952) Physics and medicine of the upper atmosphere: a study of the aeropause. University of New Mexico Press

Williams DR (2001) A historical overview of space medicine. McGill J Med 6(1)
Williams G (2016) Cardiovascular disease. In: Ernsting's Aviation and Space Medicine 5E. CRC Press, pp 385–420
Xu Y, Wang Y, Yuan J, Cheng Q, Wang X, Carson PL (2019) Medical breast ultrasound image segmentation by machine learning. Ultrasonics 91:1–9
Yeager CE (1956) High speed test flying. The Aeronaut J 60(552):785–798
Yu C, Jiang J (2020) A perspective on using machine learning in 3D bioprinting. Int J Bioprinting 6:4–11

9 Artificial Intelligence in Healthcare Systems of Low- and Middle-Income Countries: Opportunities, Challenges, and Pathways to Ethical Integration

Pedra Rabiee

Abstract

This chapter explores how artificial intelligence (AI) can help low- and middle-income countries (LMICs) overcome chronic shortages of health workers, infrastructure, and funding while safeguarding equity. After outlining the scale of the challenge—including a projected shortfall of ten million health-care workers by 2030 and 15 million premature non-communicable-disease deaths each year, 85% of which occur in LMICs—it surveys emerging AI applications from radiology triage in Ecuador to mobile decision-support tools in sub-Saharan Africa. Economic models suggest substantial efficiency gains, yet real-world pilots reveal that algorithmic success hinges on three inter-locking 'building blocks': (1) high-quality, context-specific data strategy and management; (2) ethical governance and robust regulation covering privacy, accountability, and bias; and (3) health-system integration backed by reliable connectivity, digital literacy, and sustainable funding. Case studies such as a racially biased breast-cancer histology model and South Africa's Vumacam surveillance network illustrate how ungeneralisable datasets and opaque supply chains can reproduce or intensify existing inequalities. The chapter concludes with a practical roadmap for policymakers and implementers—emphasising interoperable data standards, participatory design, continuous monitoring, and cross-sector partnerships—arguing that AI is not a panacea but, when deployed deliberately, can accelerate progress toward Universal Health Coverage and the Sustainable Development Goals without leaving vulnerable populations behind.

Keywords

Artificial Intelligence · Low- and middle-income countries · Healthcare systems · Data governance · Ethical AI

By 2030, it is estimated that there will be a shortfall of ten million healthcare workers, predominantly in low- and lower-middle-income countries, posing a significant challenge to global health systems (World Health Organization 2016). Within low- and middle-income countries

P. Rabiee (✉)
The Healthcare Leadership Academy, London, UK
e-mail: Pedra.rabiee@medics.academy

J. Malawana et al. (eds.), *Artificial Intelligence in Healthcare and Biomedical Visualization*, Biomedical Visualization 10, https://doi.org/10.1007/978-3-032-06520-9_9

(LMICs), healthcare resources are already scarce, this shortage exacerbating existing disparities in access to quality healthcare. Despite recent improvements in health outcomes and life expectancies due to rising incomes and advancements in medical technology, LMICs still face significant challenges (Bawah et al. 2016). These challenges include inadequate infrastructure, limited access to essential medical services, and a shortage of skilled healthcare professionals (Oleribe et al. 2019; Witter et al. 2022). Moreover, geographical barriers further compound the issue, with over 43% of the world's population unable to reach a healthcare facility on foot within one hour, particularly in rural areas (Weiss et al. 2020).

The COVID-19 pandemic has intensified these challenges, overwhelming already strained healthcare systems and exacerbating socioeconomic inequalities within these countries. Currently, 60% of the world's population lacks access to essential healthcare services (Labrique et al. 2018; Weissglass 2022). This is primarily due to necessary healthcare being unaffordable, where over 100 million individuals worldwide are pushed into extreme poverty due to health expenses, forcing them to survive on just $1.90 or less a day (World Health Organisation 2017). Addressing these complex issues requires innovative solutions to bridge the health gap in LMICs.

These comprehensive strategies will need to prioritise equitable access to healthcare, investment in healthcare infrastructure, and workforce development to optimise healthcare delivery and improve health outcomes in LMICs. Concurrently, the pandemic has catalysed exponential growth in health technology and its adoption within healthcare systems. Artificial intelligence (AI), in particular, holds immense promise in reshaping the trajectory towards achieving Universal Health Coverage (UHC) and the Sustainable Development Goals (SDGs) (Vinuesa et al. 2020). Most AI-based technologies are developed by and implemented within high-income countries (HICs), although now numerous LMICs have initiated explorations into integrating AI technologies into their healthcare systems, spanning from cancer prediction models to disease outbreak management (Wahl et al. 2018; Johnson et al. 2021). For instance, in Ecuador, an AI-assisted chest computed tomography was used during the pandemic as an innovative triage approach (Garzon-Chavez et al. 2021). This technology has the potential to drive game-changing improvements to address longstanding healthcare challenges and enhance service delivery within these nations.

Even though there is a huge potential for its use, there is a lack of information on how to implement and effectively scale AI solutions within healthcare systems across LMICs, especially where governance and regulatory structures of the use of these devices are still evolving (Murphy et al. 2021). Additionally, many of the AI technologies for these nations have been based on HICs' AI innovations or built by teams within HICs, which therefore requires the technology to be altered to address the unique needs of, and ensure a positive impact on, these populations.

Furthermore, it is important to note, AI will be discussed in this chapter as an additional aid for a strategy for improving healthcare—rather than THE solution to the health system challenges. As we will discuss later on, AI also has its own risks and tradeoffs that stakeholders should be aware of before accelerating towards an AI-based solution for their healthcare system. LMIC governments and stakeholders need to decide how these AI technologies will best serve the needs of their populations and their national and local health priorities.

9.1 The Complexity of AI Models: Designing Considerations

In recent years, the field of healthcare AI has predominantly utilised machine learning techniques, representing a dynamic area of ongoing research and development. Machine learning algorithms, a subset of AI, are designed to learn from data and make predictions or decisions without explicit programming. In the context of healthcare, these AI systems are engineered to estimate various outcomes, ranging from disease diagnosis to treatment response, based on patterns discerned from vast datasets. Central to the effectiveness of these AI models is their accuracy in predicting outcomes on previously unseen data, a metric that underscores their value in clinical practice (Deo 2015; Javid et al. 2022).

However, achieving optimal accuracy in these AI models within LMICs is not without its challenges. Machine learning models often face a trade-off between accuracy and complexity. This trade-off can lead to two common pitfalls: underfitting and overfitting. Underfitting occurs when an AI model is too simplistic, in terms of algorithm, to capture the intrinsic complexity of both the training data and new data, resulting in high bias. Conversely, overfitting arises when a model closely mirrors the training data but generalises poorly to new data, leading to low bias but high variance, rendering it less effective in real-world settings (Chen et al. 2017; Brynjolfsson et al. 2017; Scardoni et al. 2020).

Recognising these challenges, when developing AI models for these populations, it is increasingly emphasised to add additional dimensions to the model, particularly features that include explainability and causability. Explainability refers to the model's ability to provide understandable explanations for its predictions or recommendations, thereby demystifying 'black-box' models and enabling healthcare professionals to interpret and trust the outcomes effectively. Causability, on the other hand, involves understanding the causal relationships underlying the model's predictions, which is essential for guiding clinical decision-making and ensuring patient safety (Holzinger et al. 2019; Scardoni et al. 2020).

The integration of these additional dimensions into healthcare AI development has profound practical implications. By prioritising explainability and causability alongside accuracy and complexity, AI systems can enhance clinical decision-making, improve patient outcomes, and facilitate the adoption of evidence-based practices (Holzinger et al. 2019). Moreover, this holistic approach aligns with broader healthcare trends, such as the shift towards patient-centred care and the imperative for transparent and accountable use of technology in medicine.

9.2 Building Blocks of AI Initiatives in LMIC

When taking into account the 2030 SDGs, its fundamental backbone is to 'leave no one behind'. However, in many LMICs, access to high-quality healthcare remains a challenge for a significant portion of the population, often leading to financial hardship. Amidst this challenge, LMICs are undergoing an epidemiological transition, marked by a shift in disease patterns from communicable to non-communicable diseases (NCDs), such as heart disease, cancer, and diabetes—mirroring trends observed in wealthier nations. Yet, the burden of these NCDs weighs much heavily on LMICs, exacerbating the healthcare disparity. Approximately 15 million individuals between the ages of 30 and 69 die annually from NCDs, with a staggering 85% of these deaths occurring in LMICs (World Health Organisation 2024). This highlights the urgency of addressing healthcare accessibility, ensuring that no one is left behind in the pursuit of health equity on a global scale.

In the USA alone, integrating AI could result in $150 billion in saved healthcare costs annually by 2026 (Collier et al. 2017). The transformative impact that AI can have on the public health systems within LMICs will therefore have greater value. However, for a successful implementation and scale-up of this digital solution, it is paramount that it seamlessly integrates into the healthcare pathway (Labrique et al. 2018). According to the WHO, within their guidance on Ethics and Governance of Artificial Intelligence for Health, there are significant challenges surrounding AI implementation within LMICs, which include the lack of digitised medical and health records, to ethical and regulatory issues such as informed consent, privacy, and confidentiality (WHO 2021). Moreover, these AI technologies need to demonstrate cost-effectiveness, health system efficacy, and improved economic impacts (López et al. 2022). For this to occur, stakeholders, including leaders and policymakers, need to consider the following three building blocks when developing and scaling up an AI system:

- Data Strategy and Management
- Ethical Governance and Regulatory Compliance
- Health System Integration and Infrastructure Readiness

9.3 Data Strategy and Management

Data is the foundation upon which AI technologies operate. The effective management of healthcare data is crucial for harnessing the potential of AI to improve healthcare delivery, enhance patient outcomes, and address health disparities.

Even though AI holds great potential for addressing barriers within the healthcare system, it may actually deepen health inequalities further. For instance, to be able to train the AI algorithms, which consist of sets of coded instructions to yield specific outcomes, decisions, or recommendations, they need to provide accurate outputs appropriate to the specific population, it will require large, high-quality, unbiased datasets, which are often absent within these countries (Wahl et al. 2018; Hosny et al. 2019). For instance, a breast cancer histology AI algorithm showed bias because it reflected ethnicity instead of tumour biology. This happened because one site had more Black patients than others, affecting the AI algorithm. Such biased models can worsen existing inequalities in cancer care based on ungeneralisable datasets (Howard et al. 2021). Other notable examples are racial profiling in South Africa and labour exploitation in Venezuela (Hao and Hernandez 2022; Hao and Swart 2022). South Africa's Vumacam surveillance system repeats the pattern, tagging Black passers-by as 'suspicious' thanks to biased watch-lists. Meanwhile, the cheap Venezuelan click-workers who label data for Big Tech show how AI's benefits rest on a shaky, exploitative foundation (Hao and Hernandez 2022).

Many LMICs face frequent difficulties in acquiring complete and diverse datasets due to limited resources, fragmented information communication technology (ICT) systems, lack of interoperable electronic health records, and inadequate data management practices (Nkengasong et al. 2018; Wahl et al. 2018; Mollura et al. 2020; Circierski-Holmes et al. 2022; Seastedt et al. 2022; Oduoye et al. 2024). Taking into account the pressing realities of the lack of high-quality data availability, LMICs need to assess their data collection and management strategies to ensure that adequate data is continuously collected efficiently for AI training (Seastedt et al. 2022; Oduoye et al. 2024).

Moreover, currently, AI algorithms have been trained using data from HICs (Circierski-Holmes et al. 2022). This could lead to the technology functioning less optimally or even negatively for those who largely differ from HIC populations, as they may unknowingly be prejudicial or discriminatory towards LMICs populations. Furthermore, the algorithms are 'political by design' in that they are instilled with particular values, choices, beliefs, and norms of their developers and of those who assemble the datasets (Faraj et al. 2018; Alami et al. 2020). For example, an AI intervention may be trained with bias towards overdiagnosis of schizophrenia in African Americans, which can have detrimental consequences if used in sub-Saharan African populations (Vayena et al. 2018).

Moving forward, for LMICs interested in developing their data strategies, it is essential to adopt a structured approach that encompasses the entire lifecycle of data management for AI in healthcare. To ensure this, the following are the data management components to consider within the data management strategies:

- Data collection methods
- Data quality assurance
- Data governance frameworks
- Data sharing and interoperability
- Data accessibility and equity

These data management components are explained further in Table 9.1.

Table 9.1 shows the various data management components to consider within the data management strategies

Data management component	Description	Examples
Data collection methods	Collecting healthcare data	Electronic health records
		Mobile health applications
		Wearables
		Telemedicine platforms
Data quality assurance	Explore strategies for ensuring the quality, accuracy, and completeness of healthcare data	Data validation processes
		Data cleaning techniques
		Error detection algorithms
Data governance frameworks	Establishing data governance frameworks to manage data access, sharing, and usage	Data security policies
		Data privacy policies
		Data confidentiality policies
Data sharing and interoperability	Address challenges and opportunities related to data sharing and interoperability between different healthcare systems and organisations	Implementing standardised data formats and protocols
Data accessibility and equity	Efforts to improve data accessibility and address disparities in data availability	Collecting data from underrepresented populations and marginalised communities.

As LMICs strive to enhance their data management systems, a crucial prerequisite for the effective deployment of AI in healthcare is attention directed towards ensuring the availability of high-quality, validated data, as stated before. These datasets serve as a foundation for AI systems, enabling them to train models tailored to specific tasks, such as data pattern recognition, classification, and providing recommendations. However, as LMICs amass an abundance of data, they inevitably encounter a myriad of challenges:

1. Processing Big Data: Handling vast and complex datasets necessitates robust mechanisms for efficient processing.
2. Storing Large Amount of Data: Adequate infrastructure for the storage of substantial volumes of data is imperative for sustained AI implementation.
3. Extracting Meaningful Insights from Data: Deriving actionable insights from raw data presents a formidable hurdle, requiring advanced analytical techniques and algorithms.

To address these challenges, AI algorithms must adhere to a set of fair and transparent design principles. Interoperability emerges as a critical factor, facilitating seamless communication and interaction among diverse systems and datasets. As LMICs navigate these complexities, it is vital for governments and other stakeholders to play a pivotal role in establishing a robust policy framework that prioritises the establishment of strong foundations for data management. This framework should encompass guidance and regulations pertaining to interoperability, standardization, and explanation of both data models. Moreover, the continuous updating of AI training datasets is essential to ensure relevance and effectiveness across real-world populations.

This emphasis on data integrity and governance seamlessly transitions to the imperative of ethical governance and regulatory compliance, which is explored in the next section.

9.4 Ethical Governance and Regulatory Compliance

The rise of AI in healthcare brings forth a series of legal, ethical, and existential challenges, particularly within LMICs. While AI holds immense potential to revolutionise healthcare delivery, its development and deployment necessitate careful consideration of ethical governance and regulatory compliance (Cath 2018; Gibney 2020; Ouchchy et al. 2020; Krishnan et al. 2023). Given the diversity in socio-economic contexts, healthcare infrastructures, and regulatory frameworks across LMICs, the AI ethics research community must endeavour to develop frameworks and technical governance models that are adaptable and inclusive. This includes grappling with the global dimensions of AI policy and ensuring that principles translate into actionable rules and mechanisms that respect cultural and contextual nuances (Rotenberg 2019; ÓhÉigeartaigh et al. 2020; Schmitt 2022).

Even though there is an increase in support from funding bodies for research on the social and ethical implications of AI, there is still a lack of attention by the academic bioethics community on AI within the field of healthcare, especially within the context of LMICs (Murphy et al. 2021; Gardner et al. 2022). This gap highlights the need for a more concerted effort to understand and address the unique ethical challenges posed by AI in these settings. AI has the potential to positively impact the health of individuals directly or indirectly. On the other hand, according to Vinuesa et al. 2020, AI could equally inhibit countries in achieving all 17 SDGs, and thus further exacerbate existing patterns of health inequalities if the benefits of AI primarily support populations of the wealthiest within countries.

For instance, while AI-driven diagnostic tools can improve access to quality healthcare, they may be predominantly accessible to urban and affluent populations, leaving rural and economically disadvantaged groups underserved. As stated before, many LMICs face significant challenges in digitising their health records, which is essential data for AI to use. The lack of digital infrastructure and interoperability further compounds these challenges, creating barriers to the equitable implementation of AI technologies. This showcases that there is still an essential need to overcome the technological gap to ensure that these countries can harness the potential benefit of AI for its entire population.

Thus, it is imperative that governments collaborate with other key stakeholders to identify and address the ethical issues systematically in order to determine the areas where AI can benefit, as well as mitigate potential harms, especially for their most vulnerable populations (Murphy et al. 2021). This collaborative approach should involve international organisations, non-profits, private sector partners, and local communities to create a robust and inclusive ethical framework. It should also focus on capacity-building initiatives to enhance the digital literacy and technical skills required for effective AI deployment in healthcare.

These governance practices are paramount to the ethical management of health data and AI systems in healthcare workflows and service delivery. This entails the formulation of national AI strategies, allocation of budgets, and fostering political will and industry leadership. Additionally, guidelines for clinical and scientific validation, governance frameworks, and rights-based approaches to privacy and security are essential. The primary challenge for governance lies in harnessing AI technology and data for the collective benefit of their populations (and its healthcare systems) while ensuring responsible and ethical management.

For policymakers and governments, the overarching goal is to establish multi-level governance structures that bolster public trust, safeguard privacy and security, and foster innovation in healthcare. By navigating these complexities, LMICs can leverage AI to advance healthcare delivery while upholding ethical principles and ensuring equitable access to benefits.

9.5 Key Ethical Themes in AI-Based Healthcare Tools

As mentioned above, AI technologies within the healthcare setting in LMICs present unique ethical challenges and considerations, largely influenced by the socio-economic, technological and regulatory contexts. The implementation of AI in these regions necessitates a nuanced understanding of ethical themes, including data privacy and security, trust in AI, accountability and responsibility, and bias, all of which are critical to ensuring equitable and effective healthcare delivery. Although these issues are interconnected in many different ways, they differ in how they should be addressed.

9.5.1 Privacy and Security

Issues of privacy and data security are particularly pressing due to less robust digital infrastructure and regulatory frameworks compared to high-income countries. The collection and use of patient data by AI systems requires substantial amounts of personal health information, raising concerns about data misuse and breaches. For example, the hacking of a diagnostic laboratory database in Mumbai in 2016, which resulted in the leakage of over 35,000 patient records, underscores the vulnerabilities in data security. Patients in LMICs often lack awareness and control over how their data is used, exacerbating privacy concerns (van Panhuis et al. 2014; Alter et al. 2015; Kaewkungwal et al. 2020). Moreover, data breaches can have severe consequences, such as discrimination by employers and insurance companies based on leaked health information, further marginalising vulnerable populations (Luxton 2014; Kantarjian et al. 2015; Markowetz et al. 2014; Campolo et al. 2017).

To address these concerns, LMICs need to strengthen their data protection laws and implement robust cybersecurity measures. Policymakers should ensure that AI systems comply with these regulations and that there are clear protocols for data collection, storage, and usage. Public awareness campaigns about data privacy rights and the secure handling of personal information can also empower patients to make informed decisions.

9.5.2 Trust in AI

Building trust in AI among patients and healthcare professionals in LMICs is crucial for the successful deployment of AI technologies. Trust issues often stem from a lack of transparency and understanding of how AI systems work. For instance, the data-sharing partnership between Google DeepMind and the Royal Free London NHS Foundation Trust raised significant trust concerns due to inadequate patient consent and consultation with regulatory bodies (Powles et al. 2017; Denton et al. 2018). Such incidents highlight the need for clarity and openness in AI deployment to maintain public trust as healthcare systems move into an algorithmic age (Powles et al. 2017; Murphy et al. 2021).

In LMICs, fostering trust requires engaging with local communities, involving patients and healthcare providers in the design and implementation of AI systems, and ensuring that AI applications are culturally sensitive and contextually relevant. Training and education initiatives can help healthcare professionals understand and effectively use AI tools, while clear communication about the benefits and limitations of AI, including its development, can enhance patient trust.

9.5.3 Accountability and Responsibility for Use of AI Technologies

Determining accountability for errors and adverse outcomes related to AI in healthcare is a significant challenge in LMICs, where legal and regulatory frameworks may be underdeveloped (Sharkey et al. 2012; Siqueira-Batista et al. 2016; Mesko 2017; Powles et al. 2017; Paul et al. 2018; McBee et al. 2018). The complexity of AI algorithms makes it difficult to understand and scrutinise, complicating the process of seeking compensation or justice if harm occurs (Mesko 2017, House of Lords 2018; Nuffield Council of Bioethics 2018). Private companies often own these technologies and may limit public access for inspection (Crawford et al. 2016; Monteith et al. 2016; House of Lords. 2018). Therefore, the debate over who should be held responsible for AI errors is a difficult conversation when multiple stakeholders, including healthcare providers, AI developers, and policymakers, are involved (Sharkey et al. 2012; Paul et al. 2018; McBee et al. 2018; Murphy et al. 2021).

On one hand, healthcare professionals are legally and professionally responsible for patient care, and thus should bear responsibility for the consequences of decisions aided by AI. On the other hand, developers are responsible for ensuring the quality, safety, and effectiveness of AI technology, which includes being responsive to the needs and characteristics of specific patient populations (Hope 1989; Yuste et al. 2017; Balthazar et al. 2018; Fenech et al. 2018; O'Brolcháin 2019).

In the LMIC context, it is essential to establish clear guidelines for accountability and responsibility. Healthcare providers should be trained to critically evaluate AI recommendations and make informed decisions. AI developers should consider building accountability mechanisms into AI algorithms for black box audits to ensure that their systems are transparent, reliable, and responsive to the needs of local populations. Additionally, AI developers should also receive training on issues of accountability, privacy, and ethics. Policymakers should create regulatory frameworks that define the roles and responsibilities of all stakeholders and establish mechanisms for redress in case of harm (Paul et al. 2018; Murphy et al. 2021).

9.5.4 Biases

Addressing bias requires AI systems to reflect current ethical healthcare standards and involve a multidisciplinary and participatory approach in design and deployment. Ensuring diverse representation in AI development and training can help mitigate bias and improve the generalisability of AI output (Pasquale 2015; Mori 2017).

Bias in AI algorithms and training data is a pervasive issue that can perpetuate existing healthcare disparities in LMICs (Bowser et al. 2017; Char et al. 2018; Ching et al. 2018; Fenech et al. 2018; Howard et al. 2018). AI systems developed in high-income countries may not be generalisable to LMIC populations due to differences in demographics, disease prevalence, and healthcare practices, as well as developers being inherently influenced by their own values and implicit biases. This limits the effectiveness and accuracy of these tools and perpetuates existing biases that disadvantage certain groups within these nations (Campolo et al. 2017; Williams et al. 2018).

Addressing bias requires a concerted effort to develop and train AI systems using data that accurately represent the populations they serve. Involving local experts and stakeholders in the development process can ensure that AI tools are contextually appropriate and culturally sensitive. Additionally, continuous monitoring and evaluation of AI systems can help identify and mitigate bias, ensuring that AI contributes to reducing rather than exacerbating health inequities.

To summarise, the ethical issues surrounding AI in healthcare systems within LMICs are vast and complex. Given the relatively uncharted territory of AI in health, these challenges require tailored approaches that consider the unique socio-economic, technological, and regulatory landscapes of these regions. By fostering collaboration among governments, healthcare providers, AI developers, and local communities, LMICs can harness the potential of AI to improve healthcare delivery while upholding ethical principles and ensuring equitable access for everyone, everywhere.

9.6 Health System Integration and Infrastructure Readiness

The ubiquitous presence of smartphones in LMICs presents a ripe opportunity for integrating AI into mobile health applications, thereby enhancing healthcare accessibility and effective population engagement (Arias et al. 2024). For example, 80% of Kenyans have access to at least one simple device (Silver et al. 2018). Leveraging AI technologies, both for personal health management and within clinical settings, can potentially expand healthcare access and improve health outcomes, particularly in resource-constrained environments. However, most AI systems need at least some level of connectivity to either the internet or electricity to work (O'Donnell 2020). While the costs for broadband and connectivity have dropped significantly, they remain high in some LMICs, posing a vital barrier to implementing and integrating AI in health services (Broadband Commission for Sustainable Development 2020).

9.6.1 Connectivity

Despite the proliferation of mobile devices, reliable internet and electricity access remains uneven across many LMICs (Erku et al. 2023). Rural and remote areas often suffer the most from poor connectivity, making it challenging to deploy AI-driven health solutions effectively. Governments and stakeholders must prioritise improving infrastructure to ensure that AI technologies can be accessed by all segments of the population. This involves not only expanding broadband coverage but also making it affordable for low-income households (Broadband Commission for Sustainable Development 2020; Bajwa et al. 2021).

Currently, there are no incentives for operators to enter less attractive markets (e.g. remote areas). Policymakers and stakeholders need to make connectivity availability and affordability a priority, highlighting specific measures for underserved populations. Ensuring these populations do not miss out on the benefits of AI in their healthcare systems will also provide long-term sustainability to AI initiatives (Broadband Commission for Sustainable Development 2020). Additionally, health systems tend to suffer from technology underinvestment, and weak education systems and digital learning outcomes remain barriers to increase AI skills and uptake (Bari et al. 2023; Ahmed et al. 2023).

9.6.2 Digital Literacy and Training

The successful integration of AI into health systems in LMICs depends heavily on the digital literacy of both healthcare providers and patients. Many healthcare workers in these regions lack the necessary training to effectively utilise AI tools, which can limit the potential benefits of these technologies (Saif-Ur-Rahman et al. 2023; Fitzpatrick 2023). Investing in education and training programs is crucial to build a workforce capable of harnessing AI's capabilities.

Digital literacy initiatives should focus on:

1. *Healthcare Workers:* Providing training on the use of AI applications in clinical settings, including diagnostics, patient management, and decision support systems (Mousavi Baigi et al. 2023).
2. *Patients and Communities:* Educating the general population about the benefits and safe use of AI-driven health applications. This can help increase trust and adoption rates (Fitzpatrick 2023).
3. *Technical Skills:* Developing programs that teach coding, data science, and AI development skills to create a local workforce capable of maintaining and innovating AI technologies (Ejaz et al. 2022).

9.6.3 Integration with Existing Health Systems

For AI to be effectively integrated into health systems in LMICs, it must be compatible with existing infrastructures and workflows (Ciecierski-Holmes et al. 2022; Khan et al. 2024). This requires a careful assessment of current health systems and identifying areas where AI can add value without causing disruptions. Strategies to ensure smooth integration include:

1. *Interoperability:* Ensuring AI applications can communicate with existing health information systems to facilitate data sharing and streamline operations (Esmaeilzadeh 2024).
2. *Pilot Programs:* Implementing pilot projects to test AI solutions in real-world settings, gather feedback, and make necessary adjustments before scaling up (Nair et al. 2023; Brady et al. 2024).
3. *Local Adaptation:* Customising AI technologies to meet local needs and cultural contexts, which can improve acceptance and effectiveness (Hsu et al. 2022).

9.6.4 Sustainability and Scalability

Sustainability and scalability are critical considerations for AI initiatives in LMICs. Projects must be designed to operate within the resource constraints typical of these regions and have clear plans for scaling up successful pilots.

1. *Funding and Partnerships:* Securing funding from diverse sources, including governments, international organisations, and private sector partnerships, to support the initial deployment and ongoing maintenance of AI technologies (Gardner et al. 2022).
2. *Community Engagement:* Engaging local communities in the design and implementation of AI projects to ensure they are patient-centred by meeting local needs and have community support (Hsu et al. 2022).
3. *Monitoring and Evaluation:* Establishing robust mechanisms for monitoring and evaluating AI projects to assess their impact and identify areas for improvement (Reddy et al. 2021).

9.6.5 Addressing Basic ICT and Digital Infrastructure Needs

The reality for LMICs is that there is a lack of basic information and communications technology (ICT) and digital infrastructure needed for many AI applications to be scaled nationally. However, through other advanced technologies and the efforts of global health and development projects, this issue will be addressed in the coming years. Steps to accelerate this process include:

1. *Government Initiatives:* Governments should prioritise ICT infrastructure development in their national strategies and allocate resources accordingly.
2. *International Support:* Leveraging support from international organisations and development agencies to fund ICT projects and provide technical assistance (Vinuesa et al. 2020).
3. *Innovative Solutions:* Exploring innovative solutions such as satellite internet, community Wi-Fi initiatives, and solar-powered charging stations to overcome infrastructure challenges.

Integrating AI into health systems in LMICs holds great promise for improving healthcare access and outcomes. However, realising this potential requires addressing significant challenges related to connectivity, infrastructure, digital literacy, and system integration. By prioritising these areas and fostering collaboration among stakeholders, LMICs can build a foundation for the successful deployment of AI technologies, ensuring that all populations benefit from advancements in healthcare.

9.7 Conclusion

The promise of AI in healthcare within LMICs is immense, offering transformative potential to overcome long-standing challenges and drive significant improvements in health outcomes. However, realising this potential requires a nuanced and multi-faceted approach that addresses the unique contexts and constraints of these nations. The integration of AI into healthcare systems in LMICs must be carefully strategised, emphasising equitable access, ethical considerations, and robust regulatory frameworks.

First and foremost, the development and implementation of AI technologies in LMICs must prioritise the collection and management of high-quality, unbiased data. This involves establishing comprehensive data strategies that encompass effective data collection methods, stringent data quality assurance measures, and frameworks for data governance. Ensuring data interoperability and equitable access to AI-driven insights is crucial for maximising the benefits of these technologies across diverse healthcare settings.

Moreover, ethical governance and regulatory compliance are paramount to safeguarding patient rights and fostering trust in AI systems. This includes adhering to principles of informed consent, privacy protection, and transparency in AI decision-making processes. The integration of explainability and causability into AI models is essential for enhancing their reliability and fostering acceptance among healthcare professionals and patients alike.

Health system integration and infrastructure readiness are critical components of successful AI adoption in LMICs. Investments in digital infrastructure, workforce development, and capacity building are necessary to create an environment conducive to AI-driven innovations. Policymakers and stakeholders must work collaboratively to ensure that AI solutions align with national and local health priorities, addressing both immediate healthcare needs and long-term strategic goals.

While AI holds great promise, it is not a panacea for the healthcare challenges faced by LMICs. It should be viewed as a powerful tool that, when integrated thoughtfully and ethically, can complement existing healthcare strategies and enhance service delivery. Stakeholders must remain vigilant about the risks and tradeoffs associated with AI adoption, continuously evaluating and adapting AI systems to ensure they serve the best interests of the populations they are designed to benefit.

In conclusion, the journey towards leveraging AI in healthcare for LMICs is complex and requires a concerted effort from governments, healthcare providers, technologists, and communities. By focusing on data management, ethical governance, and health system integration, LMICs can harness the transformative power of AI to achieve UHC and make significant strides towards the SDGs. The path forward demands innovation, collaboration, and a steadfast commitment to health equity, ensuring that no one is left behind in the pursuit of better health for all.

References

Ahmed SK, Hussein S, Chandran D, Islam MR, Dhama K (2023) The role of digital health in revolutionising healthcare delivery and improving health outcomes in conflict zones. Digit Health 9:20552076231218158. https://doi.org/10.1177/20552076231218158

Alami H, Rivard L, Lehoux P, Hoffman SJ, Cadeddu SBM, Savoldelli M et al (2020) Artificial intelligence in health care: laying the Foundation for Responsible, sustainable, and inclusive innovation in low- and middle-income countries. Glob Health 16(1):52. https://doi.org/10.1186/s12992-020-00584-1

Alter GC, Vardigan M (2015) Addressing global data sharing challenges. J Empir Res Hum Res Ethics 10(3):317–323. https://doi.org/10.1177/1556264615591561

Arias A, Rickwood S (2024) Boosting healthcare capacity with AI. World Economic Forum. https://www.weforum.org/agenda/2024/01/ai-in-healthcare-could-bridge-a-significant-capacity-gap/. Accessed 19 Jun 2024

Bajwa J, Munir U, Nori A, Williams B (2021) Artificial intelligence in healthcare: transforming the practice of medicine. Future Healthc J 8(2):e188–e194. https://doi.org/10.7861/fhj.2021-0095

Balthazar P, Harri P, Prater A, Safdar NM (2018) Protecting your patients' interests in the era of big data, artificial intelligence, and predictive analytics. J Am Coll Radiol 15(3):580–586

Bari LF, Ahmed I, Ahamed R, Zihan TA, Sharmin S, Pranto AH, Islam MR (2023) Potential use of artificial intelligence (AI) in disaster risk and emergency health management: a critical appraisal on environmental health. Environ Health Insights 17:11786302231217808. https://doi.org/10.1177/11786302231217808

Bawah A, Houle B, Alam N, Razzaque A, Streatfield PK, Debpuur C et al (2016) The evolving demographic and health transition in four low- and middle-income countries: evidence from four sites in the INDEPTH network of longitudinal health and demographic surveillance systems. PLoS One 11(6):e0157281. https://doi.org/10.1371/journal.pone.0157281

Bowser A, Sloan M, Michelucci P, Pauwels E (2017) Artificial intelligence: a policy-oriented introduction. Wilson Center. https://www.wilsoncenter.org/sites/default/files/media/documents/publication/wilson_center_policy_brief_artificial_intelligence.pdf. Accessed 19 Jun 2024

Brady AP, Allen B, Chong J et al (2024) Developing, purchasing, implementing and monitoring AI tools in radiology: practical considerations. A multi-society statement from the ACR, CAR, ESR, RANZCR & RSNA. Insights Imaging 15:16. https://doi.org/10.1186/s13244-023-01541-3

Broadband Commission for Sustainable Development (2020) Reimagining Global Health through Artificial Intelligence: The Roadmap to AI Maturity. https://www.broadbandcommission.org/Documents/working-groups/AIinHealth_Report.pdf. Accessed 20 Jun 2024

Brynjolfsson E, Mitchell T (2017) What can machine learning do? Workforce implications. Science 358:1530–1534. https://doi.org/10.1126/science.aap8062

Campolo A, Sanfilippo M, Whittaker M, Crawford K (2017) AI now 2017 report. https://ainowinstitute.org/wp-content/uploads/2023/04/AI_Now_2017_Report.pdf. Accessed 19 Jun 2024

Cath C (2018) Governing artificial intelligence: ethical, legal and technical opportunities and challenges. Philos Trans A Math Phys Eng Sci 376(2133):20180080. https://doi.org/10.1098/rsta.2018.0080

Char DS, Shah NH, Magnus D (2018) Implementing machine learning in health care—addressing ethical challenges. N Engl J Med 378(11):981–983. https://doi.org/10.1056/NEJMp1714229

Chen JH, Asch SM (2017) Machine learning and prediction in medicine — beyond the peak of inflated expectations. N Engl J Med 376(26):2507–2509. https://doi.org/10.1056/NEJMp1702071

Ching T, Himmelstein DS, Beaulieu-Jones BK, Kalinin AA, Do BT, Way GP et al (2018) Opportunities and

obstacles for deep learning in biology and medicine. J R Soc Interface 15(141):20170387. https://doi.org/10.1098/rsif.2017.0387
Ciecierski-Holmes T, Singh RAM, Brenner S, Barteit S (2022) Artificial intelligence for strengthening healthcare systems in low- and middle-income countries: a systematic scoping review. NPJ Digit Med 5(1):162. https://doi.org/10.1038/s41746-022-00700-y
Collier M, Fu R, Yin L (2017) Artificial intelligence: healthcare's new nervous system: Accenture. https://www.ehidc.org/sites/default/files/resources/files/Accenture-Health-Artificial-Intelligence.pdf. Accessed 19 Jun 2024
Crawford K, Whittaker M (2016) The AI now report: the social and economic implications of artificial intelligence technologies in the near-term. White House and New York University's Information Law Institute. https://artificialintelligencenow.com/media/documents/AINowSummaryReport_3_RpmwKHu.pdf. Accessed 19 Jun 2024
Denton S, Pauwels E, He Y, Johnson W (2018) There's nowhere to hide: artificial intelligence and privacy in the fourth industrial revolution. Wilson Center, Synenergene, and the Institute for Philosophy & Public Policy. https://iapp.org/media/pdf/resource_center/ai_and_privacy.pdf. Wilson Center. Accessed 19 Jun 2024
Deo RC (2015) Machine learning in medicine. Circulation 132(20):1920–1930. https://doi.org/10.1161/CIRCULATIONAHA.115.001593
Ejaz H, McGrath H, Wong BL, Guise A, Vercauteren T, Shapey J (2022) Artificial intelligence and medical education: a global mixed-methods study of medical students' perspectives. Digit Health. 8:20552076221089099. https://doi.org/10.1177/20552076221089099
Erku D, Khatri R, Endalamaw A, Wolka E, Nigatu F, Zewdie A, Assefa Y (2023) Digital health interventions to improve access to and quality of primary health care services: a scoping review. Int J Environ Res Public Health 20(19):6854. https://doi.org/10.3390/ijerph20196854
Esmaeilzadeh P (2024) Challenges and strategies for wide-scale artificial intelligence (AI) deployment in healthcare practices: a perspective for healthcare organizations. Artif Intell Med 151:102861. https://doi.org/10.1016/j.artmed.2024.102861
Faraj S, Pachidi S, Sayegh K (2018) Working and organizing in the age of the learning algorithm. Inf Organ 28(1):62–70. https://doi.org/10.1016/j.infoandorg.2018.02.005
Fenech M, Strukelj N, Buston O. (2018) Ethical, social, and political challenges of artificial intelligence in health. Future Advocacy & Wellcome Trust. https://wellcome.ac.uk/sites/default/files/ai-in-health-ethical-social-political-challenges.pdf. Accessed 19 Jun 2024
Fitzpatrick PJ (2023) Improving health literacy using the power of digital communications to achieve better health outcomes for patients and practitioners. Front Digit Health 5:1264780. https://doi.org/10.3389/fdgth.2023.1264780
Gardner A, Smith AL, Steventon A, Coughlan E, Oldfield M (2022) Ethical funding for trustworthy AI: proposals to address the responsibilities of funders to ensure that projects adhere to trustworthy AI practice. AI Ethics 2(2):277–291. https://doi.org/10.1007/s43681-021-00069-w
Garzon-Chavez D, Romero-Alvarez D, Bonifaz M, Gaviria J, Mero D et al (2021) Adapting for the COVID-19 pandemic in Ecuador, a characterization of hospital strategies and patients. PLoS One 16(5):e0251295. https://doi.org/10.1371/journal.pone.0251295
Gibney E (2020) The battle for ethical AI at the world's biggest machine-learning conference. Nature 577(7792):609–609. Accessed 23 Jun 2024
Hao K, Hernandez A (2022) How the AI industry profits from catastrophe MIT Technol Rev. 2022. Available from: https://www.technologyreview.com/2022/04/20/1050392/ai-industry-appen-scale-data-labels/. Accessed 22 Jun 2024
Hao K, Swart H (2022) South Africa's private surveillance machine is fueling a digital apartheid. MIT Technol rev. Available from: https://www.technologyreview.com/2022/04/19/1049996/south-africa-ai-surveillance-digital-apartheid/. Accessed 22 Jun 2024
Holzinger A, Langs G, Denk H, Zatloukal K, Müller H (2019) Causability and explainability of artificial intelligence in medicine. Wiley Interdiscip Rev Data Min Knowl Discov 9(4):e1312. https://doi.org/10.1002/widm.1312
Hope M (1989) Computer-aided medicine: present and future issues of liability. Comput Law J 9(2):177–203. https://repository.law.uic.edu/cgi/viewcontent.cgi?article=1438&context=jitpl. Accessed 19 Jun 2024
Hosny A, Aerts HJWL (2019) Artificial intelligence for global health. Science 366(6468):955–956. https://doi.org/10.1126/science.aay5189
House of Lords (2018) AI in the UK: ready, willing and able? United Kingdom: authority of the house of lords. Intelligence SCoA, editor https://publications.parliament.uk/pa/ld201719/ldselect/ldai/100/100.pdf. Accessed 19 Jun 2024
Howard A, Borenstein J (2018) The ugly truth about ourselves and our robot creations: the problem of bias and social inequity. Sci Eng Ethics 24(5):1521–1536. https://doi.org/10.1007/s11948-017-9975-2
Howard FM, Dolezal J, Kochanny S, Schulte J, Chen H, Heij L et al (2021) The impact of site-specific digital histology signatures on deep learning model accuracy and bias. Nat Commun 12(1):4423. https://doi.org/10.1038/s41467-021-24698-1
Hsu YC, Huang T, Verma H, Mauri A, Nourbakhsh I, Bozzon A (2022) Empowering local communities using artificial intelligence. Patterns (NY) 3(3):100449. https://doi.org/10.1016/j.patter.2022.100449
Javaid M, Haleem A, Singh RP, Suman R, Rab S (2022) Significance of machine learning in healthcare: features, pillars and applications. Int J Intell Netw 3:58–73. https://doi.org/10.1016/j.ijin.2022.05.002

Johnson KB, Wei WQ, Weeraratne D, Frisse ME, Misulis K, Rhee K, Zhao J, Snowdon JL (2021) Precision medicine, AI, and the future of personalized health care. Clin Transl Sci 14(1):86–93. https://doi.org/10.1111/cts.12884

Kaewkungwal J, Adams P, Sattabongkot J, Lie RK, Wendler D (2020) Issues and challenges associated with data-sharing in LMICs: perspectives of researchers in Thailand. Am J Trop Med Hyg 103(1):528–536. https://doi.org/10.4269/ajtmh.19-0651

Kantarjian H, Yu PP (2015) Artificial intelligence, big data, and cancer. JAMA Oncol 1(5):573–574. https://doi.org/10.1001/jamaoncol.2015.1203

Khan SD, Hoodbhoy Z, Raja MHR, Kim JY, Hogg HDJ, Manji AAA et al (2024) Frameworks for procurement, integration, monitoring, and evaluation of artificial intelligence tools in clinical settings: a systematic review. PLOS Digit Health. 3(5):e0000514. https://doi.org/10.1371/journal.pdig.0000514

Krishnan G, Singh S, Pathania M, Gosavi S, Abhishek S, Parchani A, Dhar M (2023) Artificial intelligence in clinical medicine: catalyzing a sustainable global healthcare paradigm. Front Artif Intell 6:1227091. https://doi.org/10.3389/frai.2023.1227091

Labrique AB, Wadhwani C, Williams KA et al (2018) Best practices in scaling digital health in low and middle income countries. Glob Health 14:103. https://doi.org/10.1186/s12992-018-0424-z

López DM, Rico-Olarte C, Blobel B, Hullin C (2022) Challenges and solutions for transforming health ecosystems in low- and middle-income countries through artificial intelligence. Front Med (Lausanne) 2(9):958097. https://doi.org/10.3389/fmed.2022.958097

Luxton DD (2014) Recommendations for the ethical use and design of artificial intelligent care providers. Artif Intell Med 62(1):1–10. https://doi.org/10.1016/j.artmed.2014.06.004

Markowetz A, Błaszkiewicz K, Montag C, Switala C, Schlaepfer TE (2014) Psycho-informatics: big data shaping modern psychometrics. Med Hypotheses 82(4):405–411. https://doi.org/10.1016/j.mehy.2013.11.030

McBee MP, Awan OA, Colucci AT, Ghobadi CW, Kadom N, Kansagra AP, Tridandapani S, Auffermann WF (2018) Deep learning in radiology. Acad Radiol 25(11):1472–1480. https://doi.org/10.1016/j.acra.2018.02.018

Mesko B (2017) The role of artificial intelligence in precision medicine. Expert Rev Precis Med Drug Dev 2(5):239–241. https://doi.org/10.1080/23808993.2017.1380516

Mollura DJ, Culp MP, Pollack E et al (2020) Artificial intelligence in low- and middle-income countries: innovating global health radiology. Radiology 297(3):513–520. https://doi.org/10.1148/radiol.2020201434

Monteith S, Glenn T (2016) Automated decision-making and big data: concerns for people with mental illness. Curr Psychiatry Rep 18(12):112. https://doi.org/10.1007/s11920-016-0746-6

Mori I (2017) The one-Way Mirror: public attitudes to commercial access to health data. Wellcome Trust Journal contribution. https://doi.org/10.6084/m9.figshare.5616448.v1

Mousavi Baigi SF, Sarbaz M, Ghaddaripouri K, Ghaddaripouri M, Mousavi AS, Kimiafar K (2023) Attitudes, knowledge, and skills towards artificial intelligence among healthcare students: a systematic review. Health Sci Rep. 6(3):e1138. https://doi.org/10.1002/hsr2.1138

Murphy K, Di Ruggiero E, Upshur R et al (2021) Artificial intelligence for good health: a scoping review of the ethics literature. BMC Med Ethics 22:14. https://doi.org/10.1186/s12910-021-00577-8

Nair M, Andersson J, Nygren JM, Lundgren LE (2023) Barriers and enablers for implementation of an artificial intelligence-based decision support tool to reduce the risk of readmission of patients with heart failure: stakeholder interviews. JMIR Form Res 7:e47335. https://doi.org/10.2196/47335

Nkengasong JN, Yao K, Onyebujoh P (2018) Laboratory medicine in low-income and middle-income countries: progress and challenges. Lancet 391(10133):1873–1875. https://doi.org/10.1016/S0140-6736(18)30308-8

Nuffield Council on Bioethics (2018) Artificial intelligence (AI) in healthcare and research. https://www.nuffieldbioethics.org/publications/ai-in-healthcare-and-research. Accessed 19 Jun 2024

O'Brolcháin F (2019) Robots and people with dementia: unintended consequences and moral hazard. Nurs Ethics 26(4):962–972. https://doi.org/10.1177/0969733017742960

O'Donnell, Commentary on Harder et al (2020) Ensuring the sustainability of mHealth in low- and middle-income countries—how do we cure 'pilotitis'? Addiction 115:1061–1062. https://doi.org/10.1111/add.14986

Oduoye MO, Fatima E, Muzammil MA, Dave T, Irfan H, Fariha FNU et al (2024) Impacts of the advancement in artificial intelligence on laboratory medicine in low- and middle-income countries: challenges and recommendations—a literature review. Health Sci Rep 7(1):e1794. https://doi.org/10.1002/hsr2.1794

ÓhÉigeartaigh SS, Whittlestone J, Liu Y, Zeng Y, Liu Z (2020) Overcoming barriers to cross-cultural cooperation in AI ethics and governance. Philos Technol 33:571–593. https://doi.org/10.1007/s13347-020-00402-x

Oleribe OO, Momoh J, Uzochukwu BS, Mbofana F, Adebiyi A et al (2019) Identifying key challenges facing healthcare systems in Africa and potential solutions. Int J Gen Med 12:395–403. https://doi.org/10.2147/IJGM.S223882

Ouchchy L, Coin A, Dubljević V (2020) AI in the headlines: the portrayal of the ethical issues of artificial intelligence in the media. AI Soc 35:927–936. https://doi.org/10.1007/s00146-020-00965-5

Pasquale F (2015) The black box society: the secret algorithms that control money and information. Harvard University Press, Cambridge

Paul Y, Hickok E, Sinha A, Tiwari U, Bidare PM (2018) Artificial intelligence in the healthcare industry in India. https://cis-india.org/internet-governance/files/ai-and-healtchare-report. Accessed 19 Jun 2024

Powles J, Hodson H (2017) Google DeepMind and healthcare in an age of algorithms. Health Technol 7(4):351–367. https://doi.org/10.1007/s12553-017-0179-1

Reddy S, Rogers W, Makinen VP, Coiera E, Brown P, Wenzel M, Weicken E, Ansari S, Mathur P, Casey A, Kelly B (2021) Evaluation framework to guide implementation of AI systems into healthcare settings. BMJ Health Care Inform 28(1):e100444. https://doi.org/10.1136/bmjhci-2021-100444

Rotenberg M (2019) The AI policy sourcebook. Electronic Privacy Information Center, Epic

Saif-Ur-Rahman KM, Islam MS, Alaboson J, Ola O, Hasan I, Islam N et al (2023) Artificial intelligence and digital health in improving primary health care service delivery in LMICs: a systematic review. J Evid Based Med 16(3):303–320. https://doi.org/10.1111/jebm.12547

Scardoni A, Balzarini F, Signorelli C, Cabitza F, Odone A (2020) Artificial intelligence-based tools to control healthcare associated infections: a systematic review of the literature. J Infect Public Health 13(8):1061–1077. https://doi.org/10.1016/j.jiph.2020.06.006

Schmitt L (2022) Mapping global AI governance: a nascent regime in a fragmented landscape. AI Ethics 2:303–314. https://doi.org/10.1007/s43681-021-00083-y

Seastedt KP, Schwab P, O'Brien Z, Wakida E, Herrera K, Marcelo PGF et al (2022) Global healthcare fairness: we should be sharing more, not less, data. PLOS Digit Health 1(10):e0000102. https://doi.org/10.1371/journal.pdig.0000102

Sharkey A, Sharkey N (2012) Granny and the robots: ethical issues in robot care for the elderly. Ethics Inf Technol 14(1):27–40. https://doi.org/10.1007/s10676-010-9234-6

Silver L, Johnson C Pew Research Center Internet Connectivity Seen as Having Positive Impact on Life in Sub-Saharan Africa. 2018 Washington, DC: Pew Research Center. https://www.pewresearch.org/global/2018/10/09/internet-connectivity-seen-as-having-positive-impact-on-life-in-sub-saharan-africa-2/. Accessed 20 Jun 2024

Siqueira-Batista R, Souza CR, Maia PM, Siqueira SL (2016) Robotic surgery: bioethical aspects. Arq Bras Cir Dig 29(4):287–290. https://doi.org/10.1590/0102-6720201600040018

van Panhuis WG, Paul P, Emerson C, Grefenstette J, Wilder R, Herbst AJ, Heymann D, Burke DS (2014) A systematic review of barriers to data sharing in public health. BMC Public Health 14:1144. https://doi.org/10.1186/1471-2458-14-1144

Vayena E, Blasimme A, Cohen IG (2018) Machine learning in medicine: addressing ethical challenges. PLoS Med 15(11):e1002689. https://doi.org/10.1371/journal.pmed.1002689

Vinuesa R, Azizpour H, Leite I, Balaam M, Dignum V, Domisch S et al (2020) The role of artificial intelligence in achieving the sustainable development goals. Nat Commun 11(1):233. https://doi.org/10.1038/s41467-019-14108-y

Wahl B, Cossy-Gantner A, Germann S et al (2018) Artificial intelligence (AI) and global health: how can AI contribute to health in resource-poor settings? BMJ Glob Health 3:e000798. https://doi.org/10.1136/bmjgh-2018-000798

Weiss D, Nelson A, Vargas-Ruiz CA et al (2020) Global maps of travel time to healthcare facilities. Nat Med 26:1835–1838. https://doi.org/10.1038/s41591-020-1059-1

Weissglass DE (2022) (2022) contextual bias, the democratization of healthcare, and medical artificial intelligence in low- and middle-income countries. Bioethics 36:201–209. https://doi.org/10.1111/bioe.12927

Williams AM, Liu Y, Regner KR, Jotterand F, Liu P, Liang M (2018) Artificial intelligence, physiological genomics, and precision medicine. Physiol Genomics 50(4):237–243. https://doi.org/10.1152/physiolgenomics.00119.2017

Witter S, Sheikh K, Schleiff M (2022) Learning health systems in low-income and middle-income countries: exploring evidence and expert insights-BMJ. Glob Health 7:e008115. https://doi.org/10.1136/bmjgh-2021-008115

World Health Organization (2016) Draft global strategy on human resources for health: workforce 2030. 69th World Health Assembly. http://apps.who.int/gb/ebwha/pdf_files/WHA69/A69_38-en.pdf. Accessed 19 Jun 2024

World Health Organization (2017) World Bank and WHO: Half the world lacks access to essential health services, 100 million still pushed into extreme poverty because of health expenses. https://www.who.int/news/item/13-12-2017-world-bank-and-who-half-the-world-lacks-access-to-essential-health-services-100-million-still-pushed-into-extreme-poverty-because-of-health-expenses. Accessed 19 Jun 2024

World Health Organization (2021) Global strategy on digital health 2020–2025. https://apps.who.int/iris/handle/10665/344249. Accessed 19 Jun 2024

World Health Organization (2024) Noncommunicable diseases: mortality. https://www.who.int/data/gho/data/themes/topics/topic-details/GHO/ncd-mortality. Accessed 25 Jun 2024

Yuste R, Goering S, Arcas BAY, Bi G, Carmena JM, Carter A, Fins JJ et al (2017) Four ethical priorities for neurotechnologies and AI. Nature 551(7679):159–163. https://doi.org/10.1038/551159a

The Role of Artificial Intelligence in Workforce Adaptation and Skill Development

10

Yusuf Karmali

Abstract

This chapter on Artificial Intelligence (AI) and the required workforce adaptation and skill development addresses the pressing global healthcare workforce shortage projected to reach 18 million by 2030, exacerbated by increasing lifespans and the accumulation of chronic conditions. It explores the potential of AI to revolutionise medical practice by improving efficiency, transforming clinical roles, and increasing productivity. It presents AI's capabilities in diagnostics, treatment planning, and administrative tasks, illustrating its transformative potential. The discussion includes the current state of the medical workforce, highlighting significant shortages across various healthcare professions, and the impact of physician burnout on healthcare delivery. The chapter emphasises the need for adaptability in the medical field, underscoring the importance of interdisciplinary education and AI literacy integration into healthcare training. The chapter concludes by advocating for the incorporation of AI into medical curricula to prepare future healthcare professionals for the evolving landscape, ensuring they can harness AI's benefits while maintaining the integrity of the doctor-patient relationship.

Keywords

Artificial intelligence · Workforce · Healthcare · Artificial intelligence literacy

10.1 Introduction

Globally, we are predicted to be short of 18 million healthcare workers by the year 2030 (World Health Organization 2016). The result of this will be significant unmet healthcare demands in both the developed and developing world. Additionally, increasing life spans and subsequent accumulation of chronic comorbidities have made managing patients more complex. Medical knowledge is currently doubling every 73 days, making it hard for clinicians to keep on top of current medical evidence (Densen 2011). Despite the lengthy training times of doctors and other healthcare professionals, the third leading cause of death is medical error (Makary and Daniel 2016).

Artificial Intelligence (AI) has the promise to revolutionise medicine, bringing in more efficient patterns of working, new and transformed clinical roles, and increased productivity within a labour-intensive field. AI additionally has the potential to lead to new drug discoveries, safer medical care, earlier diagnosis, and improved

Y. Karmali (✉)
Medics.Academy, Kings College Hospital NHS Trust, London, UK
e-mail: yusuf.karmali@medics.academy; yusuf.karmali1@nhs.net

J. Malawana et al. (eds.), *Artificial Intelligence in Healthcare and Biomedical Visualization*, Biomedical Visualization 10, https://doi.org/10.1007/978-3-032-06520-9_10

health outcomes with populations living longer lives with fewer comorbidities. However, without a workforce ready to implement this technology effectively and safely, many of the promises of AI will never be realised. This chapter will examine the current state of the medical workforce before discussing how AI may disrupt the existing paradigm. It will then aim to discuss the need for adaptability, the role of interdisciplinary education, and strategies for integrating AI literacy into healthcare training.

10.2 The Current State of the Medical Workforce

The World Health Organisation (WHO) projected the global medical workforce shortage will be short of 18 million healthcare workers by 2030 (World Health Organization 2016). This was before the COVID-19 pandemic and so the number could be higher given treatment delays, longer waiting lists, and unmet health demand generated by the pandemic. A different study using data from 2019 posited an even higher number—suggesting we are currently 6.4 million doctors, 30.6 million nurses, 3.3 million dentists, and 2.9 million pharmacists short of meeting the standard of universal healthcare across the globe (Collaborators 2022). Whilst this shortage is more acute in lower-income and middle-income countries (LMICs), economically developed countries are also affected. The Association of American Medical Colleges (AAMC) has projected that the United States of America (US) could be short of up to 86,000 doctors by 2036 (Dall et al. 2024). The United Kingdom is projected to be short of up to 250,000 healthcare staff by 2030 (The King's Fund 2018). The NHS in England (NHSE) has recently released its workforce plan to address this, but a breakdown of the funding shows that this could be incredibly difficult to achieve given fiscal constraints. Indeed, the implications of the workforce plan would imply 1 in 11 people in the UK would be employed by the NHS.

Currently doctors must complete a primary medical qualification and be on a medical register to practice medicine. Different countries have varying practices, for example in the United States of America (USA), a primary medical qualification may only be obtained as a postgraduate degree, while in the United Kingdom (UK), a medical degree may be obtained through either a five-year undergraduate degree or a shorter four-year postgraduate degree (The BMA 2024). In the UK the minimum standards expected for doctors graduating from medical school are outlined by the General Medical Council (GMC)'s 'Outcome for Graduates' document (General Medical Council 2020). They are employed by healthcare providers (hospitals, GP practices, etc.) and typically undergo training programmes that are designed within its 'Generic Competency Framework' (General Medical Council 2017). In the UK, training a consultant (i.e. specialist) is estimated to cost more than £500,000 while training a general practitioner (family physician) is thought to cost almost £400,000 (Anderson et al. 2021).

Doctors are not the sole healthcare providers for patients, they work as part of a multidisciplinary team with other healthcare professionals, including nurses, pharmacists, paramedics, occupational therapists, physiotherapists, speech and language therapists, and healthcare assistants to name just a few. As evidenced by the WHO workforce report, across the globe, staff shortages are present in all these fields, leading to stretched healthcare services (World Health Organization 2016). The impact of the workforce crisis is an unmet demand for healthcare across the globe. In LMICs, it has been estimated that 8.6 million deaths could be averted with adequate investment in healthcare coverage and healthcare systems (Kruk et al. 2018). To meet this unmet demand in healthcare, two possible strategies could be employed—increase the number of healthcare workers or make existing healthcare workers more productive. AI has the potential to increase the productivity of existing healthcare workers, while also making it more cost-effective to train future healthcare workers.

10.3 Staff Burnout

An underappreciated concern amongst the medical workforce is physician burnout. Estimates of physician burnout vary greatly depending on the study, ranging from 0% to 80% (Rotenstein et al. 2018). A study in the USA found that 46% of physicians reported at least one symptom of burnout, and also revealed that doctors were more likely to be burnt out than the local US population (Shanafelt et al. 2012). Recent longitudinal studies suggest that the prevalence of physician burnout is increasing (Ortega et al. 2023). It is currently unclear of the long-term effect of the COVID-19 pandemic on burnout, as this is a relatively recent phenomenon, however, current evidence suggests that in the short term, the pandemic worsened burnout (Martin et al. 2023). Physician burnout imposes significant costs on clinicians, patients, and healthcare systems. A meta-analysis of studies found an association between burnout and patient safety (Garcia et al. 2019). Burnout is associated with reduced staff productivity (Dewa et al. 2014b). Within the US, physician burnout is estimated to cost $4.6 billion a year, demonstrating a significant cost to healthcare systems (Han et al. 2019). Those who are burnt out are more likely to retire early or limit working hours, thereby reducing the number of full-time equivalent doctors to treat patients (Dewa et al. 2014a). Additionally, longitudinal studies have demonstrated an increase in staff turnover for primary care physicians suffering from burnout (Willard-Grace et al. 2019).

Several factors have been identified to cause physician burnout. Cognitive load theory provides one explanation. As patients become increasingly complex, with multiple morbidities, physicians' *intrinsic load* (i.e. inherent complexity of the task) has increased. However, *extraneous load,* i.e. the way in which information is presented, has also increased over time. When data is presented in an incoherent, disorganised format, physicians utilise additional working memory to complete a task, increasing their overall cognitive load. Seventy percent of clinicians said in a survey using electronic healthcare records (EHR) added stress to their working lives. Indeed, this was found to be an independent predictor of burnout amongst clinicians (Gardner et al. 2018). In addition to cognitive load theory, physicians also cite long working hours, excessive bureaucracy, insufficient pay, working conditions, and a loss of clinical autonomy as reasons for burnout (Yates 2020).

The overall picture of the healthcare workforce is an understaffed, stretched, and burnt-out. This culminates in increased risk of mistakes, worsening healthcare outcomes for patients, and increased stress on healthcare systems. If we are to meet the challenges of universal healthcare, to improve healthcare within both developed countries and LMICs, then a radical change is needed.

10.4 The Need for Adaptation

AI has the potential to transform the way we practice medicine. It is already better at carrying out tasks in several clinical settings. These wide-ranging activities include triaging, diagnostic imaging, and dermatological examination, to name a few (Weidman et al. 2025; Salinas et al. 2024). It is likely to soon be used in treatment planning, and perhaps may provide the key to unlocking the holy grail of medicine: personalised treatments. AI has potential applications in virtually every specialty. Within pathology, there is evidence that computer vision algorithms can diagnose histological slides more accurately than human pathologists in a variety of tumour types. In 2021, the Food and Drug Administration in the US (FDA) licensed Paige Prostate, an AI software, to detect prostate cancer (Shafi and Parwani 2023). It works by applying its machine learning algorithm on histopathology slides to identify the most likely area of malignancy on this slide, allowing the pathologist to assess this area more quickly, therefore improving productivity. Computer vision extends to radiology, whereby there is ample evidence that it is effective in reading scans across a multitude of imaging modalities (Najjar 2023). The power that visualization technologies possess extends to cardiology, whereby there is now evidence that AI can improve diagnosis within 2-D echocardiographic images (Alsharqi et al. 2018). A big promise is the speed at which AI can interpret echocardiographic images, which is particularly important in patients with acute cardiac pathologies (such as acute coronary syndromes or acute heart failure) where prompt management is important to preserve myocardial function.

Computer vision is not the only way AI may revolutionise medicine. Genetic testing, while significantly cheaper than before, remains an expensive test to do. AI can help prioritise the specific genes to test by feeding phenotypic information into deep neural networks (Hsieh et al. 2019). Endoscopy performed by gastroenterologists can be augmented by computer-aided diagnosis, by assisting in the optimal site for biopsy of conditions like Barrett's Oesophagus (de Groof et al. 2020). Not only can AI improve diagnostics, but it can also improve treatment planning for patients in a variety of fields. Machine learning models can help predict the likelihood of cirrhotic patients developing hepatocellular carcinoma (HCC). It can also predict the likelihood of patients with HCC's response to trans-arterial chemoembolization (TACE) (Kröner et al. 2021). Additionally, there is evidence that AI can improve donor-recipient matching in patients requiring liver transplants, albeit more work is required to validate these models (Ayllón et al. 2018). Multimodal machine learning has been used to combine multiple datasets (genetic biomarkers, biochemical markers, imaging characteristics, and clinical features) to classify which patients should have operative management vs conservative management for patients with pancreatic cysts (Springer et al. 2019). Within radiation oncology, there is emerging evidence that deep neural networks may be able to support treatment planning, although this work is still very early (Jarrett et al. 2019).

AI can help improve non-clinical tasks that clinicians do, too. Indeed, the American College of Physicians (ACP) has recognised the negative consequences of excessive administrative tasks and is keen to liberate clinicians from such tasks (Erickson et al. 2017). AI has the potential to reduce cognitive load on clinicians by reducing extraneous load. For example, it can rapidly gather and organise data, such as a patient's blood tests or physiological parameters, and bring this in a ready-to-read format for the clinician to enact (Gandhi et al. 2023). Additionally, improvements within natural language processing (NLP) mean digital scribes can reduce the clerical burden clinicians face when encountering a patient (Quiroz et al. 2019). There is some evidence that the use of digital scribes in real-world practice reduces the time that clinicians spend on EHRs (Rotenstein et al. 2024). A small study has also suggested that use of virtual scribes may be associated with improvement in physician burnout, although it should be noted that half of the clinicians in this study discontinued scribe use (Stephens et al. 2022). Large language models (LLMs) such as ChatGPT from OpenAI, Gemini (previously Bard) from Google, and Claude by Anthropic have only recently gained mass market traction. LLMs are a form of generative AI that produces original text. They function by examining extensive text datasets to predict and produce language patterns for a range of tasks. One study demonstrated using written patient vignettes that ChatGPT may perform as well, or better, than doctors at writing discharge summaries, demonstrating the proof-of-concept that LLMs may be used within clinical workflows (Clough et al. 2024). Additionally, LLMs can transform patient discharge summaries to make them more patient-friendly (Zaretsky et al. 2024). An AI specifically trained within a medical context may perform better than ChatGPT at these tasks, although it should be noted that a large portion of healthcare information exists outside of electronic medical records, and some human oversight is likely to be needed (Ando et al. 2022).

Away from specific tasks, there is increasing evidence that AI can outperform doctors and medical students on written examinations. ChatGPT (GPT4) can pass the USMLE and can provide clinical reasoning as to why it has selected its preferred answer, as well as an explanation as to why other answers are incorrect (Shieh et al. 2024). This is not just limited to American exams, but also extends to Italian residency exams (Scaioli et al. 2023) and the UK's Membership of the Royal College of Physicians (MRCP) written exams (Maitland et al. 2024). The results suggest that LLMs may be able to contribute as a clinical decision aid in some circumstances. The most recent release of ChatGPT, GPT4o, is multimodal, meaning it has visual intelligence in addition to its text-based intelligence. This, accompanied by its natural language capabilities, expands the possible use of the technology. At the time of writing this, GPT4o has only just been rolled out, but one could imagine a multimodal AI with training on medical signs (say, images of dermatological lesions), with an LLM incorporated into it. It could ask a patient about their symptoms, examine their skin through its computer vision, before giving a recommended set of investigations or differential diagnosis. This promises to be a powerful technology in addition to the narrower AIs that were previously described.

Only a few use-cases from the literature have been described above, but it is evident that AI will transform many of the tasks that clinicians undertake, and in the future may be able to deliver medical consultations. Doctors should be aware that if AI were to practice like an autonomous physician, it would only need to be as good as the *worst* doctor on the medical register of a particular country to have a licence to practice. To be considered *average,* it would only need to be performing at the level of the median physician. Given the pace at which AI is developing, it is likely that it will outperform the *best* doctors in certain tasks within their respective fields soon (Masters 2019). The question that beckons then is at what point do we harness the power of AI and begin its deployment, and how do we implement this technology in a safe and effective manner. AI promises to transform the doctor-patient relationship; indeed, it may even supplant the doctor within this relationship, causing redundancies across the sector. How can clinicians adapt to this new world, whereby they are no longer the all-knowing gods of the patient–doctor relationship? Where do humans need to hone their skills?

In the past, when new technologies emerged, clinicians have adapted and changed their practice. Indeed, technology has fundamentally transformed several specialties over the last few decades. The advent of computed tomography and ultrasonography led to the development of a whole new specialty: radiology. Radiology itself has innovated to include procedural skills in the relatively new field of interventional radiology (Murphy and Soares 2005). The genome revolution has transformed the role clinical geneticists play, from being clinicians able to spot a rare disease by looking at someone, to now applying genome-wide testing to accurately diagnose and treat patients (Tromans and Barwell 2022). Radiotherapy techniques have improved over time to allow oncologists to offer Gamma Knife Radiosurgery (Monaco et al. 2012). Surgeons have begun to employ robotics in clinical practice in a variety of different operations ranging from endometriosis to nephrectomies (Morrell et al. 2021). Exciting developments within immunotherapy have allowed haematologists to expand their arsenal of treatment options for patients with blood cancers (Noh et al. 2020). The role of cardiology was transformed with the advent of the biomechanical stent, allowing percutaneous coronary intervention to become the mainstay of treatment for patients with ischaemic heart disease, one of the biggest causes of mortality globally (Scafa Udrişte et al. 2021).

The central reason these technologies gained traction is that they *empowered* clinicians to deliver more comprehensive care and expand the scope of what they could offer patients, leading to better health outcomes. Whilst clinicians were in the driving seat of these technologies, we successfully translated these technologies into clinical practice. Training programmes had to be changed, new specialties were developed, and effective stakeholder engagement meant the successful rollout of these new technologies. AI promises to augment clinicians too, whether it be optimising a treatment for a patient or suggesting areas to biopsy. However, in contrast to previous technological developments, it is fundamentally different from previous technologies because it has the potential to challenge physician autonomy.

The doctor-patient relationship is a thousand-year-old relationship that has been at the heart of clinical practice and has evolved over time from a paternalistic model to a shared decision-making model (Kaba and Sooriakumaran 2007). The development of the internet and digital health tools has changed the nature of the relationship already, giving patients further information and more autonomy. The prospect of artificial intelligence inserting itself into clinical practice could profoundly further change this relationship. A patient may be able to put their symptoms into an LLM and get a probable diagnosis to take to the clinician, further empowering patients within the shared decision-making model that already exists. Conversely, clinicians using AI may struggle to explain how AI operates in a black box, and we do not understand how it makes decisions. This explainability is core to the patient–doctor relationship. Will patients be willing to trust a computer for the choice of a cytotoxic medication with potentially lethal effects, if it cannot explain why a particular course of treatment is beneficial? Will physicians be happy to take an AI's recommendation if the physician remains liable for the choices it makes?

Scipion et al. undertook a scoping review to identify barriers to clinicians using AI (Scipion et al. 2025). Key barriers they identified include performance concerns about AI accuracy and reliability, effort-related challenges with integrating AI into specific workflows, and inadequate training and technical support. Beyond these technical factors, clinicians experience hesitancy driven by fears of job displacement in primary care and loss of clinical autonomy. Other barriers include legal and ethical concerns ranging from patient safety and misdiagnosis to data privacy issues to liability uncertainties. Clinicians are worried about AI potentially undermining patient-clinician interactions or reducing trust in decisions if they are made by AI. Additional barriers include questions about AI conclusiveness and evidence-based reliability, and limited clinician involvement in AI development and implementation processes. These barriers are context-dependent, with their impact varying significantly across primary, secondary, and tertiary care settings (Scipion et al. 2025).

To ensure effective diffusion of AI technologies across healthcare systems, doctors and other clinicians will need to understand how AI may impact their clinical workflows. Additionally, doctors will need to understand how the technology works, its pitfalls, practical and ethical implications of AI within the context of healthcare.

10.5 Integrating Artificial Intelligence into the Medical Curriculum

In the UK, the GMC's Outcomes for Graduates demonstrates no significant specific mention of AI. Within the US, there is no formal testing of AI in healthcare within the US Medical Licensing Exam (USMLE 2025). The UK is soon to pilot its equivalent—the UK medical licensing assessment (UKMLA)—and again, there is no formal examination of AI within its curriculum. There are currently few plans from medical schools on integrating AI literacy into the curriculum (Grunhut et al. 2021). Despite this, students are aware that AI is an important thing to learn about and are keen to learn more about its applications within healthcare (Sit et al. 2020). This phenomenon is not just found in UK medical students but has been replicated in surveys in Australia (Stewart et al. 2023) and Saudi Arabia (Alwadani et al. 2024). Post-graduate doctors in the UK appear to be optimistic about the use of AI, feeling that it will lead to reduced workload and improve their training. However, they are concerned by the lack of formal AI training within their current curricula and would support additional development of AI in their education (Banerjee et al. 2021). A systematic review with an associated cross-sectional survey completed in 2022 found that a plurality of physicians across the globe, in multiple different disciplines (dermatology, pathology, radiology, psychiatry, general practice, gastroenterology) are positive about the ascent of AI within their respective fields (Chen et al. 2022). Clinicians expect AI to release them from mundane aspects of the job, allowing them to spend more time with their patients and deploy their expert knowledge. Chen et. Al.'s subsequent survey of 758 medical students and physicians found that more than three-quarters of clinicians would be keen to use AI. This review also found that there is a lack of AI knowledge amongst clinicians, which must be rectified if we are to ensure safe and effective implementation (Chen et al. 2022). Lastly, there is evidence that medical students are keen to learn about topics allied to AI, such as clinical informatics; however, they often do not know where or how to pursue learning such subjects or careers within these fields (Banerjee et al. 2015).

To begin to rectify the current lack of AI literacy amongst clinicians, and subsequently improve the safe deployment of AI, educational institutions must look to incorporate AI literacy into both the undergraduate and postgraduate curricula. Rather than simply being the end-user of this powerful technology, clinicians must engage with their role as a core stakeholder and engage with AI to ensure it is appropriately embedded in clinical workflows, while ensuring the technology meets the high standards clinicians would expect. When adopting new technologies, clinicians have traditionally not needed to build them personally, but they must grasp the core principles of how these technologies function, their advantages and risks, and the methods for safe implementation in clinical practice. For example, a radiologist needs to know how a CT scanner works, the scientific principles underlying the technology, and understand when they are useful and not. Additionally, they must appreciate the risks and benefits of this technology and understand when it would be more appropriate to use a different imaging. They must also be able to interpret the output of the images created by the scanner. However, it is not expected that radiologists know how to build or develop CT scanners from scratch. The same principle could be applied to clinical decision aids, which are widely used in clinical practice. Doctors regularly use a variety of scoring tools, such as the Glasgow-Blatchford score, to predict the need for medical intervention in upper gastrointestinal bleeding (Laursen et al. 2012). Clinicians need to be able to apply this tool, know its components and the data surrounding its implementation, and ensure that they can appreciate the pitfalls of clinical scoring tools. However, they do not necessarily need to know how to make a clinical scoring tool to deliver care to patients. Similarly, doctors do not necessarily need technical AI skills—i.e. they do not need to know how to code or build AI models. However, to successfully implement AI into clinical practice, clinicians must have a fundamental understanding of how it works, its advantages and disadvantages, and when these tools are useful in clinical practice.

Accrediting medical bodies have yet to develop a framework for integrating artificial intelligence in the medical curriculum. Liaw et al. have proposed six competency domains clinicians require to successfully implement AI into their clinical practice: foundational knowledge, critical appraisal, medical decision making, technical use, patient communication, and having an awareness of unintended consequences (Liaw et al. 2022). Russell et al. have proposed a similar set of competencies and subcompetencies following interviews with subject matter experts (Russell et al. 2023). They reiterated the need for foundational knowledge and identified the need for clinicians to be aware of the social and ethical implications of AI. Again, successfully using AI to enhance clinical encounters is featured, as does being able to evaluate the evidence base for AI interventions. Clinicians should be expected to understand how AI will change specific workflows within the wider healthcare team. Underpinning the Russell et al. framework is having an awareness of practice-based learning and improvement using AI-based tools.

10.5.1 Foundational Knowledge

During the preclinical phase of medical education, dedicated time should be allocated to essential aspects of health informatics and AI. The foundation of AI and ML is data; clinicians must therefore be trained to understand mathematical and statistical principles relevant to AI. Important mathematical principles related to AI, such as linear algebra and calculus, could become mandatory prior to admission to medical school. In the USA, students sit the medical college admission test (MCAT), while many prospective applicants in the UK, New Zealand, and Australia sit the Universities Clinical Aptitude Test (UCAT), prior to admission to medical school. Incorporating algebra and statistics into these admission tests could help select prospective clinicians who would excel at some of the foundational knowledge required for AI. Because AI works by making probabilistic outcomes based on a dataset, clinicians need to understand the contributions data science and clinical informatics have made in developing AI-healthcare products. Once in medical school, clinicians will need to develop knowledge of data structures, big data, and understanding how this applies to healthcare. Students will need to learn about building and curating quality datasets that may be used within AI and learn techniques related to data cleaning and visualisation (Paranjape et al. 2019).

After building on a solid foundation related to data science, clinicians must be able to at least define basic terms within the field and have an appreciation of the different types of AI that currently exist. In particular, clinicians should familiarise themselves with the commonest types of machine learning algorithms that apply to healthcare, including supervised learning, unsupervised learning, deep learning, and reinforcement learning (Bajwa et al. 2021). Additional areas of machine learning that clinicians must be aware of include NLP and LLMs that have been popularised with the advent of ChatGPT by OpenAI and will undoubtedly have an impact on healthcare (Thirunavukarasu et al. 2023). The goal for foundational knowledge should be for clinicians and healthcare workers to gain literacy within AI rather than proficiency (Kolachalama and Garg 2018). AI is a rapidly developing field, and it is likely that new machine learning techniques will be discovered in the future. Students grounded with foundational knowledge related to AI will be better placed to navigate the inevitable changes that will come (Paranjape et al. 2019). Additionally, with an understanding of the core principles of AI, clinicians will then be able to envision the types of tasks that are suitable for AI. This should empower innovative clinicians to envision and implement novel applications of the technology, tailoring it to their specific clinical needs and contexts.

There have been successful pilots demonstrating that students can gain some confidence in understanding the basics of AI. One pilot demonstrated that with just 10 h of study, students applying a machine learning algorithm to detect breast cancer felt more confident with the principles of ML (Fan et al. 2020). A number of academic institutions like Stanford University and Duke University are building programmes related to AI in Healthcare, but this is not yet widespread amongst educational institutions (Paranjape et al. 2019).

10.5.2 Critical Appraisal

A core part of the medical curriculum is being able to critically appraise medical literature to ensure that a truly evidence-based approach translates into practising clinical medicine. These critical appraisal skills need to be adapted when interpreting papers related to AI (Faes et al. 2020). Applying critical appraisal skills to AI and ML enables readers to assess the reliability of study findings and determine their generalisability, reproducibility, and clinical relevance. Given AI commonly operates in a 'black box', it is imperative that clinicians can evaluate clinical studies, appreciate patient outcomes, and ensure it is clear when it is appropriate to deploy an AI tool. Some of the key questions relating to critical appraisal include evaluating the model developed and examining the ML methodology the authors may have used. For example, a key question that clinicians must ask when appraising an AI paper is the use of data when used to train the model in question. Were the training data, test data, and validation data all separate? Without understanding some of the fundamentals of AI, it will be hard for non-experts to effectively appraise AI papers. Faes et al. have produced a good guide for clinicians seeking to appraise ML models (Faes et al. 2020).

Workshops and seminars should equip medical students with the ability to critically appraise ML models. However, to practically deliver critical appraisal skills, a part of coursework within medical school curricula could be to write a critical appraisal on a selected ML paper. Journal clubs across hospitals should be encouraged to foster a learning of culture amongst healthcare clinicians.

10.5.3 Ethical, Legal, and Regulatory Implications

Currently, medical students are expected to learn about medical ethics. Clinicians should be aware of the basic principles of autonomy, justice, beneficence, and non-malfeasance that inform everyday clinical practice. These ethical concepts are then built upon so that clinicians can understand legal frameworks that apply to healthcare (e.g. the Mental Capacity Act 2005 in the UK). Clinical practice becomes difficult without understanding the ethical, legal, and regulatory context in which doctors are allowed and licensed to practice medicine. AI currently poses several significant ethical and societal challenges. First, AI systems often function as 'black boxes', meaning their decision-making processes are opaque and difficult for operators to interpret or explain. This lack of transparency poses challenges in understanding precisely how an AI arrives at its outputs or recommendations. Bias is another significant concern related to AI. Developing unrepresentative samples could mean AI products are only effective on select groups. If not actively countered, baking in real-world bias into algorithms will lead to widening health disparities, undermining trust in healthcare institutions, and worsening health outcomes for select populations. There are additional significant concerns related to data security, privacy, and accountability with this emerging technology (Tang et al. 2023).

Clinicians using AI-enhanced products must understand the ethical implications and potential drawbacks of using AI. Ethics seminars should be built upon to include these newer concerns related to AI in clinical practice. While much regulation related to AI is evolving, the FDA has begun to approve some AI tools. Clinicians must understand the way in which they may become liable for decisions made by an AI.

10.5.4 Clinical Practice

After understanding the appropriate context to use AI, and appreciating the advantages and disadvantages of AI products, clinicians must obtain technical literacy. Many clinicians find EHR to be troublesome and an independent cause of burnout, but AI will likely operate through a digital interface, perhaps through an EHR. Therefore, some basic training in digital health may equip clinicians with key skills, reduce burnout, and increase productivity (Wald et al. 2014). Obtaining basic digital health literacy will help with the transition to AI literacy.

When it comes to specific AI products, much of the technical information should sit with the developers of these products. Nonetheless, becoming AI-literate will help with the facilitation of implementing these new technologies (Liaw et al. 2022). Clinicians must understand how to use the specific product. Throughout the clinical years of medical school, while students are applying their pre-clinical knowledge, they should also seek to learn about case studies of practical AI examples in the field. They should aim to try out using these tools to gain some experience in using an AI tool to deliver healthcare.

It is inevitable AI will make mistakes, and clinicians need to be able to detect when these occur. Clinicians must be aware of the principle of automation bias, i.e. a tendency to over-reliance on automation. Ensuring doctors do not succumb to this is particularly important in a world where increasing time pressures are adding to clinical workloads (Khera et al. 2023). Ways to counter automation bias in existing decision support systems relate to their design and implementation (Goddard et al. 2012). If clinicians can understand the reasons why a decision support system has made its recommendation, they are more likely to use a tool appropriately. This is naturally harder with AI systems that operate in a black box, but some of the work pertaining to explainable AI may ease this in the future. Additionally, ensuring clinicians remain accountable for their decisions may also reduce automation bias, although the evidence for this is mixed. Training clinicians in the pitfalls of a specific decision support system has also been shown to reduce complacency bias (Goddard et al. 2012).

10.5.5 Building Clinical AI Leaders

While all doctors need to know about how AI will impact healthcare and be equipped to navigate this change, some will undoubtedly be interested in developing these skills further. This represents an opportunity to develop leaders within AI in healthcare. This is important to facilitate interdisciplinary learning, bridging the gap between medicine and computer science. Developing healthcare leaders with technical AI skills, who are grounded in clinical principles, and understand the patient–doctor interface would be an invaluable asset to the institutions tasked with steering the future of healthcare. Select medical students should be offered the combined courses with academic exposure, such as MB/PhDs, with the PhD component in artificial intelligence in healthcare, to allow them to get to grips with some of the technical skills related to AI. Those interested in ensuring effective implementation of AI could pursue MD/MBAs (Kolachalama and Garg 2018). Away from formal degrees, a wider range of short courses would allow those with an interest in AI to further develop their skills with micro-accreditation. All specialty programmes should provide continuing professional development (CPD) or continuing medical education (CME) credits for learning about specialty-specific applications of AI. For doctors in the post-graduate phase, the development of residency programmes and fellowships with these specific interests could be of benefit.

The NHS has undertaken early work to introduce posts for those with an interest in AI. It has begun implementing recommendations from the Topol review, a review aimed at equipping the healthcare workforce for the digital future (Topol 2019). The wide-ranging review recommended Guys and St Thomas NHS Foundation Trust (GSTT) to develop a year-long fellowship in Clinical Artificial Intelligence. It has developed a curriculum to accompany its fellowship (Deng et al. 2024). Healthcare providers should seek to develop posts like this, to help develop a generation of doctors who have the practical ability to develop and produce AI products (Fig. 10.1).

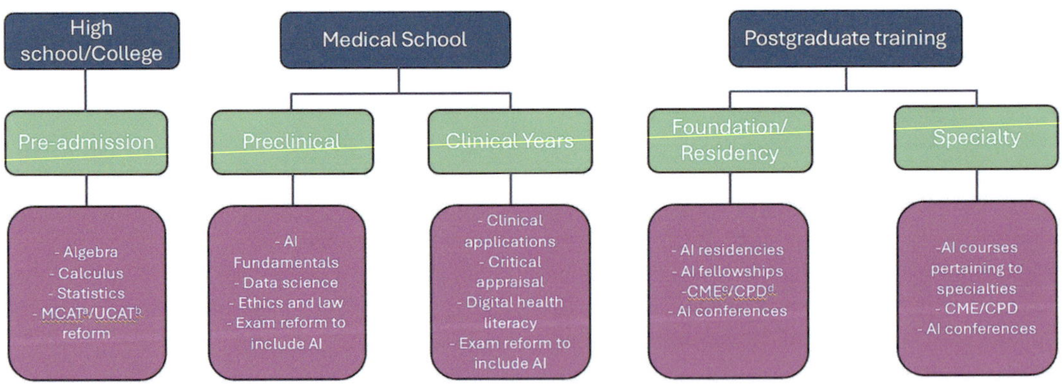

Fig. 10.1 A schematic diagram illustrating where components of an AI curriculum would fit across different aspects of medical training[a]MCAT Medical College Admission Test[b]UCAT University Clinical Aptitude Test[c]CME Continuing medical education[d]CPD Continuing professional development

10.6 Challenges to Implementing AI with the Medical Curriculum

There are several challenges to implementing AI within the medical curriculum. Firstly, AI does not appear within medical licensing exams (such as the USMLE or UKMLA). Much of medical school education is aimed at ensuring students can pass this as well as achieve core competencies as outlined by accrediting bodies (e.g. outcomes for graduates by the GMC/entrustable professional activities in the USA). While academics have made some propositions for a framework to pursue AI literacy, these have yet to gain traction with those who set medical curricula. This makes it hard for educational providers to determine the required depth or breadth for medical students in AI literacy. Medical school is already a lengthy endeavour with limited time available for these additional competencies to be obtained. Some studies cite faculty resistance to change as another barrier (Russell et al. 2023). Additionally, it is likely that the medical faculty does not currently have the expertise to deliver such a profound curriculum change. Medical schools must broaden their faculty to include data scientists and AI experts to deliver sessions related to AI.

To address some of these challenges, key stakeholders must recognise the need to integrate AI within the healthcare curriculum. Indeed, some bodies are starting to do this. The Canadian Association of Radiologists (CAR) has released a white paper on AI in Radiology (Tang et al. 2018). CAR advocates integrating clinical informatics, computer science, and statistics courses within residency programmes in radiology. Other training organisations, such as the Royal College of Physicians (RCP) in London, or the Royal College of General Practitioners (RCGP), are responsible for governing post-graduate training programmes within their respective specialties. However, there have been no reports on how they envision the future of training to integrate AI literacy. Additionally, regulators like the GMC in the UK and AMA have yet to produce their own frameworks for understanding how AI should fit within the medical curriculum. Programmes like those built by smaller organisations like the GSTT Clinical AI Fellowship need to be studied and replicated with a view to scale across the country.

10.7 Artificial Intelligence and Medical Education

While a core function of AI will be the improved productivity and clinical performance of the existing workforce, AI, in combination with other technologies, may be used to help scale medical education, increasing the number of doctors produced. Given the current projected shortfall of healthcare workers, we need to think of ways to rapidly and efficiently scale medical education. If we are to scale medical education across the world, new medical schools must be built, and this requires significant capital, labour, and infrastructure. AI may be able to play a role in selecting students for medical school. Large language models (LLMs), like GPT-4 from OpenAI, Claude from Anthropic, and Gemini from Google have the potential to transform medical education (Abd-Alrazaq et al. 2023). LLMs could speed up the deployment of medical schools by improving the speed and reducing the cost at which new medical schools develop their own curricula. They could help lecturers develop lesson plans, generate new learning materials, and provide marking rubrics.

An essential benefit of AI is its ability to personalise desired products or outcomes to a specific individual's needs. In the context of medical education, LLMs have the potential to create personalised study plans for learners. It is not hard to imagine an LLM built to test an individual's knowledge and then provide detailed explanations until the learner is able to understand, before providing additional new questions in areas the student struggled. LLMs can create personalised learning materials and build up a learner's knowledge base focussing on areas of weakness of learners. Geeky Medics, a medical-education company based in the UK, has been using ChatGPT to simulate OSCE stations for its members (Geeky Medics 2024). The chatbot can voice different histories to the practicing student. Additionally, it can then quiz you on your differential diagnosis and perform viva questions to help test one's knowledge. This technology would be hugely beneficial for disparate communities that struggle to meet up for OSCE practice. Additionally, LLMs could draw on its natural language processing and clinical reasoning to engage in Socratic questioning with learners (Thirunavukarasu et al. 2023).

LLMs could also plausibly be used within the assessment of medical students and within postgraduate exams. A pre-trained LLM on 'optimal answers' and a marking rubric could provide marks for students and offer feedback, reducing the time educational staff spend marking work, and reducing costs. In time, dynamic exams, i.e. an exam that changes in difficulty as the student answers, could push students to find areas where they excel. In theory, LLMs could undertake viva voce in the future to ensure that students have deeper understanding of their topics than answering simple best answer questions which commonly become an exercise in pattern recognition. Current evidence suggests that LLMs are not at the standard of humans in assessment yet (Khademi 2023), but given the speed at which LLMs are being deployed and progressing, it is possible to see the potential use case.

Much of the usual caveats when discussing AI apply to its use in medical education. Because LLMs produce a probabilistic answer based on the input, they quite often lack expert knowledge and when pushed on topics they may 'hallucinate'. This means they make up answers that are not true. Relying on LLMs to educate future doctors without necessary safeguards and persistent review of the models could lead to students learning false or incorrect information. Widespread use of AI within academia may lead to its potential abuse by students. Students could use LLMs to write academic papers or reflective pieces rather than creating their own original work. By encouraging the use of LLMs for learning there is the possibility of academic dishonesty by students. For these reasons, robust educational studies must be designed to evaluate how we can effectively implement LLMs within medical education.

10.8 Recommendations for Future

To successfully implement workforce adaptation, institutions need to quickly move and begin to develop the necessary steps. The GMC, and equivalent organisations across the world should seek to build on existing work highlighted in this chapter. A consultation with medics, academics, computer scientists, data scientists, ethicists, and other subject matter experts should help regulatory bodies determine a framework that medical schools and other educational providers can use to deliver these programmes. Once developed, medical schools must work with science, technology, engineering, and mathematics (STEM) departments at their respective universities to recruit faculty who could build content to fit this educational framework. Close interdisciplinary collaboration between the STEM and medical departments will be required. If medical schools are struggling to find the necessary talent, then collaborating across universities and building shared content should be encouraged. With the advent of the internet era and the development of virtual teaching, this should be easier to facilitate. Exams must also change to reflect curricular transformation. The USMLE, UKMLA, and equivalent exams should have questions related to mathematics, data science, and AI. Additional assessments in the form of reflective essays, coursework, and practical projects related to AI could demonstrate competency with this new technology. Those governing training programmes should seek to collaborate with leaders in clinical AI, to build the postgraduate clinical training programmes. Employers must grant a degree of flexibility to motivated leaders who may choose to undertake a secondment for those who want to pursue opportunities within AI, while carefully balancing service provision. As mentioned, the NHS has good form in this, promoting less than full-time training (LTFT) and out of programme experiences (OOPEs).

Expanding these further could help greatly. Countries could learn from the NHS in this regard. Lastly, institutions from LMICs should seek to collaborate with leaders within these fields to begin scaling programmes in their respective countries.

Further research is also required on how we can use AI to deliver medical education itself. While there have been numerous pilots and innovative ideas outlined, there are limited robust educational studies to demonstrate its effectiveness in improving educational outcomes. Its impact on reducing administrative time within an educational setting has also not been explored.

10.9 Conclusion

Globally, we are short of healthcare workers, which has a significant negative impact on both economically developed and less economically developed countries. In addition to this, the current healthcare workforce is suffering significant burnout, causing adverse outcomes for patients, healthcare workers, and the systems in which they work. AI has the potential to both improve the productive capacity of healthcare workers through inventions like digital scribes, but also to augment and empower the way in which clinicians treat their patients. However, to truly recognise the promise AI has, we require significant changes to the undergraduate and postgraduate medical curriculum to equip the medical workforce with the appropriate skills. This chapter has drawn on previous work to reiterate the need for a novel framework that will equip clinicians with skills to effectively implement this potentially transformational technology. Accrediting bodies, such as the GMC in the UK, in association with health employers and specialist societies, need to work in tandem with doctors and computer scientists to begin integrating artificial intelligence into the medical curriculum. Interdisciplinary education is key. Lastly, while clinicians need to work with AI to improve healthcare outcomes, we can and should consider utilising artificial intelligence itself to enhance medical education.

References

Abd-Alrazaq A, Alsaad R, Alhuwail D, Ahmed A, Healy PM, Latifi S, Aziz S, Damseh R, Alabed Alrazak S, Sheikh J (2023) Large language models in medical education: opportunities, challenges, and future directions. JMIR Med Educ 9:e48291

Alsharqi M, Woodward WJ, Mumith JA, Markham DC, Upton R, Leeson P (2018) Artificial intelligence and echocardiography. Echo Res Pract 5:R115–r125

Alwadani FAS, Lone A, Hakami MT, Moria AH, Alamer W, Alghirash RA, Alnawah AK, Hadadi AS (2024) Attitude and understanding of artificial intelligence among Saudi medical students: an online cross-sectional study. J Multidiscip Healthc 17:1887–1899

Anderson M, O'neill C, Macleod Clark J, Street A, Woods M, Johnston-Webber C, Charlesworth A, Whyte M, Foster M, Majeed A, Pitchforth E, Mossialos E, Asaria M, Mcguire A (2021) Securing a sustainable and fit-for-purpose UK health and care workforce. Lancet 397:1992–2011

Ando K, Okumura T, Komachi M, Horiguchi H, Matsumoto Y (2022) Is artificial intelligence capable of generating hospital discharge summaries from inpatient records? PLoS Digit Health 1:e0000158

Ayllón MD, Ciria R, Cruz-Ramírez M, Pérez-Ortiz M, Gómez I, Valente R, O'grady J, De La Mata M, Hervás-Martínez C, Heaton ND, Briceño J (2018) Validation of artificial neural networks as a methodology for donor-recipient matching for liver transplantation. Liver Transpl 24:192–203

Bajwa J, Munir U, Nori A, Williams B (2021) Artificial intelligence in healthcare: transforming the practice of medicine. Future Healthc J 8:e188–e194

Banerjee R, George P, Priebe C, Alper E (2015) Medical student awareness of and interest in clinical informatics. J Am Med Inform Assoc 22:e42–e47

Banerjee M, Chiew D, Patel KT, Johns I, Chappell D, Linton N, Cole GD, Francis DP, Szram J, Ross J, Zaman S (2021) The impact of artificial intelligence on clinical education: perceptions of postgraduate trainee doctors in London (UK) and recommendations for trainers. BMC Med Educ 21:429

Chen M, Zhang B, Cai Z, Seery S, Gonzalez MJ, Ali NM, Ren R, Qiao Y, Xue P, Jiang Y (2022) Acceptance of clinical artificial intelligence among physicians and medical students: a systematic review with cross-sectional survey. Front Med (Lausanne) 9:990604

Clough RAJ, Sparkes WA, Clough OT, Sykes JT, Steventon AT, King K (2024) Transforming healthcare documentation: harnessing the potential of AI to generate discharge summaries. BJGP Open 8, BJGPO.2023.0116.

Dall T et al (2024) The complexities of physician supply and demand. The Association of American Medical Colleges. Available at: https://www.aamc.org/media/75236/download?attachment (Accessed: 05 August 2025)

De Groof AJ, Struyvenberg MR, Van Der Putten J, Van Der Sommen F, Fockens KN, Curvers WL, Zinger S, Pouw RE, Coron E, Baldaque-Silva F, Pech O, Weusten B, Meining A, Neuhaus H, Bisschops R, Dent J, Schoon EJ, De With PH, Bergman JJ (2020) Deep-learning system detects neoplasia in patients with barrett's esophagus with higher accuracy than endoscopists in a multistep training and validation study with benchmarking. Gastroenterology 158:915–929.e4

Deng A et al (2024) FCAI Clinical AI curriculum 3.2, NHS Fellowship in Clinical AI. Available at: https://gsttcsc.github.io/assets/docs/FCAI_Curriculum_v3.2.pdf. (Accessed: 05 August 2025)

Densen P (2011) Challenges and opportunities facing medical education. Trans Am Clin Climatol Assoc 122:48–58

Dewa CS, Jacobs P, Thanh NX, Loong D (2014a) An estimate of the cost of burnout on early retirement and reduction in clinical hours of practicing physicians in Canada. BMC Health Serv Res 14:254

Dewa CS, Loong D, Bonato S, Thanh NX, Jacobs P (2014b) How does burnout affect physician productivity? A systematic literature review. BMC Health Serv Res 14:325

Erickson SM, Rockwern B, Koltov M, Mclean RM (2017) Putting patients first by reducing administrative tasks in health care: a position paper of the American college of physicians. Ann Intern Med 166:659–661

Faes L, Liu X, Wagner SK, Fu DJ, Balaskas K, Sim DA, Bachmann LM, Keane PA, Denniston AK (2020) A clinician's guide to artificial intelligence: how to critically appraise machine learning studies. Transl Vis Sci Technol 9:7

Fan KY, Hu R, Singla R (2020) Introductory machine learning for medical students: a pilot. Med Educ 54:1042–1043

Gandhi TK, Classen D, Sinsky CA, Rhew DC, Vande Garde N, Roberts A, Federico F (2023) How can artificial intelligence decrease cognitive and work burden for front line practitioners? JAMIA Open 6

Garcia CL, Abreu LC, Ramos JLS, Castro CFD, Smiderle FRN, Santos JAD, Bezerra IMP (2019) Influence of burnout on patient safety: systematic review and meta-analysis. Medicina (Kaunas) 55

Gardner RL, Cooper E, Haskell J, Harris DA, Poplau S, Kroth PJ, Linzer M (2018) Physician stress and burnout: the impact of health information technology. J Am Med Inform Assoc 26:106–114

GBD 2019 Human Resources for Health Collaborators (2022) Measuring the availability of human resources for health and its relationship to universal health coverage for 204 countries and territories from 1990 to 2019: a systematic analysis for the Global Burden of Disease Study 2019. Lancet 399:2129–2154

Geeky Medics (2024) Virtual patients for OSCE preparation | AI patients | geeky medics, Prepare for OSCEs with our virtual patients. Available at: https://geekymedics.com/ai-simulated-patients-for-osce-preparation/ (Accessed: 06 October 2025)

General Medical Council (2020) Outcomes for graduates guidance – GMC, General Medical Council. Available at: https://www.gmc-uk.org/education/standards-guidance-and-curricula/standards-and-outcomes/outcomes-for-graduates/outcomes-for-graduates (Accessed: 05 August 2025)

General Medical Council (2017) Generic professional capabilities framework - the essential generic capabilities needed for safe, effective and high quality medical care in the UK - General Medical Council - General Professional Capabilities Framework. Available at: https://www.gmc-uk.org/education/standards-guidance-and-curricula/standards-and-outcomes/generic-professional-capabilities-framework (Accessed: 05 August 2025)

Goddard K, Roudsari A, Wyatt JC (2012) Automation bias: a systematic review of frequency, effect mediators, and mitigators. J Am Med Inform Assoc 19:121–127

Grunhut J, Wyatt AT, Marques O (2021) Educating future physicians in artificial intelligence (AI): an integrative review and proposed changes. J Med Educ Curric Dev 8:23821205211036836

Han S, Shanafelt TD, Sinsky CA, Awad KM, Dyrbye LN, Fiscus LC, Trockel M, Goh J (2019) Estimating the attributable cost of physician burnout in the United States. Ann Intern Med 170:784–790

Hsieh TC, Mensah MA, Pantel JT, Aguilar D, Bar O, Bayat A, Becerra-Solano L, Bentzen HB, Biskup S, Borisov O, Braaten O, Ciaccio C, Coutelier M, Cremer K, Danyel M, Daschkey S, Eden HD, Devriendt K, Wilson S, Douzgou S, Đukić D, Ehmke N, Fauth C, Fischer-Zirnsak B, Fleischer N, Gabriel H, Graul-Neumann L, Gripp KW, Gurovich Y, Gusina A, Haddad N, Hajjir N, Hanani Y, Hertzberg J, Hoertnagel K, Howell J, Ivanovski I, Kaindl A, Kamphans T, Kamphausen S, Karimov C, Kathom H, Keryan A, Knaus A, Köhler S, Kornak U, Lavrov A, Leitheiser M, Lyon GJ, Mangold E, Reina PM, Carrascal AM, Mitter D, Herrador LM, Nadav G, Nöthen M, Orrico A, Ott CE, Park K, Peterlin B, Pölsler L, Raas-Rothschild A, Randolph L, Revencu N, Fagerberg CR, Robinson PN, Rosnev S, Rudnik S, Rudolf G, Schatz U, Schossig A, Schubach M, Shanoon O, Sheridan E, Smirin-Yosef P, Spielmann M, Suk EK, Sznajer Y, Thiel CT, Thiel G, Verloes A, Vrecar I, Wahl D, Weber I, Winter K, Wiśniewska M, Wollnik B, Yeung MW, Zhao M, Zhu N, Zschocke J, Mundlos S, Horn D, Krawitz PM (2019) Pedia: prioritization of exome data by image analysis. Genet Med 21:2807–2814

Jarrett D, Stride E, Vallis K, Gooding MJ (2019) Applications and limitations of machine learning in radiation oncology. Br J Radiol 92:20190001

Kaba R, Sooriakumaran P (2007) The evolution of the doctor-patient relationship. Int J Surg 5:57–65

Khademi A (2023) Can ChatGPT and bard generate aligned assessment items? A reliability analysis against human performance. arXiv preprint arXiv:2304.05372.

Khera R, Simon MA, Ross JS (2023) Automation bias and assistive AI: risk of harm from AI-driven clinical decision support. JAMA 330:2255–2257

Kolachalama VB, Garg PS (2018) Machine learning and medical education. NPJ Digit Med 1:54

Kröner PT, Engels MM, Glicksberg BS, Johnson KW, Mzaik O, Van Hooft JE, Wallace MB, El-Serag HB, Krittanawong C (2021) Artificial intelligence in gastroenterology: a state-of-the-art review. World J Gastroenterol 27:6794–6824

Kruk ME, Gage AD, Joseph NT, Danaei G, García-Saisó S, Salomon JA (2018) Mortality due to low-quality health systems in the universal health coverage era: a systematic analysis of amenable deaths in 137 countries. Lancet 392:2203–2212

Laursen SB, Hansen JM, Schaffalitzky De Muckadell OB (2012) The Glasgow Blatchford score is the most accurate assessment of patients with upper gastrointestinal hemorrhage. Clin Gastroenterol Hepatol 10:1130–1135.e1

Liaw W, Kueper JK, Lin S, Bazemore A, Kakadiaris I (2022) Competencies for the use of artificial intelligence in primary care. Ann Fam Med 20:559–563

Maitland A, Fowkes R, Maitland S (2024) Can ChatGPT pass the MRCP (UK) written examinations? Analysis of performance and errors using a clinical decision-reasoning framework. BMJ Open 14:e080558

Makary MA, Daniel M (2016) Medical error—the third leading cause of death in the US. BMJ 353:i2139

Martin B, Kaminski-Ozturk N, O'hara C, Smiley R (2023) Examining the impact of the Covid-19 pandemic on burnout and stress among U.S. nurses. J Nurs Regul 14:4–12

Masters K (2019) Artificial intelligence in medical education. Med Teacher 41:976–980

Monaco EA, Grandhi R, Niranjan A, Lunsford LD (2012) The past, present and future of Gamma Knife radiosurgery for brain tumors: the Pittsburgh experience. Expert Rev Neurother 12:437–445

Morrell ALG, Morrell-Junior AC, Morrell AG, Mendes JMF, Tustumi F, Lg DE-O-E-S, Morrell A (2021) The history of robotic surgery and its evolution: when illusion becomes reality. Rev Col Bras Cir 48:e20202798

Murphy TP, Soares GM (2005) The evolution of interventional radiology. Semin Intervent Radiol 22:6–9

Najjar R (2023) Redefining radiology: a review of artificial intelligence integration in medical imaging. Diagnostics (Basel) 13

Noh JY, Seo H, Lee J, Jung H (2020) Immunotherapy in Hematologic Malignancies: Emerging Therapies and Novel Approaches. Int J Mol Sci 21

Ortega MV, Hidrue MK, Lehrhoff SR, Ellis DB, Sisodia RC, Curry WT, Del Carmen MG, Wasfy JH (2023) Patterns in physician burnout in a stable-linked cohort. JAMA Netw Open 6:e2336745

Paranjape K, Schinkel M, Nannan Panday R, Car J, Nanayakkara P (2019) Introducing artificial intelligence training in medical education. JMIR Med Educ 5:e16048

Quiroz JC, Laranjo L, Kocaballi AB, Berkovsky S, Rezazadegan D, Coiera E (2019) Challenges of developing a digital scribe to reduce clinical documentation burden. NPJ Digit Med 2:114

Rotenstein LS, Torre M, Ramos MA, Rosales RC, Guille C, Sen S, Mata DA (2018) Prevalence of burnout among physicians: a systematic review. JAMA 320:1131–1150

Rotenstein L, Melnick ER, Iannaccone C, Zhang J, Mugal A, Lipsitz SR, Healey MJ, Holland C, Snyder R, Sinsky CA, Ting D, Bates DW (2024) Virtual scribes and physician time spent on electronic health records. JAMA Netw Open 7:e2413140

Russell RG, Lovett Novak L, Patel M, Garvey KV, Craig KJT, Jackson GP, Moore D, Miller BM (2023) Competencies for the use of artificial intelligence-based tools by health care professionals. Acad Med 98:348–356

Salinas MP, Sepúlveda J, Hidalgo L, Peirano D, Morel M, Uribe P, Rotemberg V, Briones J, Mery D, Navarrete-Dechent C (2024) A systematic review and meta-analysis of artificial intelligence versus clinicians for skin cancer diagnosis. NPJ Digit Med 7(1):125

Scafa Udriște A, Niculescu AG, Grumezescu AM, Bădilă E (2021) Cardiovascular stents: a review of past, current, and emerging devices. Materials (Basel) 14

Scaioli G, Lo Moro G, Conrado F, Rosset L, Bert F, Siliquini R (2023) Exploring the potential of ChatGPT for clinical reasoning and decision-making: a cross-sectional study on the Italian Medical Residency Exam. Ann Ist Super Sanita 59:267–270

Scipion CEA, Manchester MA, Federman A, Wang Y, Arias JJ (2025) Barriers to and facilitators of clinician acceptance and use of artificial intelligence in healthcare settings: a scoping review. BMJ Open 15:e092624

Shafi S, Parwani AV (2023) Artificial intelligence in diagnostic pathology. Diagn Pathol 18:109

Shanafelt TD, Boone S, Tan L, Dyrbye LN, Sotile W, Satele D, West CP, Sloan J, Oreskovich MR (2012) Burnout and satisfaction with work-life balance among US physicians relative to the general US population. Arch Intern Med 172:1377–1385

Shieh A, Tran B, He G, Kumar M, Freed JA, Majety P (2024) Assessing ChatGPT 4.0's test performance and clinical diagnostic accuracy on USMLE STEP 2 CK and clinical case reports. Sci Rep 14:9330

Sit C, Srinivasan R, Amlani A, Muthuswamy K, Azam A, Monzon L, Poon DS (2020) Attitudes and perceptions of UK medical students towards artificial intelligence and radiology: a multicentre survey. Insights Imaging 11:14

Springer S, Masica DL, Dal Molin M, Douville C, Thoburn CJ, Afsari B, Li L, Cohen JD, Thompson E, Allen PJ, Klimstra DS, Schattner MA, Schmidt CM, Yip-Schneider M, Simpson RE, Fernandez-Del Castillo C,

Mino-Kenudson M, Brugge W, Brand RE, Singhi AD, Scarpa A, Lawlor R, Salvia R, Zamboni G, Hong SM, Hwang DW, Jang JY, Kwon W, Swan N, Geoghegan J, Falconi M, Crippa S, Doglioni C, Paulino J, Schulick RD, Edil BH, Park W, Yachida S, Hijioka S, Van Hooft J, He J, Weiss MJ, Burkhart R, Makary M, Canto MI, Goggins MG, Ptak J, Dobbyn L, Schaefer J, Sillman N, Popoli M, Klein AP, Tomasetti C, Karchin R, Papadopoulos N, Kinzler KW, Vogelstein B, Wolfgang CL, Hruban RH, Lennon AM (2019) A multimodality test to guide the management of patients with a pancreatic cyst. Sci Transl Med 11

Stephens J, Kieber-Emmons AM, Johnson M, Greenberg GM (2022) Implementation of a virtual asynchronous scribe program to reduce physician burnout. J Healthc Manag 67:425–435

Stewart J, Lu J, Gahungu N, Goudie A, Fegan PG, Bennamoun M, Sprivulis P, Dwivedi G (2023) Western Australian medical students' attitudes towards artificial intelligence in healthcare. PLoS One 18:e0290642

Topol E (2019) The Topol review: preparing the healthcare workforce to deliver the digital future. Available at https://topol.hee.nhs.uk/. (Accessed 10/05/2025)

Tromans E, Barwell J (2022) Clinical genetics: past, present and future. Eur J Hum Genet 30:991–992

The King's Fund (2018) The health care workforce in England: Make or break? | The Kings Fund. Available at: https://www.kingsfund.org.uk/insight-and-analysis/reports/health-care-workforce-england (Accessed: 05 May 2025)

The BMA (2024) Medical training pathway, The British Medical Association. Available at: https://www.bma.org.uk/advice-and-support/studying-medicine/becoming-a-doctor/medical-training-pathway#:~:text=for%20more%20information.-,The%20foundation%20programme%20%2D%20postgraduate%20medical%20training,Run%2Dthrough%20training%20programmes (Accessed: 05 August 2025)

Tang A, Tam R, Cadrin-Chênevert A, Guest W, Chong J, Barfett J, Chepelev L, Cairns R, Mitchell JR, Cicero MD, Poudrette MG, Jaremko JL, Reinhold C, Gallix B, Gray B, Geis R (2018) Canadian Association of Radiologists White Paper on artificial intelligence in radiology. Can Assoc Radiol J 69:120–135

Tang L, Li J, Fantus S (2023) Medical artificial intelligence ethics: a systematic review of empirical studies. Digit Health 9:20552076231186064

Thirunavukarasu AJ, Ting DSJ, Elangovan K, Gutierrez L, Tan TF, Ting DSW (2023) Large language models in medicine. Nat Med 29:1930–1940

Usmle (2025) USMLE® content outline, USMLE Content outline. Available at: https://www.usmle.org/sites/default/files/2022-01/USMLE_Content_Outline_0.pdf (Accessed: 05 August 2025)

Wald HS, George P, Reis SP, Taylor JS (2014) Electronic health record training in undergraduate medical education: bridging theory to practice with curricula for empowering patient- and relationship-centered care in the computerized setting. Acad Med 89:380–386

Weidman AC, Malakouti S, Salcido DD et al (2025) A machine learning trauma triage model for critical care transport. JAMA Netw Open 8(6):e259639. https://doi.org/10.1001/jamanetworkopen.2025.9639

Willard-Grace R, Knox M, Huang B, Hammer H, Kivlahan C, Grumbach K (2019) Burnout and health care workforce turnover. Ann Fam Med 17:36–41

World Health Organization (2016) Global strategy on human resources for health: workforce 2030

Yates SW (2020) Physician stress and burnout. Am J Med 133:160–164

Zaretsky J, Kim JM, Baskharoun S, Zhao Y, Austrian J, Aphinyanaphongs Y, Gupta R, Blecker SB, Feldman J (2024) Generative artificial intelligence to transform inpatient discharge summaries to patient-friendly language and format. JAMA Netw Open 7:e240357–e240357

Conclusion

Arian Arjomandi Rad and Robert Vardanyan

Reflections on the Journey Through AI in Healthcare

As we conclude this exploration into the transformative potential of Artificial Intelligence and biomedical visualization in healthcare, it is essential to reflect on the profound themes and insights that have emerged. This book has illuminated the remarkable ways in which AI has reshaped diagnostics, education, surgical training, and healthcare delivery. These advancements demonstrate AI's capacity to address long-standing challenges while unlocking unprecedented opportunities. From empowering underserved communities to reimagining the frontiers of space medicine, AI's applications span an extraordinary spectrum, underscoring its growing significance in shaping the future of medicine.

The journey through these pages reveals not only the technical advancements of AI but also the human narratives interwoven within this technological revolution. At its core, AI in healthcare is a narrative about solving critical problems—extending lives, reducing disparities, and equipping practitioners to meet the ever-evolving demands of their field. Yet, it is also a cautionary tale, reminding us of the ethical responsibilities and collaborative efforts required to ensure that technological progress aligns with humanistic values. This balance between innovation and ethics will define the next era of AI in medicine.

Key Takeaways and Implications

Addressing Complex Challenges

The global healthcare landscape faces a convergence of crises that demand innovative solutions. Workforce shortages, aging populations, and the exponential growth of medical data present unique challenges that traditional methods struggle to overcome. AI offers solutions that are not merely incremental but transformative. By automating routine tasks, enhancing diagnostic precision, and optimizing resource allocation, AI alleviates critical pain points across healthcare systems. These innovations are not confined to affluent nations; they have transformative potential in low- and middle-income countries, where resource scarcity often limits access to care.

Unlocking New Frontiers

AI's ability to analyze vast datasets and uncover actionable insights has revolutionized healthcare delivery in unexpected ways. For example, in regions with limited infrastructure, AI-driven telemedicine has provided new lifelines for patients who would otherwise remain unseen.

A. Arjomandi Rad
Department of Cardiothoracic Surgery, John Radcliffe Hospital, Oxford University Hospitals NHS Foundation Trust, Oxford, UK

R. Vardanyan
Department of Neurosurgery, John Radcliffe Hospital, Oxford University Hospitals NHS Foundation Trust, Oxford, UK

J. Malawana et al. (eds.), *Artificial Intelligence in Healthcare and Biomedical Visualization*, Biomedical Visualization 10, https://doi.org/10.1007/978-3-032-06520-9

Beyond Earth, in the domain of space medicine, AI has demonstrated its capacity to safeguard astronaut health and deliver solutions in remote and unforgiving environments. These advancements reinforce AI's role as a universal enabler of healthcare innovation, pushing the boundaries of what is achievable in both terrestrial and extraterrestrial settings.

The Ethical Imperative

While the promise of AI is vast, its implementation must be grounded in ethical principles. Algorithmic bias, data privacy, and the accountability of AI-driven decisions remain critical concerns that must be addressed. This book has underscored the importance of transparency, inclusivity, and equity in AI development, ensuring that these technologies benefit all segments of society without exacerbating existing disparities. It is only through responsible stewardship of AI that its full potential can be realized without compromising trust and fairness.

The Human Element

Despite its transformative potential, AI cannot replace the empathy, intuition, and moral judgment that healthcare professionals bring to their work. The integration of AI must complement, not substitute, the human touch that is so integral to patient care. As practitioners adopt AI-driven tools, they must also retain their commitment to the art of medicine, ensuring that technology enhances rather than diminishes the doctor-patient relationship. This interplay between human expertise and technological augmentation will remain central to the success of AI in healthcare.

A Vision for the Future

The future of healthcare is one where AI and biomedical visualization seamlessly integrate into every aspect of medical practice, research, and education. It is a future where technology and humanity coexist in harmony, driven by a shared commitment to improving health outcomes. To achieve this vision, stakeholders across disciplines must collaborate, innovating responsibly and ensuring that AI's benefits reach even the most marginalized populations.

Advancing Education and Research

AI's role in education and research cannot be overstated. By equipping future generations of clinicians with AI literacy and fostering interdisciplinary collaboration, we can prepare the healthcare workforce to navigate the complexities of an AI-driven ecosystem. Simultaneously, AI-powered research will continue to uncover groundbreaking discoveries, pushing the boundaries of what is possible in medicine. For example, machine learning models capable of predicting rare diseases from limited datasets are beginning to reshape diagnostic paradigms, offering hope where traditional approaches fall short.

AI-enhanced simulations and virtual reality training environments are also transforming medical education. Trainees now have access to lifelike scenarios that allow for iterative learning without risk to patients. These innovations ensure that clinicians are better prepared to deliver high-quality care in an increasingly complex medical landscape.

Bridging Gaps and Expanding Access

From telemedicine to remote monitoring, AI has already begun to dismantle geographical and logistical barriers to care. These technologies have enabled underserved regions to access diagnostic tools and specialist expertise, leveling the playing field for patients worldwide. As these technologies mature, they hold the potential to democratize healthcare access, ensuring that quality care is no longer a privilege but a universal right. Expanding access to AI-driven solutions will require sustained investment, regulatory support, and a commitment to addressing disparities at their root.

Promoting Collaboration Across Disciplines

The successful integration of AI into healthcare will depend on collaboration among technologists, clinicians, policymakers, and ethicists. No single discipline holds all the answers, but together they can navigate the complexities of AI adoption. This book has illustrated how such collaborations have already yielded transformative results, from predictive analytics in disease management to ethical frameworks that safeguard patient autonomy. By fostering dialogue across these domains, we can ensure that AI serves the collective good.

Closing Thoughts

This book has provided a window into the transformative potential of AI and biomedical visualization in healthcare, offering a balanced perspective that celebrates its achievements while critically examining its limitations. As we look ahead, the responsibility lies with clinicians, researchers, policymakers, and technologists to navigate this new era thoughtfully and collaboratively.

AI has the power to redefine what is possible in healthcare. By embracing its potential responsibly, we can create a future where innovation and compassion coexist, ensuring that the benefits of AI extend to every patient, every community, and every corner of the world. This is not just the future of medicine—it is the future of humanity.